Women's Mental Health in Primary Care

Women's Mental Health in Primary Care

Kathryn J. Zerbe, MD

Jack Aron Professor in Psychiatric Education
Training and Supervising Psychoanalyst
The Menninger Clinic
Topeka, Kansas

W.B. SAUNDERS COMPANY

A Division of Harcourt Brace & Company
Philadelphia London Toronto Montreal Sydney Tokyo

W.B. SAUNDERS COMPANY

A Division of Harcourt Brace & Company

The Curtis Center
Independence Square West
Philadelphia, Pennsylvania 19106

Library of Congress Cataloging-in-Publication Data

Women's mental health in primary care / Kathryn J. Zerbe.

p.   cm.

ISBN 0–7216–7239–6

1. Women—Mental health.   2. Primary care (Medicine).   I. Title.
   [DNLM: 1. Women's Health. 2. Mental Health. 3. Primary Health
   Care.   WA 309 Z58w 1999]

RC451.4.W6Z47 1999   616.89′0082—dc21

DNLM/DLC   98–7959

WOMEN'S MENTAL HEALTH IN PRIMARY CARE   ISBN 0–7216–7239–6

Printed in the United States of America

Last digit is the print number: 9   8   7   6   5   4   3   2   1

For Kelli

Preface

The complete answer is not to be found on the outside, in an outward mode of living. This is only a technique, a road to grace. The final answer, I know, is always inside. But the outside can give a clue, can help one to find the inside answer. One is free, like the hermit crab, to change one's shell.

Anne Morrow Lindbergh, 1955, p. 35.

This is a book for practicing clinicians. It is designed to help those in the primary care specialties—family practice, internal medicine, pediatrics, and obstetrics/gynecology—increase their "comfort zone" in working with the array of mental health issues in patients who present every week in a busy medical practice.

Every clinician should know that psychiatric problems require a huge amount of health care dollars. If patients are untreated, overall medical costs rise exponentially.

By the year 2020, depression is projected to be the second leading cause of death. Depression, alcohol misuse, bipolar disorder (manic-depressive illness), schizophrenia, and anxiety disorders are already among the top 10 causes of disability. In *The Global Burden of Disease: Summary*, psychiatric disorders are demonstrated to play a central but until now almost invisible role in causing disability and impaired health across all cultures and countries (Murray and Lopez, 1996). In all likelihood, the measures of disease burden will gradually change funding and health care policies, but the clinician will still be left with the often unsettling, puzzling questions about how to intervene with an individual patient in a practical way.

In this book, I hope that my readers will have a greater array of tools and principles that are not too prescriptive but nonetheless helpful in offering patients concrete advice, empathic concern, and personal strategies about their emotional concerns and psychological struggles. In essence, my aim is to integrate the latest pharmacologic and psychotherapeutic approaches to assist readers in treatment planning.

On an individual basis in a primary care situation, the care of a patient with a psychiatric problem can be uniquely rewarding but can also cause management challenges. A patient struggling with an emotional issue finds it difficult to comply with treatment; she may have trouble adjusting to life experiences; and she is often perplexing to the clinician, both diagnostically and therapeutically. For these reasons, I have tried to help clinicians recognize how patients with psychiatric problems present in the real world of practice. I have also included *Additional Guidelines for the Primary Care Clinician* in each chapter to assist in the beginning of effective and useful intervention. The intent is not to make the primary care clinician a psychiatrist or a mental health professional, rather it is to increase the understanding of the patients' emotional needs that lie just beneath the surface, which can so often interfere with the overall quality of life and your suggestions for medical treatment.

Partnering with women in mental health care requires more than medication management. Although each chapter offers recommendations for state-of-the-art psychopharmacologic management of the major disorders (e.g., anxiety disorders, depression, posttraumatic stress disorder, and complicated bereavement) you are likely to treat, you will find that professional satisfaction can be derived from understanding, to some extent, the patient's psychological world and partnering with her so that she can achieve a fuller quality of life.

Most men and women are now more knowledgeable and assertive than ever before when it comes to health care. Their activism and involvement are changing the way medicine is practiced. Consequently, I have included in each chapter a list of recommendations in the patient guidelines section to help women and their family members understand, and to some extent more effectively deal with, the problems that have impeded a more joyful, fulfilling life.

The primary care clinician or the care extender in your office can copy these recommendations and hand them to the patient as a way of saying, "Here are some ways you might consider working with the struggles you face." Emphasis is placed on the role of medications, the most common side effects, the various psychotherapeutic strategies that are likely to help, and ancillary support systems (e.g., classes at women's health cooperatives, support groups for particular disorders or diagnoses) that can also be effective. The goal, of course, is to encourage the patient to feel empowered in her partnership with you, her primary clinician, and to make one small step toward the management of mental illness. Millions of patients do not receive the treatment that could save them from much suffering, not because it is unavailable but because they are fearful and ashamed to seek it out. In the treatment of psychiatric disorders, the stigma of mental illness remains our most formidable foe.

Although this book is written primarily for practicing primary care clinicians, I also hope to reach residents, medical students, and other clinicians who could benefit from guidelines about "what to do next" when working with and beginning the treatment of a patient with a psychiatric problem. Since referral to a psychiatrist or other mental health specialist is, of course, warranted in many situations, it also is reviewed. The emphasis is on what the primary care clinician can and should reasonably be able to do with the array of mental health concerns that inevitably arise. Because contemporary medicine is increasingly a team approach involving care extenders—advanced registered nurse practitioners, physician's assistants, social workers, and so forth—suggestions are also made about how to use ancillary professionals to improve quality of care, reduce cost, and help patients feel heard and understood.

In each chapter, I include an annotated bibliography for both patients and clinicians. The resources for patient sections are designed as another potential means to involve the patient and to help the clinician reach out and say, "Here are some books about patients who have had a situation similar to your own. You might want to take a look. Learning from the experience of others will help you gain courage and strength to face your own difficulties. And, I am interested in what you learn." The patient references are not meant to be inclusive, but rather to serve as a starting point to involve the patient and to increase compliance.

You might question why a practicing psychiatrist and psychoanalyst would choose to write a text that addresses the gender differences that have an impact on the diagnosis of psychiatric disorders and the etiology, prevalence, and treatment of issues facing women. Actually, it has been enormously gratifying to work with primary care clinicians who are so attuned to the "inner life" of their patients. In part, this interest occurs because many primary care clinicians intuitively sense the toll taken by disrupted relationships, interpersonal conflicts, unresolved losses, catastrophic traumas, and other life experiences that thwart the overall quality of life, increase physical disease, reduce compliance, and cause relapse. Although the developments in pharmacotherapy and psychotherapy, including cognitive-behavioral, psychophysiologic, and psychodynamic, are essential and integrated into the overall plan of this book, most primary care clinicians naturally embrace the view that one must treat the soul as well as the body to help any person heal (Andreasen, 1996).

All clinicians, regardless of specialty, actually start from the same place—on the outside—with a manifested symptom. We then gradually work our way to the inside—to fully grasp the situation in which the patient is found. Intrinsically, the release a patient finds from formidable psychiatric symptoms and her capacity for resilience also have the power to transform the clinician. When the patient is shown the way to disentangle herself from her most vexing life experiences, she becomes free to change. Ultimately, so do we.

References

Andreasen N: Body and soul [editorial]. *Am J Psychiatry* 1996; 153:589–590.
Lindbergh AM: *Gift from the Sea.* New York, Signet Books, 1955.
Murray CJL, Lopez AD: *The Global Burden of Disease: Summary.* Boston, World Health Organization and Harvard University, 1996.

Acknowledgments

Several years ago a talented primary care physician, who had recently completed residency, observed how common emotional problems were in her practice but found no single, practical guide to the literature on women's mental health. I will always be grateful for that insight, which was so related to a parallel problem of my own: How can contemporary psychiatry, which has so much to offer patients, speak to the actual concerns that other specialists have about patient care? So often it seems that clinicians—with whom I have collaborated while treating patients with eating disorders, depression, anxiety, and the like—want to know more than just the latest pharmacologic treatments. Their interest in and appreciation for the psychologic world of their patients have challenged me not only to think more about how a psychiatrist can be helpful but also to begin to place some of those thoughts on paper. I will always be indebted to those primary care clinicians who have shared the dilemmas they encounter in practice every day and who have expressed a desire to integrate insights garnered from biologic, cognitive-behavioral, and psychodynamic psychiatry to help their patients better cope and grow.

As is the case with most clinicians, my patients have been—and continue to be—my finest teachers. The privilege of talking to other human beings about their private world on a daily basis is a sacred experience. It has illuminated for me, time and time again, the human capacity to be resilient, creative, and adaptive, even in the face of life's most perplexing problems. The lessons my patients have taught me about how they have faced and, in many cases, gained victory over emotional difficulties form the basis of the patient guidelines section in each chapter of this book. These lessons are forever woven into the fabric of my practice.

I especially wish to thank a marvelous group of colleagues for agreeing to review, comment on, and provide thoughtful suggestions for further reading on various sections of this book: Kelli Holloway, MD; Mae Sokol, MD; Peter Parks, PhD; Faye Heller, ARNP, CST; Marci Bauman-Bork, MD; Deborah Steinberg, MD; Robert Conroy, MD; Alice Brand Bartlett, MLS; Judith Bernstein, MSW, LCSW; Jane Alford, MSW, LSCSW; and Janice Bingle, MD. I am also indebted to a far-flung, energizing network of colleagues and friends who have provided me generous encouragement and support over the years. I particularly wish to thank Jon Allen, PhD; Sharon Nathan, PhD; Sam Bradshaw, MD; James McCrory, MEd; Laura Rung, MD; Carol Nadelson, MD; Leah Dickstein, MD; Joel Yager, MD; Wayne Timan, BS; and Pauline Powers, MD.

I will always treasure my memories of working with the late Stuart Averill, MD, Mary Cerney, PhD, and Cotter Hirschberg, MD. To a large extent, each of these individuals underscored that even in an era when forces oppose careful listening and attunement to nuances, an understanding of the patient always comes first.

I am especially grateful to my extraordinarily competent and talented administrative assistant, Janice Bays, who provided invaluable assistance and boundless confidence at every stage of this project. Mary Ann Clifft, MS, and Philip Beard, MDiv, MA, have energetically and devotedly edited the entire manuscript with attention to detail and tact.

The seemingly indefatigable, meticulous staff of The Menninger Clinic professional library—Alice Brand Bartlett, MLS; Lois Bogia, MS; Nancy Bower; Andrea Burgett, BA; Krista Comly; Shawna Conroy; Lizabeth Stamati; Judy Kash, MALS; Don Pady, MLS; Marcelline Schott, MLS—located all manner of references and citations with the highest degree of kindness, professionalism, and dedication.

None of us could have done our work or enjoyed it half as much without the keen intelligence, clever wit, and sincere friendship of the administrator of the Karl Menninger School of Psychiatry and Mental Health Sciences, Susan Smith, MPA.

For all kinds of support, I am grateful to the colleagues, faculty members, students, and support staff of The Menninger Clinic and The Topeka Institute for Psychoanalysis. The Jack Aron Endowed Chair in Psychiatric Education provided me with the editorial assistance and time for writing the final chapters of this book.

I also wish to thank Ray Kersey, my editor at W.B. Saunders Company, for his enthusiastic support of this project, from nascent idea to completion, and to the entire team at W.B. Saunders who brought the book into its final form: Cass Stamato, Sally Grande, Marie Gardocky-Clifton, Denise LeMelledo, Mary Anne Folcher, and Beverly Braunlich.

I have been particularly blessed by a loving and supportive family. In my case, the choice of a career in psychiatry was the natural amalgamation of years of "shadowing" my late father, as he compassionately practiced primary care medicine, and of observing my mother's penchant for "talking with anybody about practically anything," especially their troubles. Even though my father and I would often joke about her "kitchen counseling" sessions, we were, in fact, witnessing a master in the art of listening. She remains one of the best soothers of other people's psyches that I know. Deepest gratitude is also due to my ebullient Uncle "Skip" Schreckengaust, who continues to provide ardent support and sage advice, no matter what the undertaking. By growing up in a small town in Pennsylvania, I learned firsthand the importance of having an extended family network—a concept I stress throughout the book in fostering the health and well-being of individuals. Over the years Charles and Doris Myers, Bob and Peggy Trace, Bob and Betty Bishard, and Peg Muhleman have been particular sources of inspiration by their countless acts of good will and spiritual example. Beth and Dale Holloway have been the encouraging presence and reassuring voices every person needs. Carlene Benson is more of a sister than a best friend. Kelli Holloway, MD, loyally and enthusiastically supported me throughout the long period of preparation of the manuscript. Her integrity, quiet intellect, and genuineness have been pivotal to this creative process, so it is to Kelli that I dedicate this book.

NOTICE

Medicine is an ever-changing field. Standard safety precautions must be followed, but as new research and clinical experience broaden our knowledge, changes in treatment and drug therapy become necessary or appropriate. Readers are advised to check the product information currently provided by the manufacturer of each drug to be administered to verify the recommended dose, the method and duration of administration, and the contraindications. It is the responsibility of the treating physician, relying on experience and knowledge of the patient, to determine the dosages and the best treatment for the patient. Neither the publisher nor the editor assumes any responsibility for any injury and/or damage to persons or property.

THE PUBLISHER

Contents

Chapter 1

Anxiety Disorders

Anxiety disorders are the most prevalent psychiatric disorders. Occurring two to three times more frequently in women than in men, they influence quality of life, lead to costly medical workups, and cause general deterioration in overall health and well-being. Clinicians often do not realize the impact of these disorders. A survey of the most comprehensive epidemiologic data available on psychiatric illnesses found an 11.3% incidence of anxiety disorders in the population (27 million people), which far exceeded the 6.4% incidence of alcohol and drug abuse (10 million people) and the 6.0% incidence of affective disorders (about 10 million people) (Regier et al., 1984, 1988).[1] The economic impact of anxiety disorders totals approximately $47 billion dollars (DuPont et al., 1996b).[2] Fortunately, anxiety disorders are highly treatable conditions for the majority of sufferers.

Appropriate diagnosis and increased availability of low-cost outpatient services reduce the social and economic costs of anxiety disorders. To manage anxiety disorders in a primary care practice, clinicians must recognize both overt and veiled manifestations of the illness, understand some of their beguiling aspects, rule out medical conditions that mimic them, and have a working knowledge of the pharmacologic and psychosocial treatment options that are now available. Because anxiety disorders affect women more often than men, this chapter focuses on management of these conditions in women.

Symptoms of anxiety often motivate women to seek medical and psychiatric care. They are a leading cause of women's disproportionate consumption of minor tranquilizers and other psychotropic agents (Balter et al., 1974; Baum et al., 1988; Yonkers and Ellison, 1996). A number of factors may contribute to a woman's experience of anxiety, which often involves feeling "sick" or ineffectual and precludes her from seeking help in a timely, straightforward way. These factors include disappointments and frustrations in personal and professional life, low self-esteem, lack of a sense of mastery, struggles with autonomy and authenticity, aftereffects of unsatisfying adult relationships, bereavement or anticipated bereavement (Shear and Mammen, 1997), and physical care of family members, particularly parents and children. In our society, it may be more acceptable, and even desirable, for women to think of themselves as passive and weak, and they may report symptoms more frequently.

Even though symptoms of anxiety bring women of all ages to physicians, little is known about the underlying genetic, neurobehavioral, and psychosocial

---

[1]This NIMH-funded project involved a five-city survey of the incidence of mental health problems. The anxiety data combined panic attacks, panic disorders, agoraphobia, and generalized anxiety disorders to arrive at the 11.3% figure. It did not include phobias, which were found to affect 7% of the population.

[2]Direct costs (e.g., medical services, short-term hospitalization, physician services, prescription drugs) total $11 billion (23%). Indirect costs (e.g., lost productivity, worker absenteeism, disability, non–health-care-related costs) total $36 billion (76%).

mechanisms that appear to affect women uniquely. Genetic studies have shown that familial lineage plays a role (Kendler, 1993; Kendler et al., 1992, 1993; Shear et al., 1993), but anxiety is best understood as an end result of interactions among heredity, biology, and environment.

Women require special consideration when it comes to treating anxiety. Pharmacologic treatment must take into account their smaller weight and body size, menstrual cycle, and use of contraceptives. Psychotherapeutic approaches should consider particular psychosocial stressors that complicate the diagnostic picture as well as the treatment.

WHY PATIENTS DO NOT SEEK HELP FOR ANXIETY

Some patients find it painful to seek help for anxiety. Prominent reasons are a sense of personal defect, lack of knowledge, fear of having an emotional problem, and inaccurate evaluation. In addition to describing these reasons, this section provides suggestions for addressing patients' reluctance and embarrassment.

Sense of Personal Defect

The stigma of having a psychological problem precludes many patients from seeking help. Emotional problems are viewed as a sign of personal weakness. A patient may even prefer to blame a physical problem rather than to blame herself for a "weak will." She avoids seeking help because she believes she must face the issues by herself. If she is able to overcome her initial reluctance, she may not follow through on taking prescribed medications out of fear of dependence or because "I want to get better on my own."

Initial strategies for helping women seek treatment for anxiety include greater public awareness through patient education. Review with your patient the model of anxiety as an interaction between biologic (e.g., genetic) and psychological (e.g., stress) factors. Explain how individuals with a genetic predisposition to anxiety, when exposed to stress—which is ubiquitous in life—often learn a maladaptive response to stress.

Each of the anxiety disorders is characterized by the need to *worry excessively.* Reframe this symptom as the woman's tendency to be highly *attuned* to her environment and to the needs of others, especially loved ones. Emphasize how the tendency to develop anxiety may actually serve as an adaptive survival advantage for some people. For example, women in primitive cultures who wandered far from home were often in mortal danger, as were their children. The hypersensitive or overdeveloped "alarm system" some women possess may be a residual of what was once a way to preserve their own lives and the lives of their young. This explanation may be a useful and supportive metaphor ("Your anxiety thermostat is set a little too high") for women who tend to degrade themselves for having anxiety. It can later be used to introduce the value of pharmacotherapy, which helps to "damp down without shutting off" the very valuable anxiety alarm system.

Many patients are reluctant to disclose their difficulties, so the physician must be specific when asking about them (Higgins, 1996). Because patients feel greater anguish in having a psychiatric rather than a medical diagnosis, they sometimes become angry when their primary physician suggests that they have an emotional illness. No matter how effective the treatment is or potentially can be, an alienated patient will not return. If an anxiety disorder is suspected, the physician must provide a great deal of education about the disorder and its treatment to reduce any shame the patient may feel.

Although most authorities emphasize that multiple factors contribute to anxiety disorders, which consequently require an integrated treatment approach involving drug therapy and psychosocial intervention, patients may first be approached with the knowledge that anxiety disorders are biologically based. Psychosocial tools can help them gain a sense of mastery and control over their lives (DuPont et al., 1996a). Demystifying the condition by explaining that it is simply exaggerated normal anxiety helps patients begin to identify thought patterns that may escalate into full-blown, paroxysmal anxiety attacks. Helping a patient develop a sense of humor about her fears and referring her to the growing self-help literature are particularly useful adjuncts to treatment. They enhance the patient's collaboration with her physician and help her develop a sense of personal mastery over the illness.

Inaccurate Evaluation

In the evaluation of the anxious patient, medical conditions that result in a presentation of anxiety must always be ruled out (Wise and Griffies, 1995). Drugs of abuse (e.g., amphetamines, cocaine), caffeine, and alcohol all can precipitate anxiety attacks. In addition, medical illnesses may engender particular stressors that lead to uneasiness, worry, and even panic. Patients with anxiety disorders spend a considerable amount of time and resources in the primary care setting, but appropriate treatment reduces the duration of impairment and unnecessary costs to the patient and the health care system (Katon and Kleinman, 1980; Zerbe, 1995).

Although numerous medical conditions mimic anxiety (Table 1–1), some disorders in particular must be ruled out in women. Coronary conditions such as angina pectoris, dysrhythmias, valvular disease (especially mitral valve prolapse), and congestive heart failure are frequently accompanied by dread and apprehension. Because coronary disease has been underdiagnosed in women (Clark et al., 1994; Judelson, 1994; Wenger, 1994), sensitivity to gender-related issues can help the clinician to accurately differentiate cardiac symptomatology from the acute anxiety of panic disorder (Katon, 1996).

Other medical "mimics" to which women are preferentially predisposed are hyperthyroidism, systemic lupus erythematosus, and anemia. In addition, respiratory conditions such as asthma, chronic obstructive pulmonary disease, and pneumonia may cause acute anxiety symptoms. It is noteworthy that smoking predisposes people to these respiratory conditions. Although overall smoking rates have declined since 1974, the rates for teenage females are increasing fastest. Both age and smoking status should be carefully considered in the differential diagnosis of anxiety disorders.

Unless asked directly by the physician, women tend to avoid mentioning medications they are taking. The list of drugs known to precipitate anxiety is

Table 1–1. **Medical Conditions Associated with Symptoms of Anxiety: Differential Diagnosis**

Cardiovascular disease
  Angina pectoris
  Congestive heart failure
  Myocardial infarction
  Mitral valve prolapse—a.k.a. circulatory neurasthenia (DaCosta's syndrome, soldier's heart, hyperdynamic beta-adrenergic circulatory state)
  Chest pain of unknown origin and normal coronary arteries (80% of affected persons ultimately diagnosed with panic disorder, depression, or both)
  Arrhythmia
Pulmonary disease
  Chronic obstructive pulmonary disease
  Pulmonary embolism
  Physical exertion/hyperventilation
  Asthma
Endocrine disease
  Hyperthyroidism/hypothyroidism
  Cushing's disease
  Diabetes mellitus
  Carcinoid syndrome
  Hypoglycemia
  Pheochromocytoma
  Hypercalcemia/hypocalcemia
  Hyperadrenalism
Collagen vascular disease
  Systemic lupus erythematosus
Dermatologic disease
  Psoriasis/eczema
  Atopic dermatitis
  Pruritus
  Self-excoriations
Hematologic disease
  Vitamin B_{12} deficiency
Gastrointestinal disease
  Irritable bowel syndrome
  Ulcerative colitis
  Peptic ulcer
Neurologic disease
  Headache, particularly migraine
  Demyelinating diseases
  Epilepsy (complex partial seizures)
  Dementia
Pharmacologic agents
  Thyroid replacement
  Bronchodilators
  Decongestants
  Digitalis (toxicity)
  Corticosteroids
  Cocaine, cannabis, or other hallucinogen intoxication
  Nicotine and alcohol withdrawal
  Sedative hypnotic withdrawal or paradoxic reaction
  Antituberculosis agents
  Stimulants, particularly caffeine

long, and it is imperative to ask the patient what she takes. *All* prescribed and over-the-counter medications should be noted. Women who use nonsteroidal antiinflammatory agents, steroids, psychostimulants for dieting, and pseudo-ephedrine compounds for allergies or upper respiratory infections may present with a subthreshold or full-blown anxiety attack because of medication side effects. Be sure to inquire about the use of caffeinated beverages and foods (e.g., chocolate), because even small amounts in some at-risk persons can precipitate or exaggerate anxiety.

DIAGNOSING ANXIETY: THE CHALLENGE OF RECOGNITION

Making an accurate diagnosis of an anxiety disorder is a formidable challenge in a primary care setting. Unlike patients who seek out a psychiatrist or other mental health professional because they worry too much, or seem agitated or irritable, or are having problems in relationships or at their jobs, primary care patients tend to view the problem as organically based. They *resist* the idea that they may have an emotional disorder, and they may become angry with you for even suggesting it! They also may ignore therapeutic suggestions (Higgins, 1996; Lieberman, 1996; Stoudemire, 1996). It therefore behooves the primary care clinician to listen carefully for the excessive worry, unrealistic fear, and anticipatory anxiety that can accompany situational or social settings (Brown et al., 1994; Hirschfeld, 1995; Liebowitz, 1993; Rosenbaum et al., 1995; Zerbe, 1995).

Although some clinicians find it useful to delineate the patient's particular anxiety disorder (Table 1–2), treatment can be recommended after making an "in-the-ballpark" diagnosis. Most patients benefit from supportive psychotherapy and newer medications, which are effective for a range of anxiety disorders. Moreover, most patients with an anxiety disorder have another comorbid psychiatric condition: Depression, alcoholism, and more than one anxiety disorder are the norm rather than the exception for both sexes (Boulenger and Lavallee, 1993; DuPont, 1995; Stahl, 1993). Indeed, it is now considered rare for a patient to present with a "pure culture" of only one anxiety disorder diagnosis (Goldenberg et al., 1996), in part because the most common symptoms overlap. Tables 1–3 and 1–4 point out the similarities and differences in some of the anxiety disorders.

For practical purposes, empathize with the *misery* the anxious person experiences most days of her life. For her, life is continually unsettling, as if she is on trial every moment or is preparing for the ultimate examination. As she anticipates failure and bewilderment, her heart pounds as she ruminates about what she will say or do next. Viewing her future as truly rife with danger at every step, the anxious person remains hypervigilant, tense, and insecure in most situations.

Sometimes the anxious patient turns to her child or significant other to relieve her heightened state of negative arousal, because such attachments help her to feel safe or more in control. This heightened autonomic arousal leads to some of the somatic complaints that are particularly prominent in the patient with generalized anxiety disorder or panic disorder (see Tables 1–3 and 1–4). However, sometimes the discrete episodes of anxiety become so intense that patients believe they are actually "going crazy" or will die. In reality, these patients are not psychotic, and reassuring them that they are not experiencing a cataclysmic event alleviates much of their suffering.

Table 1–2. **Most Common Anxiety Disorders Among Women**

Generalized anxiety disorder (GAD)

GAD is a syndrome of excessive worry and tension which commonly has its onset in childhood or early adulthood. It is a chronic condition, often lasting a lifetime, but is highly treatable. Patients with GAD do not have the distinguishing features of panic, avoidance, obsessions and compulsions, or social phobia only. GAD is particularly common among women.

Panic

Panic is a paroxysm of sudden fear accompanied by physiologic symptoms such as palpitations, chest pain, choking, vertigo, trembling, shaking, and a fear of catastrophe or emotional decompensation. Psychosensory disturbances (e.g., distortion in light or sound intensity) are also common. Typically, panic attacks last only a few seconds or a few minutes. They are three times as common in women as in men.

Social phobia

The fear of humiliation or embarrassment, leading to avoidance, is known as social phobia. Once thought to be more common in men than in women, social phobia now appears to affect more women, perhaps because more women are entering the workforce or seeking treatment.

Obsessive-compulsive disorder (OCD)

Obsessive-compulsive disorder is characterized by obsessions (repetitive intrusive, unwanted, and disturbing thoughts, often with aggressive or sexual content) and compulsions (repeated, seemingly senseless rituals used to ward off anxiety associated with obsessions). Women with OCD tend to be older at age of onset than men, to have more depression and anorexia, and to suffer from compulsive washing. Some cases of OCD begin in the postpartum period, probably as a result of changing hormone levels. OCD spectrum disorders pertaining to women include compulsive buying, premenstrual dysphoric disorder, body dysmorphic disorder, and binge eating disorder.

Agoraphobia

Fear or panic associated with being away from a safe person or safe place is called agoraphobia. It can be understood as "adult separation anxiety" because the fear erupts when the patient is alone in an unfamiliar place. The patient is terrified of a sudden loss of control, death, or emotional catastrophe.

Phobia

Avoidance of an experience or situation because of fear or panic is a phobia. Some of the most common phobias are fear of heights and fear of small animals or reptiles (e.g., rodents, snakes).

Posttraumatic stress disorder (PTSD)

Anxiety that results from severe stress leads to chronic anxiety syndrome, and is characterized by reliving the stress, nightmares, and increased arousal has been termed PTSD. Symptoms may worsen during the luteal phase of the menstrual cycle. PTSD may result from childhood trauma, sexual abuse, incest, rape, or other life-threatening events (see Chapter 6).

The onset of an anxiety disorder frequently occurs after a major life event (e.g., loss of a spouse, physiologic stress resulting from physical illness), but 33% of patients with diagnosed panic disorder have some recurrent panic attacks in their sleep, and about 4% of patients have more attacks while they are sleeping than when awake. In fact, some patients first experience the illness with a panic

Table 1–3. **Anxiety Symptoms: Similarities**

Generalized Anxiety Disorder	Panic Disorder
Shortness of breath	Shortness of breath
Palpitations	Palpitations
Sweating	Sweating
Dizziness, lightheadedness	Dizziness, lightheadedness
Gastrointestinal complaints	Gastrointestinal complaints
Hot flashes, chills	Hot flashes, chills
Trembling or shaking	Trembling or shaking

attack that interrupts their sleep. Although this occurrence is unusual, it frequently leads to extensive medical workups, particularly of the cardiovascular system, because the patient awakens believing she is having a heart attack. This presentation can be a diagnostic red herring in primary care! Moreover, it demonstrates that the actual pathophysiology underlying anxiety is still unknown.

RISK FACTORS TO ASSESS BEFORE BEGINNING TREATMENT

In addition to making the diagnosis of anxiety, the primary care clinician should be prepared to intervene in regard to the following frequently encountered comorbid risk factors: depression, addiction, suicidal behavior, genetic and family factors, preoccupation with physical disease, anger, shame, and life events (including trauma). Their significance is often underestimated, but it is vitally important to address them to facilitate the patient's recovery. Clinicians understandably seek to achieve parsimony and homogeneity in practice, preferring to believe that they treat definitive entities that respond to concrete, scientifically valid therapeutics. In fact, diagnostic categories, like the clinical presentations themselves, often overlap. They are beguiling because they paradoxically suggest

Table 1–4. **Anxiety Symptoms: Differences**

Generalized Anxiety Disorder	Panic Disorder
Essential feature: excessive worry	Essential feature: worry that a panic attack will come "out of the blue"
Muscle tension, aches, soreness	Paresthesias
Restlessness	Depersonalization/derealization
Easy fatigability	Sensory disturbances
Dry mouth	Chest pain, chest discomfort
Excessive tension, "on edge" feeling	Choking
Irritability	May lead to excessive restriction in woman's life (e.g., agoraphobia)
Frequent urination	
"Lump in the throat"	

effective, straightforward illnesses which, on further reflection, lack concrete boundaries.

Depression

There is now a compelling body of literature linking anxiety with depression (Marshall, 1996; Regier et al., 1984, 1988; Roy-Bryne, 1996; Stahl, 1993). However, there is significant heterogeneity in the spectrum of anxious and depressed patients. One likely reason for this diversity is related to a complex dysregulation of the neurotransmitters. Although current attention focuses on the pivotal role of serotonin, several other systems (dopamine, norepinephrine, and gamma-aminobutyric acid [GABA]) also mediate emotions and mental illness.

When the neurotransmitter systems are disrupted or destabilized because of stress, medication restores their "homeostatic setpoint" (Petty et al., 1996). The behavioral effects of any drug are mediated via neural networks with multiple interactions. The "selective serotonin receptors" are not completely specific to serotonin but affect other biogenic amine systems in the brain. It is currently believed that the neurotransmitters are more numerous and complex than once thought. Consequently, the psychophysiology and pathophysiology of depression and anxiety are best understood clinically as the end result of an amalgam of interacting, but as yet incompletely understood, systems (Greist, 1996).

This clarification suggests why patients experience a variety of symptoms that differ dramatically from individual to individual. In practice, the selective serotonin reuptake inhibitors (SSRIs) currently used are safe and effective agents for the treatment of panic disorder (Klein, 1996), generalized anxiety disorder (Lucki, 1996), obsessive-compulsive disorder (OCD) (Pigott, 1996), social phobia (Jefferson, 1996; Marshall, 1992), and posttraumatic stress disorder (Davidson and van der Kolk, 1996).

Mixed depression and anxiety are frequently encountered in the primary care setting. Although the depression component can be life-threatening and therefore warrants treatment, anxiety is less likely to be recognized for the multiple disabilities it causes. When anxiety and depression occur together, greater functional impairment results. Prognosis is poor unless the syndrome is recognized, therapy is initiated, and compliance is maintained (Shear and Mammen, 1997; Stahl, 1993; Stokes, 1993). Treatment attenuates the interpersonal, vocational, and medical costs; early diagnosis, in particular, can further reduce human suffering and cost by allaying concerns about medically unexplained somatic symptoms that often lead to expensive workups.

Family practitioners often observe that anxious patients seek them out, complaining of fatigue, exhaustion, irritability, poor sleep, and frequent somatic difficulties. When entertaining the possibility of anxiety or mixed anxiety-depression syndrome, it is important to elicit family members' observations (especially those of the significant other). *People who are close to the patient are often the first to notice a change in function or mood.* They may make statements such as, "Doctor, she gets so mad at little things nowadays; she seems jittery and edgy. She is restless at night."

Employing an SSRI or a tricyclic antidepressant (TCA) may initially increase anxiety and agitation. These drugs share similar activating properties (Yonkers and Ellison, 1996). Your patients will nevertheless be reassured when you voice your belief that the syndrome is a common and highly treatable medical illness (Ballenger, 1997). Enhance compliance by providing support, advice to take the medication with food, and reassurance that side effects usually diminish. Your aim is to help the patient to feel well, not just better (Pollack, 1993), and several trials may be necessary to find the best drug. Emphasize that *choices* for pharmacologic treatment are available to the patient, including anxiolytics, TCAs, monoamine oxidase inhibitors (MAOIs), SSRIs, azapirones, or combinations. Highlight the advantages and disadvantages of each class and the reasons for your recommendations (see "Guidelines for Pharmacotherapy"). A combination of medication and psychotherapy also shortens the course of this illness and increases the patient's sense of mastery and self-worth. It is also likely to lower the relapse rate. Most studies demonstrate that cognitive-behavioral therapy, psychodynamic therapy, or both are integral to an enhanced sense of well-being and recovery from anxiety and depression (Barlow, 1992; Bergin and Garfield, 1994; Craighead et al., 1994; Milrod et al., 1996, 1997; Street and Barlow, 1994).

Your patient may feel that she is not a good enough caregiver (Shear and Mammen, 1997) or is personally weak. Emphasis on her role in making choices about treatment and conveying respect for her cooperative participation reinforce her tendency to follow recommendations and become involved in her own recovery. Above all, *emphasize that the syndrome is unlikely to go away on its own accord; the tendency for relapse without treatment is high* (Keller and Hanks, 1995).

Addiction

About 15% of patients with an anxiety disorder also have a substance abuse disorder (DuPont, 1997). More common is the substance-abusing patient who also has an anxiety disorder (see Chapter 4). As previously stated, anxiety disorders are a leading cause of women's disproportionate consumption of benzodiazepines and other psychotropic agents.

In the office setting, you can usually differentiate patients whose principal problem is anxiety from those whose principal problem is substance abuse by their attitude toward taking medication. As DuPont has pointed out, *patients who are addicted tend to want higher doses of prescribed medication* (DuPont, 1995, 1997; DuPont et al., 1996a). They are fearless and tend to seek out substances. With an anxious patient, you may prescribe a moderate dose of a benzodiazepine (e.g., clonazepam, 1–4 mg/day) in divided doses and achieve good stabilization. Those patients who suffer from addiction, however, are likely to tell you that the medication is helping—but only up to a point. They may even demand that you increase the dose of the drug; and frequently they will seek treatment from multiple health care providers, who unknowingly prescribe more benzodiazepines.

In contrast, *anxious patients worry about taking medication.* They are fearful of many things—meeting new challenges, having medical illnesses, caring adequately for their families or friends—and particularly about taking medication, even if it is prescribed and helpful. They must be reminded that the TCAs and SSRIs, now considered first-line drugs in the treatment of anxiety, are nonaddicting. Many physicians have avoided prescribing benzodiazepines because of the potential for addiction, although these medications can often benefit patients with a primary diagnosis of anxiety who do not have an abuse problem (see "Guidelines for Pharmacotherapy"). Short-term use is encouraged.

Obtaining a lifetime history of substance use and anxiety helps you to determine whether the patient abused alcohol or drugs before the onset of anxiety. Contrary to popular medical mythology, few people drink to "treat" their anxiety (DuPont, 1997), but successful management of anxiety may have an impact on alcohol consumption. When anxiety and substance abuse disorder occur in the same person, both conditions need thorough assessment and treatment. Although you may not feel expert in providing a full range of therapeutic options, you can be aware of community resources and make an appropriate referral. The primary provider who is cognizant of local 12-step fellowships (e.g., Alcoholics Anonymous, Narcotics Anonymous), residential treatment programs, and mental health professionals with expertise in drug and alcohol treatment is a major resource and supportive figure for such patients.

Unrecognized substance abuse is a major problem among women (see Chapter 4). Clinicians may fall victim to reverse gender bias when they fail to consider addiction in the differential diagnosis of female patients. Treatment of this most painful and debilitating problem begins only when it is recognized and emphasized as the life-threatening disorder it truly is.

If you must choose whether to treat the anxiety or the addiction first, prioritize addiction treatment. DuPont's clinical maxim (1997) bears frequent repeating to the patient, her significant other, and her family, and even to your support staff: "Addiction is a progressive and potentially fatal disease. Leaving addiction untreated, even briefly, is hazardous to the patient's life".

Suicidal Behavior

There is a high incidence of suicidal thinking and suicide attempts among anxious patients, particularly those with panic disorder. Although professionals recognize the risk of suicide in patients with depression, bipolar disorder, or eating disorders, they underestimate this risk in adult patients with anxiety disorders. Yet these patients experience anxiety as unbearable! Thoughts of suicide can wax and wane, but usually are alleviated once treatment has begun. The behavior appears to be more frequent in women than in men, particularly in women who are single, divorced, or widowed (Allgulander and Lavori, 1991; Johnson and Weissman, 1990).

To avert suicide, the primary care physician should consult a mental health clinician who has expertise in providing a safe environment (e.g., hospitalization), interacting with the legal system if commitment is necessary, suggesting a range of social support, recommending psychopharmacotherapy, and evaluating the patient's coping skills and interpersonal conflicts. At the same time, the primary care physician should remain involved in the overall care of the patient, expressing optimism about long-term resolution of problems and providing support to both the patient and her family.

Genetic Factors and the Role of the Family

Working with the entire family is an entrée into primary and secondary prevention of anxiety. Diagnosis of an anxiety disorder in one member alerts the clinician to potential problems with anxiety in other family members. Familial genetic factors play a significant etiologic role (30%–40%) in anxiety disorders (Kendler, 1993; Kendler et al., 1992, 1993) and are even more important (65%–80%) in bipolar illness and schizophrenia.

Women with anxiety disorders have been reported to be less warm and emotionally available to their children (Sable, 1991; Shear and Mammen, 1997). Mothers with untreated anxiety disorders, therefore, are likely to have children who also have psychological difficulties, presumably because of disruptions in the mother-child relationships. Attachment and nurturance obviously are impeded by a parenting style that is colored by an anxious temperament or severe anxiety symptoms. These constitutional predispositions may include irritability, criticism, negativity, lack of awareness of the child's age-appropriate separation and autonomous behaviors, and preoccupation with physical health.

The social incapacitation of the anxious woman often goes unrecognized. When a young mother is struggling with a severe generalized anxiety disorder or social phobia, she is probably reluctant to reach out for those community or interpersonal relationships that can sustain her. An agoraphobic patient who is housebound usually turns to her mate or her child to deal with her separation anxiety; this obviously has long-lasting effects on the functioning of the child, who may refuse to go to school (school phobia) or play with peers, and on the marital relationship (Quadrio, 1984; Sable, 1991; Shear et al., 1993). Indeed, interpersonal problems and limited companionship outside the home are highly correlated with symptoms of anxiety in women, but not in men (Shear and Mammen, 1997; Shear et al., 1993).

Preoccupation with Physical Disease

Anxious patients focus on their bodies. They worry about becoming ill, often to the point of obsession with their symptoms, which can result in somatization disorder. Even experts have a hard time distinguishing between generalized anxiety disorder or panic disorder and somatization disorder (see Chapter 8).

The very nature of the autonomic arousal associated with panic disorder and generalized anxiety triggers the physical symptoms of chest pain, palpitations, shortness of breath, and dizziness—and these symptoms overlap with somatization. However, patients with generalized anxiety or panic tend to report such symptoms more frequently than do those with somatization. Anxious patients also tend to localize symptoms to one or two body systems (Brawman-Mintzer and Lydiard, 1996; Kennerley, 1996; Shear and Mammen, 1997). Somatization begins in younger women and tends to be chronic. Patients who somatize are frequently dissatisfied with their physician, in contrast to anxious patients, who seek out caretaking, comfort, and reassurance. Anxious patients commonly recall childhood fears and have a history of childhood anxiety. They report more "stressful" life events. Nevertheless, their life patterns are often marked by achievement, particularly before the onset of the bona fide anxiety disorder. Social interaction and role functioning are severely curtailed only *after* onset. Patients with somatization tend to have been brought up in chaotic families, lead chaotic lives, and as a group are less successful.

Episodes of Anger

Women, particularly mothers, often become distressed by their anger; they worry especially that it may have a harmful effect on their children. Anger attacks and anxiety have been correlated in the psychiatric literature; such attacks occur in patients with generalized anxiety disorder, panic disorder, posttraumatic stress disorder, or depression (Shear and Mammen, 1997; Shear and Weiner, 1997). Hypothesized to represent a variant of panic disorder, anger attacks are accompanied by rapid onset of overwhelming emotion and autonomic arousal. These symptoms respond to antidepressants. If a female patient complains of increased anger or irritability, be sure to rule out anxiety, depression, and a mixed anxiety-depression syndrome.

Shame in Seeking Help

Each of the previously discussed risk factors should be considered as a diagnostic caveat when a patient requests help. However, anxiety often goes untreated or undertreated because patients view their symptoms with shame and therefore do not seek help at all or at least not specifically for those symptoms. For example, women with OCD often carry out their rituals in private. Individuals with social phobia succumb to professional backsliding or fail to accept promotions because they are so incapacitated that they cannot make a speech or even talk to colleagues for "fear of humiliation" (Menninger, 1995).

Clinicians are therefore challenged to make therapies more acceptable and more accessible. Most are familiar with the newsworthy case of the housebound agoraphobic patient who finally seeks help after years of an increasingly narrow and stultifying existence. She begins to "live, as if for the first time," after a course of an SSRI, a TCA, or a benzodiazepine is initiated—a seemingly "miraculous cure." Regardless of the origin of a particular anxiety disorder, however, effective treatment is precluded until the patient musters the *courage* to step forward and confide her problem to a clinician who can intervene with reassurance and education about these common and highly treatable conditions. One's own power as a healer to help the patient engage in treatment must never be underestimated. In many cases, this support is truly lifesaving.

Life Events and Trauma

A significant minority of persons who experience loss develop pathologic reactions resembling anxiety or depression. The primary care physician must be able to intervene during the time of bereavement or catastrophic loss (see Chapter 9) by listening empathically and attentively. Patients will not discuss their feelings unless given permission to talk, and even a few minutes of face-to-face interaction can help them feel less alone and more cared for by the doctor. Some women experience acute loss as a traumatic separation. Elderly persons are particularly prone to anxiety and depression after the death of a spouse with whom they have spent most of their lives. Women who have had to deal with a medical catastrophe in their own life or the life of a loved one (see Chapter 9) are also prone to experience the anlage of anxiety.

Murrey and colleagues (1993) found that 48.5% of their sample of women with anxiety disorders had a history of childhood sexual abuse. Although sexual abuse has most frequently been linked with posttraumatic stress disorder, these investigators also found high rates of panic disorder, OCD, and depression in this group. Moreover, samples of battered women (Herbst, 1992), Vietnam war veterans (Furey, 1991), and victims of political persecution (Fornazzari and Freire, 1990) also have indicated an increased incidence of anxiety.

Anxiety may be prolonged and potentiated if there is a dearth of caretaking in the environment. In such cases, patients should be encouraged to reach out for support. Try to "put yourself in the patient's shoes." There is a human tendency to avoid or deny the grief a patient is experiencing because it forces you to see the limits of your own skills as a healer and to come to grips with your own mortality. Patients accurately pick up cues from their environment that say, "I'm sympathetic to you, but I don't want to talk about it." Safe places where difficult issues can be discussed (e.g., groups for survivors, counseling and psychotherapy situations, women's peer groups, brief one-on-one dialogues with the physician or care extender) are life affirming and symptom attenuating. The treatment principle is *to inquire and not turn away* from the patient, who benefits enormously when another human being listens seriously to her anguish and pain.

LISTEN TO YOUR OWN FEELINGS: A HELPFUL GUIDE TO THE PATIENT'S EXPERIENCE

Anxious patients tend to make others feel anxious as well. When you talk with them in the consulting room, you may also feel a sense of alarm or worry, frustration about how best to proceed, or irritability that their symptoms seem to follow no straightforward pattern. Anxious patients can also be dependent and may be experienced as draining or needy. They seek a reliable source of security and will test that out in the therapeutic relationship. Anxiety is the mental state concerned with the experience of fear and danger, and therefore it can be very uncomfortable for both the patient and the clinician.

To make progress, the patient needs to take responsibility for her own difficulties over time, which means that the clinician should not have a "monopoly on anxiety" (Renik, 1995, p. 126) that blocks therapeutic progress. Although it is essential that clinicians acknowledge their own feelings and humanity, growth means that the patient must, with time, identify and become aware of what causes her anxiety.

Ideally both patient and physician learn about themselves in the treatment process and become more comfortable and accepting of their vulnerabilities and failings. They also must tap into their strengths and harness their sense of resiliency in the face of adversity. Situations once perceived as dangerous or threatening when "judgment was immature and information incomplete" (Renik, 1995, p. 130) can be mastered when they are openly discussed and rationally assessed. Psychotherapy provides the opportunity to become more familiar with one's mental life. In this safe, secure setting, the patient reasonably and realistically confronts outmoded dangers in the presence of an accepting human being.

REPRODUCTION AND CHILDBEARING

The postpartum period is a high-risk time for the onset of psychiatric illness, particularly anxiety and depression. One series of case reports described a range of anxiety syndromes that occur during pregnancy, particularly in the first and last trimesters (Sichel et al., 1993b). There remains a great need for recognition and treatment of these disorders, particularly because postpartum anxiety disorders have been identified less often than postpartum depression (see Chapter 11).

Panic disorder, OCD, and generalized anxiety disorder have been reported in the postpartum period (Sichel et al., 1993a, 1993b). Both neurophysiologic and psychosocial factors may play an etiologic role. New mothers naturally experience a host of concerns about the well-being and care of their babies. A continuum of worries abounds, ranging from the overall care and safety of the infant to obsessional preoccupation about harm, disease, and one's competency as a mother. Some anxious mothers have difficulty breast-feeding, which may have adverse effects on the infant's health and the bond between mother and infant.

Sichel and associates (1993b) hypothesized that the rapid decline of estrogen and progesterone after birth has an adverse affect on serotonergic functioning, leading to the acute onset of OCD in some patients. Because their patients responded well to an SSRI, they speculated that an interaction between rapidly changing reproductive hormone levels and a predisposition to psychiatric disorders, rather than an individual's adjustment to motherhood, may underlie obsessive-compulsive thoughts and actions in the puerperium.

With respect to panic disorder, some studies show a consistent improvement during pregnancy and a worsening after delivery (Cohen et al., 1993; Yonkers and Ellison, 1996). Many women with panic attacks complain of concomitant premenstrual worsening. Progesterone elevation during the later luteal phase of the cycle causes chronic hyperventilation, which may lead to panic in vulnerable groups. Klein (1996) argues that the decrease in hyperventilation after progesterone withdrawal provokes panic; panic then triggers a "suffocation alarm system," which may have offered some advantage in natural selection. Women with a sensitive alarm system who had the panic diathesis might hypothetically have been more able to protect themselves and their children when placed in life-threatening situations.

PATIENT GUIDELINES FOR COPING WITH ANXIETY

1. Learn as much as you can about anxiety disorders and methods of treatment (see "Resources for the Patient"). This knowledge base will help you see that you are not alone and that anxiety is one of the most undertreated medical and psychological problems. Learning as much as you can about the subject from informed clinicians and from other patients will also help you develop new strategies for dealing with your problems.
2. Recognize that the physical symptoms you experience, such as rapid breathing, nausea, muscular tension, and headaches, are signs of your body's readiness for action in a dangerous environment. Sometimes individuals unwittingly increase their tendency to heighten anxiety and panic by thinking they are "going crazy" or "about to die." If this happens, take a few deep breaths and remind yourself that you are not in real physical or psychological danger. Try to break the spiral that leads to increased anxiety by diverting your attention to another activity.
3. Remember that anxiety is a normal and an expected response to stress that is common to all human beings. Physical and psychological changes that you

experience are actually adaptive in times of danger. Anxiety helps each of us to cope with certain stressors (e.g., preparing for a test). Try to think positively about your problems with anxiety; that is, view them as your body's attempt to prepare you for a "fight or flight" response to a misperceived threat.

4. Identify the psychological stressors in your life that make you feel more anxious. Research has demonstrated that anxious persons tend to "catastrophize" situations. In other words, they think the worst is bound to occur, based on past experience and their heightened alertness to feared situations. Confront your tendency to see a crisis around every corner. When you find yourself worrying about a problem, remember that this thinking style not only does not help to solve the problem but actually can increase anxiety.

5. Increase your belief in yourself and develop a repertoire of skills that help you feel strong and competent. These can be essential tasks in overcoming anxiety. Many authorities believe that women are especially prone to developing anxiety disorders because they have fewer coping strategies and a greater tendency than men to feel inadequate and self-blaming. To enhance your sense of mastery and improve your coping strategies, seek out classes or groups offered at your local mental health center or women's treatment cooperative. This will counter your tendencies to feel demoralized and to employ maladaptive strategies in anxiety-provoking situations.

6. Realize that there is a family pattern to anxiety disorders. Learn about your own family history and be sure to tell your therapist and primary care provider about it. Because anxious parents tend to have children who also struggle with anxiety, you will want to become familiar with how you may be communicating anxiety in your family. Creating a safe, secure base for children is essential for a sound and maturing parent-child relationship (Bowlby, 1969, 1980; Winnicott, 1965).

7. Refuse to blame yourself for not being perfect or for "passing on something bad" to your family. Although genetic factors seem to play a significant role in anxiety disorders, researchers also believe that environment is a crucial factor. Women, in particular, tend to blame themselves for family difficulties. Counter this tendency in yourself. Try to confront situations that scare you, such as meeting new people, facing separations, or dealing with health-related concerns. Remember that your own anxiety can increase the vulnerability to anxiety in your loved ones, and that everyone can benefit from keeping stress at a manageable level.

8. Identify stressful life events. For many people, anxiety disorders can be traced to an acute loss, a past catastrophic or threatening event (e.g., car accident), or a physical or emotional separation from significant people. For many, psychodynamic (exploratory) therapy to examine the multiple psychological causes involved in this vulnerability to anxiety may be useful. Exploratory psychotherapy may be helpful alone or in combination with medication or cognitive-behavioral therapy.

9. Work on your interpersonal relationships, seek out confidants, and increase your opportunities to network with others. Vulnerability to anxiety and depression increases with reduced levels of social support. Having more resources of this kind buffers the individual from the vicious cycle of anxiety

that is initiated when important ties to others are disrupted (e.g., when a child begins school).

10. Deal with your anger. Anxious people tend to avoid conflict because of the overwhelming fear that it will disrupt an important relationship. Becoming increasingly assertive and less conflicted about the healthy expression of anger helps relieve anxiety. The goal is to have an increased ability to acknowledge and tolerate strong feelings, particularly those related to anger, separation, and loss.

11. Use exercise as an outlet whenever possible. Although some anxious people feel worse when they exercise, this is not true for the majority. Find the level of activity that you can tolerate and gradually increase it. When you feel anxiety coming on, turn to your routine of walking, running, weight lifting, or relaxation exercises to help achieve calmness.

12. Learn about and use relaxation exercises. Members of your health care team can suggest some highly effective ways to improve your capacity to relax. There are also a number of self-help resources and public workshops aimed at increasing your personal repertoire of strategies to manage anxiety. Over the past 20 years, research studies have proved these methods to be effective for many patients.

13. Practice your problem-solving skills whenever you can. Define what worries you and what it involves. Brainstorm about possible solutions, and by all means incorporate suggestions from other people. You may even find it helpful to rank the list of solutions and plan how you will put them to use. Should one solution not bring about the desired outcome, try another. Problem solving of this nature provides the structure to break out of the cycle of unproductive worry. And *targeting the tendency to worry* appears to be one of the most important steps in overcoming anxiety.

14. Do not automatically rule out taking medication as a part of treatment. For many people with an anxiety disorder, medication is a safe, effective, and essential component of treatment. The most frequently provided medications for anxiety, the benzodiazepines, act rapidly and usually are quite safe if taken for just a brief period. Although these medications may be addicting, they are a first-line treatment for some people. Some patients safely use benzodiazepines for long periods without becoming addicted. Many others are helped in the long term by the older, less expensive tricyclic antidepressants (TCAs), such as desipramine, or by the newer selective serotonin reuptake inhibitors (SSRIs), such as fluoxetine.

15. Be willing to try different medications if the first one is not effective. Researchers now believe that anxiety probably arises from an imbalance of neurotransmitters, chemicals in the brain that help to carry messages between brain cells. The neurochemical serotonin stabilizes anxiety, which is a brain-based dysfunction. Over the past 10 years, research has also clearly demonstrated the effectiveness of the TCAs and SSRIs for treating the broad range of anxiety disorders: generalized anxiety disorder, panic disorder, phobia, social phobia, obsessive-compulsive disorder, and posttraumatic stress disorder. This now means that new options are available to you, and if one medication is not successful, others can be tried.

16. Work with your physician or therapist to develop those skills and life changes

that may minimize the need for medication, but realize that stopping medication may not be possible. Anxiety is now being viewed as a long-term disorder, and a significant number of patients need some form of treatment over the course of their lives.

17. Take the anxiety disorder seriously and work to find the treatment option that best suits you. Without treatment, demoralization sets in. Over time, depression follows. In the past, clinicians and patients tended to minimize the misery, economic cost, and personal toll of these disorders. Only now are we beginning to recognize and understand how living with anxiety can destroy a person's morale.

18. Establish a relapse prevention plan for yourself. Because anxiety tends to be a recurrent, long-term problem, even with the most appropriate individualized treatment plan, symptoms can reoccur or come "out of the blue." After you are in good control of your anxiety problem, anticipate situations that might be problematic. Develop a contingency plan of breathing and relaxation exercises, or consider ways of distracting yourself when you are caught off guard.

ADDITIONAL GUIDELINES FOR PRIMARY CARE CLINICIANS

The following goals and strategies are recommended as ways to facilitate the recognition and treatment of anxiety in primary care.

1. Recognize symptoms of anxiety. Learn to suspect its presence in an array of patient presentations.
   a. Although anxiety can mimic or exacerbate various medical conditions, it can also be a result or expression of those same disorders (see Table 1–1). Women with a medical condition who are comorbid for anxiety and depression have lower levels of functioning and poorer quality of life than do patients with medical disorders alone.
   b. Psyche and soma are always intertwined. The connection between body and mind means clinically that a neat distinction between psychiatric and medical causes of anxiety is impossible. The excessive noradrenergic activity in the locus caeruleus that may underlie panic disorder is no less real than the excessive thyroid hormone secreted in hyperthyroidism. Some patients with "psychic" anxiety may induce an angina attack simply by ruminating on a disturbing thought.
   c. The patient's use of stimulants should be assessed. Cigarettes, coffee, carbonated beverages, chocolate, or alcohol may be used as "comfort tools" in response to stress when, in fact, they induce excessive anxiety as they are metabolized. Be sure to inquire about the patient's use of these agents when taking her history.

2. Educate the patient that anxiety is a real but treatable illness. Clarify that it is often a long-term condition.
   a. Early identification improves prognosis. Primary care providers are in a unique position to recognize untreated anxiety disorders, because patients often avoid the stigma of seeing a mental health specialist (Lieberman, 1996).

b. Studies of the long-term course of anxiety disorder are sobering. For many patients, the condition is not trivial or self-limiting. The primary care physician must not only diagnose but also be prepared to treat many patients over the long haul, trying available pharmacologic agents and cognitive-behavioral methods.

c. Anxiety is more common than depression. Most patients turn to their primary care provider first, even though they are likely to deny having anxiety. The disorder may be masked by a host of physical and/or psychological symptoms (Brawman-Mintzer and Lydiard, 1996). Reassure these patients that they have a bona fide but highly treatable condition.

d. Patients should be commended for coming forward and sticking with treatment. Even if you decide to refer a patient to a psychiatrist or other mental health professional, your continuing support and encouragement are invaluable aids in management and tertiary prevention (Kennerley, 1996).

3. Learn basic psychotherapeutic techniques of problem solving, relaxation, and exposure therapy, but do not hesitate to refer the patient to a mental health specialist if there is no improvement.

a. Incorporating some basic cognitive-behavioral and relaxation methods into your practice (see below and Chapter 7 for some examples) can improve compliance and relieve suffering. A number of studies have shown that primary care professionals can be highly successful in helping anxious patients manage symptoms by demonstrating a range of cognitive-behavioral techniques in the office and by having patients follow up with "homework assignments" (Barlow, 1988, 1994; Bergin and Garfield, 1994; Craig and Dobson, 1995; Craighead et al., 1994; Kennerley, 1996).

b. In some cases, anxiolytic medications can be avoided (Catalan and Garth, 1985) by using problem-solving techniques; in other cases, a combination of medication and cognitive-behavioral therapy will act adjunctively. For some patients, particularly those who decline drug therapies or who should avoid drugs (e.g., pregnant women), relaxation therapies or cognitive-behavioral methods can reduce anxiety to manageable levels and thus enhance quality of life significantly (Shear and Mammen, 1997; Street and Barlow, 1994).

c. Some patients have psychological issues that predispose them to development of anxiety disorders. These issues include personality problems, disturbances in interpersonal relationships, difficulty with defining and tolerating strong emotions (especially anger and feelings of abandonment), and unconscious conflicts about separation, anger, and sexuality. For such patients, psychodynamic psychotherapy is highly effective and useful, especially when the patient is motivated to want to learn more about the predisposing causes of her difficulties (Gabbard, 1992; Milrod et al., 1997; Zerbe, 1990).

4. Educate the patient about the range of available treatments.

a. There are now three highly effective and specific treatment modalities for anxiety disorders: (1) medication (Rosenbaum and Pollock, 1994; Rosenbaum et al., 1995, 1996); (2) cognitive-behavioral therapy (Barlow, 1988, 1992, 1994; Bergin and Garfield, 1994); and (3) psychodynamic treatment

(Gabbard 1992; Milrod et al., 1997; Shear and Weiner, 1997). Because psychiatry is still in its infancy in selecting which interventions work for particular groups or subtypes of anxious patients, it is impossible to know at initial intake which interventions will benefit a specific patient. However, with respect to the anxiety disorders, the major problem confronting generalists and specialists alike is recognizing the conditions and maximizing the usefulness of treatments that are already available (Rosenbaum, 1997).

  b. In practice, the primary care clinician should be aware of each modality in a general way and should be able to explain the rationale for its use to the patient. Moreover, the role of unconditional support and long-term follow-up for the patient cannot be minimized.

  c. Clinicians are in a privileged position to hear the patient's concerns and voice; the skills they bring to the relationship help many women come forward who otherwise would suffer in silence. Considerable professional satisfaction derives from making the diagnosis of anxiety and helping patients, who may be riddled with shame about their disorder or who face unabated suffering without treatment, to confront this disabling symptom effectively (Ballenger, 1989, 1997).

5. Learn the indications for recommending psychodynamic therapies.

  a. The primary care clinician should consider referring to psychodynamically oriented therapists those patients who do not respond to short-term treatment with cognitive-behavioral therapy and/or medications. Psychodynamic psychotherapy helps patients solidify connections with attachment figures, which alleviates anxiety and links episodes of tension (or even panic) to long-standing characterologic issues and defensive patterns (Milrod et al., 1996). The result is increased assertiveness, less apprehensiveness, and fewer conflicts when faced with inevitable separations, anger, and sexuality (Milrod et al., 1996; Shear and Weiner, 1997).

  b. Psychodynamic therapy is particularly recommended for patients who are curious to learn more about themselves and to develop insight into the unconscious factors that contribute to their anxiety. Today, many health care plans limit the number of visits to a psychotherapist. The patient then must forgo exploration, and maximum integration of modalities is not achieved (Menninger, 1995). Ultimately, dynamic therapy may be cost-effective when it is part of an integrated treatment program that includes medication to address the neurophysiologic component of symptoms (Gabbard, 1992). Some patients whose insurance does not cover psychotherapy may be willing to pay out of pocket, particularly if they experience a beneficial, synergistic effect between medication and insight-oriented psychotherapy.

  c. Psychodynamic therapy provides a new opportunity for a more appropriate, accepting human relationship. As described, anxious patients are often ashamed of their symptoms, expect ridicule and abandonment from clinicians, and are highly conflicted about expressing intense feelings, particularly anger. Psychodynamic therapy supports the patient by restoring "meaning to the symptoms" and "presenting a more appropriate object relationship to be internalized" (Gabbard, 1992, p. A10).

GUIDELINES FOR OFFICE-BASED, SHORT-TERM COGNITIVE-BEHAVIORAL INTERVENTIONS

The following cognitive-behavioral strategies, which have been found effective in controlled clinical trials (Barlow, 1988, 1992, 1994; Brown et al., 1993; Craske et al., 1994), are suggested for office use in providing integrated treatment. Clinicians who have a special interest in treating patients with particular anxiety disorders (e.g., phobia, social phobia) are referred to the specific books and articles listed in the "Resources for the Clinician" section at the end of this chapter.

1. Breathing retraining
   a. Hyperventilation and the unpleasant symptom of anxiety have been linked. Teach the patient to breathe diaphragmatically by having her place one hand on her chest and the other hand on her abdomen. Instruct her to breathe deeply, so that her lower hand moves up and down more than her upper hand.
   b. Ask the patient to hyperventilate while being supervised by you or a care extender, so that she can learn to recognize the role of hyperventilation in the development of symptoms.
   c. Have the patient practice in the office. Breathing retraining involves helping the patient set a comfortable pace of 8 to 10 breaths per minute. Encourage the patient to use this technique during stressful periods in her day-to-day work. Women may resist this suggestion because it seems inappropriate or awkward in the workplace. Deal with their reluctance by stating that some authorities now believe that improper thoracic breathing contributes to the higher incidence of panic attacks in women than in men (Klein, 1996).

2. Cognitive restructuring
   a. As noted previously, anxious patients tend to catastrophize events and to think in terms of black and white (all-or-none categories). Cognitive restructuring aims at correcting misappraisals of events or physical sensations.
   b. Help the patient recognize situations in which she anticipates a disastrous, traumatic outcome. Counter her tendency to catastrophize by showing her how she is most likely overestimating the probability of danger and exaggerating negative or frightening aspects of an experience.
   c. Take time to listen to the patient. You must get her to talk before you can be successful in presenting the therapy or cognitive exercises. Women who are given time to express their fears in the office of a kind and concerned practitioner are in a better position to confront their errors in thinking. Your nonverbal acceptance of the patient may be particularly crucial. Be sure to add that the patient is showing courage by coming forward and mastering her difficulties.
   d. Point out that in our society women tend to be highly critical of themselves. Confront the tendency to believe that a single mistake makes one a bad person (dichotomizing response) or an incompetent person (exaggeration response).
   e. Stress that the tendency to catastrophize is a symptom of anxiety that can be mastered.

3. Guided imagery and relaxation
    a. A wide range of relaxation exercises is available for women. To encourage a sense of mastery and competence in the female patient with anxiety, suggest that your patient take advantage of group relaxation training available at women's health cooperatives or through local educational events. Some excellent programs are now available in smaller towns and cities at community colleges, hospitals, and mental health clinics. One technique described for the treatment of insomnia (see Chapter 7) can also be applied to the anxious patient. Another technique is outlined below. This frequently employed relaxation exercise can be reviewed by you or your care extender. Prescribe this exercise as you would a medication. That is, have it written down and give it as a homework assignment when your patient leaves the office.
    b. To increase compliance and make sure the exercise is being carried out, ask your care extender to call the patient within a week of her office visit. Although this aspect of patient management takes a bit more time, it is highly cost-effective because it ensures that the patient is involved in the recovery process. This augurs well for a favorable prognosis in patients with anxiety disorders.

Sample Relaxation Exercise

- Have the patient sit in a comfortable position. At home, have her locate a quiet spot (e.g., a favorite chair).
- Suggest that her body is becoming as relaxed as possible. Have her focus on inhaling slowly, sometimes repeating a soft word or phrase as she breathes.
- As she exhales, ask the patient to bring to mind a soothing image or word.
- Continue to repeat the cycle, each time breathing slowly and using the diaphragm. Continue for at least a few moments.

Have the patient *practice* this technique three times a day for at least 10 minutes per session. Stress the advantage of developing the skill so that it can be used in anxiety-provoking situations.

4. Situational exposure
    a. The most common problem women with anxiety face is avoidance of the anxiety-provoking situation. In some cases, taking aversive action can lead to agoraphobia. A key to addressing the problem is graduated exposure to the circumstances that arouse the anxiety. Unfortunately, many women do not tell the clinician that they are avoiding certain situations (e.g., speaking in public, going shopping) because they feel embarrassed and misunderstood. If the patient is able to tell you about this most distressing and limiting symptom, she has already taken the most important first step in confronting a problem situation.
    b. To help the patient avoid initial failure, work with her to develop a contingency plan if she cannot get as far as the first step. For example, she may not be able to think about giving a speech in public, but perhaps she could practice speaking in front of a mirror at home. After this substitute first step is accomplished and rehearsed, she can proceed to the next step until her goal is reached.

GUIDELINES FOR PHARMACOTHERAPY

Excellent pharmacologic treatments for the anxiety disorders have been identified and investigated over the past few decades. With the increasing emphasis
on cost containment and symptom-targeted treatment, use of pharmacologic
agents will continue to grow in the coming years. Particularly as more patients
with anxiety are recognized and treated, the majority of them will benefit from
the available categories of highly efficacious drugs.

Tricyclic Antidepressants

Although initially prescribed for depression, the TCAs also are useful for
treating panic disorder, mixed anxiety and depression, and generalized anxiety.
The two most well-established tricyclic antipanic drugs are imipramine and
clomipramine; others that show promise are desipramine and nortriptyline.
Weight gain is a bothersome side effect for many women. A sizable minority
(30%) cannot tolerate the anticholinergic side effects or central nervous system
stimulation of the TCAs.

Monoamine Oxidase Inhibitors

These medications have been provided traditionally for the treatment of
depression, particularly atypical depression and refractory depression. They are
also very helpful in the treatment of various anxiety syndromes, including panic
attack, phobia, generalized anxiety, and social phobia (Jefferson, 1996, 1997).
The most widely accepted irreversible MAOI for panic attack is phenelzine
(45–90 mg/day). The safer and more tolerable reversible inhibitors of monoamine
oxidase (RIMAs) moclobemide and brofaromine have been employed successfully to treat social phobia and panic disorder. They are not yet available in the
United States. Because of the potential for fatal hypertensive crises (necessitating
dietary restrictions of tyramine-containing foods) and the less consequential but
uncomfortable effects of weight gain, insomnia, and sexual dysfunction, the
MAOIs typically are not used until after safer, more tolerable agents have been
tried (Rosenbaum, 1992; Rosenbaum et al., 1996).

Selective Serotonin Reuptake Inhibitors

Most experts now prefer SSRIs rather than TCAs as the first-line treatment
of anxiety disorders. In most patients, side effects of the SSRIs are limited.
However, a significant number of women complain of jitteriness, nausea, or
inhibited sexual desire and delayed orgasm (see Chapter 13). For these women,
the risk-benefit ratio needs to be weighed. The clinician may decide to initiate
a trial of a TCA if the patient does not respond to or has side effects from the
SSRIs. For patients with panic disorder, begin with a very low dose of an SSRI
and titrate upward slowly. For patients with OCD, you may start with a moderate
dose, but frequently a maximal dose is needed for optimal treatment (e.g.,
fluoxetine 60–80 mg/day). Open clinical trials also support SSRIs in the treatment
of some socially phobic patients. Although more definitive information is needed,

fluvoxamine and sertraline have been shown to decrease social anxiety (Jefferson, 1996; Marshall, 1994; Rosenbaum and Pollock, 1994).

High-Potency Benzodiazepines

Because antidepressants have a delayed onset of effect (often several weeks) and potentially deleterious side effects, high-potency benzodiazepines must be considered as a first-line treatment for generalized anxiety disorder, panic disorder, and social phobia. Because patients with a history of substance abuse can misuse these effective medications, some clinicians avoid these agents when they are appropriate and needed (Catalan and Garth, 1985; DuPont, 1995, 1997).

Benzodiazepines are able to quickly reduce anxiety to tolerable levels, thereby enhancing overall compliance with therapy. Additional benefits include safety (high therapeutic index). Consider the use of high-potency benzodiazepines when the patient has significant anticipatory anxiety, panic attacks, or incapacitating social phobia. These medications are effective in emergencies but may also be considered for long-term use. Clonazepam (0.5–2.5 mg/day) is gaining widespread acceptance for maintenance treatment of the anxiety disorders because of its long half-life and lesser tendency to be addicting than alprazolam (Davidson, 1997).

If you decide to discontinue a benzodiazepine, titrate downward slowly to avoid recurrent anxiety and/or withdrawal and the precipitation (in rare cases) of seizures or psychoses. Virtually all patients can be tapered from benzodiazepines successfully if sufficient time is given (Rosenbaum et al., 1996). When properly administered, a benzodiazepine has only a minimal risk of addiction, although the clinician should always be mindful of the potential for abuse.

Azapirones

This newer class of anxiolytics is successful in the treatment of generalized anxiety. These medications have not been found effective for panic disorder, social phobia, or OCD. These partial serotonin agonists are nonsedating and do not appear to induce tolerance, physical dependence, or withdrawal, making them popular medications in primary care. However, they tend not to be as effective as the other agents, except in anxious patients who are medically ill (Stoudemire, 1996). They must be used for *at least* 1 week to achieve their antianxiety effect and cannot be used to taper off benzodiazepines. Common side effects include dizziness, nausea, headache, and jitteriness. The dosage range for buspirone is 5 to 60 mg/day (average, 20 mg/day); it should be given on a thrice-daily schedule because of its relatively short half-life.

Beta-blockers

The primary role for beta-blockers (e.g., propranolol, atenolol) is for the treatment of social phobia. By curtailing peripheral symptoms (e.g., sweating, palpitations, tremors), beta-blockers reduce the experience of anxiety. Propranolol (20–40 mg) or atenolol (50–100 mg) taken several hours before a performance is effective in reducing stage fright (Marshall, 1992). Atenolol has the advantages of once-daily dosage and less likelihood of bronchial constriction. It does not cross the blood-brain barrier, making it less likely to cause depression or sleepiness.

GUIDELINES FOR TREATING THE PREGNANT PATIENT

1. Nonpharmacologic alternatives are the preferred first-line treatments for anxiety disorders in women of childbearing age. Although it appears that teratogenic risks of the standard antianxiety medications listed previously are small (the same 2–3% incidence of major malformation in pregnant women who take any medication), the physician does bear the medical and legal risk should an untoward event occur (Cohen et al., 1989).
2. The risk of teratogenesis from medication is probably much lower than the risk associated with a high level of maternal anxiety, or with exacerbation of an anxiety disorder, or the risk of symptoms from medication withdrawal. When this risk-benefit profile is discussed with patients, many women opt to continue their medication. You may comfortably advise a mother-to-be that a series of case reports (Sichel et al., 1993a; Yonkers and Ellison, 1996) of women taking medication during pregnancy has shown no ill effects to the fetus.
3. Conservative treatment means that the lowest possible dose of a medication should be used, to provide as much protection as possible to the fetus. Sometimes increasing the use of cognitive-behavioral therapies helps the patient reduce or even discontinue medication during pregnancy, particularly during the first trimester.
4. If a medication must be used, fluoxetine or a TCA is preferred. Large numbers of case follow-ups over time suggest that untoward effects are minimal. Oral cleft palate has been associated with in utero exposure to benzodiazepines, but an absolute risk has not been proved.
5. By the second half of pregnancy, when increased intravascular volume leads to decreased absorption and/or enhanced capacity of metabolism, higher doses of medication may be needed.
6. During labor and delivery, antidepressants may be continued to minimize the risk of relapse. Benzodiazepine dosage should be reduced to prevent fetal intoxication or withdrawal symptoms in the newborn. Treatment of anxiety disorders in pregnant patients may require specialty consultation, because new options are likely to evolve quickly and influence standards of care.

Contraceptive Use and Premenstrual Anxiety

1. Psychotropic drugs can affect the efficacy of oral contraception (Yonkers and Ellison, 1996; Yonkers and Gurguis, 1995). Drug levels can vary over the course of the menstrual cycle, and the drugs themselves can interact with contraceptives. Changing the dose of contraceptive sometimes decreases anxiety or depression. A few case reports have linked levonorgestrel (Norplant) with the onset of major depression and panic disorder (Wagner and Berenson, 1994).
2. A growing body of literature suggests that anxiety disorders (e.g., panic attacks) may worsen premenstrually (Yonkers and Ellison, 1996). The clinician

therefore must be aware of potential iatrogenically induced (e.g., by a contraceptive) or menstrually related syndromes when evaluating women with anxiety (see Chapter 11).

SUMMARY

Anxiety disorders are the most prevalent psychiatric disorders, and they occur two to three times more frequently in women than in men. They take a high toll on the sufferer's family and professional life, as well as on her overall health and well-being. However, their substantial morbidity has been underappreciated. Clinicians and patients alike tend to underestimate the misery associated with anxiety disorders. There is also an incomplete understanding of new psychopharmacologic and psychotherapeutic techniques that can help the majority of sufferers.

Emphasis must be placed on accurately evaluating the anxious patient and sorting out those medical conditions that mimic anxiety. However, many patients do not seek help because they lack knowledge and are afraid of the stigma associated with the disorder. Targeting the patient's low self-esteem, her sense of shame, and particularly her need to worry is a useful counseling adjunct. Other crucial considerations that require evaluation are comorbidity (e.g., depression, substance abuse), genetic factors, family roles, and preoccupation with physical disease. The high incidence of suicide requires special attention. The postpartum period may be a high-risk time for the onset of an anxiety disorder, perhaps because of the shifting hormone levels of the patient.

Integrated treatment of anxiety now offers relief to most patients with anxiety disorders. However, late data underscore that these patients are likely to need long-term therapy. There is a significant tendency for relapse without ongoing treatment. The primary care clinician plays a pivotal role in making the diagnosis of anxiety, engaging the patient in cost-effective pharmacotherapy and psychotherapy, and teaching about the long-term nature of the illness and the need for treatment.

In this chapter, guidelines are offered for both patients and clinicians. Patients are encouraged to take an active role in understanding and determining the optimal treatment for their specific anxiety disorders. Clinicians are encouraged to engage patients in treatment from the outset. The physician plays a pivotal role in a number of areas: helping the patient sort out stressful life events that precipitate attacks, encouraging the practice of problem-solving skills that ameliorate anxiety, and discovering conflictual situations that trigger paroxysms of catastrophic thinking and autonomic cascades (i.e., episodes of hyperarousal) in the patient. A multidimensional treatment approach of this kind helps most women with anxiety disorders not only to find relief but also to attain an enhanced sense of well-being and competency in their lives.

The treatment of patients with anxiety disorders can be gratifying. A wide range of treatment options is available, and the patient usually is appreciative of the clinician's efforts. With treatment, patients often comment that pernicious symptoms are controlled, permitting full engagement in life for the first time in many years. By recognizing anxiety and supporting the patient in treatment, therefore, the primary care clinician can positively affect the quality of life for both the patient and her family. In addition, health care costs ultimately are reduced, and mortality may actually decline as a result of successful intervention.

Resources for the Patient

Bemis J, Barrada A: *Embracing Fear: Learning to Manage Anxiety and Panic Attacks.* Center City, MN, Hazelden, 1994.
> *Although primarily devoted to helping patients with anxiety recognize and work through their difficulties by regular practice in confronting the phobic stimulus, this book describes in detail many easy-to-use techniques to help patients with anxiety get past their "stuck points." The authors emphasize adhering to goals, practicing every day, dealing with setbacks, and consolidating achievements. Virtually every woman with anxiety could benefit from the practical steps and helpful tools suggested for tolerating stress and minimizing discomfort in phobic or anxiety-triggering situations, or such as going to restaurants, driving alone, flying.*

Gold MS: *The Good News about Panic, Anxiety, and Phobias: Cures, Treatments, and Solutions in the New Age of Biopsychiatry.* New York, Bantam, 1990.
> *This comprehensive book approaches the diagnosis and treatment of anxiety disorders from a primarily biologic perspective. Readers are presented with excellent information about what has been learned in the past 20 years to clarify diagnosis and to differentiate anxiety from medical conditions. Gold includes some simple behavioral steps and relaxation exercises to augment what he believes to be a breakthrough in the treatment of the anxiety disorders, namely, psychopharmacology.*

Marshall JR: *Social Phobia: From Shyness to Stage Fright.* New York, Basic Books, 1994.
> *The paralyzing effects of social phobia have come to light in the past decade. This book offers a number of case histories of people who, despite accomplishment in some areas, were desperately lonely and led limited lives because of their fear in group, social, and interpersonal situations. Marshall details the presentation of social phobia over the life cycle and outlines effective treatment modalities. He believes that many socially phobic patients attempt to self-medicate with alcohol and drugs. Women with social phobia will find in this book that they are not alone in their concerns about performance, scrutiny at work, loneliness, sexual intimacy, and physical preoccupation with the body (e.g., blushing, making eye contact). Parents will profit from the section devoted to social fears in children and how to differentiate normal anxiety from bona fide social phobia.*

Ross J: *Triumph over Fear: A Book of Help and Hope for People with Anxiety, Panic Attacks, and Phobias.* New York, Bantam, 1994.
> *This easy-to-read, factual, and comprehensive volume written by the president of the Anxiety Disorders Association of America offers hope and effective tools for patients who suffer from anxiety. First tackling the discrimination that people with mental disorders face, the author then describes "the many faces of anxiety"—meaning the many undiagnosed, but potentially treatable, anxious conditions. Lacing her writing with clinical examples of men and women who have benefited from medication and psychotherapy in their recovery, the author emphasizes how those who suffer from an anxiety disorder can develop their own self-help programs. Although not a substitute for psychotherapy or pharmacotherapy, this book offers a unique combination of moving case histories and practical advice to bring relief from anxiety, sometimes in a relatively brief time.*

Resources for the Clinician

Barlow DH: *Anxiety and Its Disorders: The Nature and Treatment of Anxiety and Panic.* New York, Guilford, 1988.
> *For the clinician who treats a number of patients with anxiety disorders, this book is*

a comprehensive overview of diagnosis and treatment. Written by a pioneer in the use of cognitive-behavioral therapy for anxiety, the volume includes principles and practical points for office management. For those who wish to learn even more behavioral techniques, see Craske MG, Meadows EA, Barlow DH: Therapist's Guide for the Mastery of Your Anxiety and Panic II and Agoraphobia Supplement, Albany, Graywind Publications, 1994.

Milrod BL, Busch FN, Cooper AM, et al.: *Manual of Panic-Focused Psychodynamic Psychotherapy.* Washington, DC, American Psychiatric Press, 1997.

In relatively few pages, these authors describe the rationale for offering psychodynamic psychotherapy to selected patients with panic. They describe positive outcomes based on long-term research in the field. Credence is placed in the psychological underpinning of many symptoms, and the authors include their own treatment protocols for working with anxious patients. This sensitive guide is a boon for the practitioner who is interested in taking a deeper look at the meaning and personal history underlying the symptom.

Shear MK, Weiner K: Psychotherapy for panic disorder. *J Clin Psychiatry* 1997; 58(Suppl 2):38–43.

For many patients, short-term treatments do not offer a favorable long-term outcome. These authors studied the benefit of nondirected, emotion-focused treatment for panic. They describe guidelines to aid patients in "focused unfolding" of their panic attacks. The result is an intervention that involves patient education, daily monitoring of panic episodes, and exploring and recalling the emotions triggered at the time of panic. The authors believe that their approach has the "added benefit of targeting general anxiety and depressive symptoms and addressing psychological problems that may contribute to long-term vulnerability to panic attacks" (p. 43). For the one fourth of patients who do not respond to medications or cognitive-behavioral therapy alone or in combination, knowledge of this approach is helpful. Referral to a psychotherapist with these psychodynamic skills is recommended.

The following supplements to the quarterly journal *Bulletin of the Menninger Clinic* offer overview articles by experts on particular anxiety disorders. They are the result of symposia presented at the annual meetings of the American Psychiatric Association. Although written with mental health professionals in mind, they are a comprehensive resource for the generalist as well. Each issue includes psychodynamic perspectives, cognitive-behavioral therapy, psychopharmacology, comorbidity, and an integrated treatment approach.

1. *Integrated Treatment of Panic and Social Phobia* 1992;56(Suppl A).

2. *Fear of Humiliation: Integrated Treatment of Social Phobia and Comorbid Conditions* 1994;58(Suppl A). Also published as Menninger WW (ed.): *Fear of Humiliation: Integrated Treatment of Social Phobia and Comorbid Conditions*. Northvale, NJ, Jason Aronson, 1995.

3. *Coping with Anxiety: Integrated Approaches to Treatment* 1995;59(Suppl A). Also published as Menninger WW (ed.): *Coping with Anxiety: Integrated Approaches to Treatment*. Northvale, NJ, Jason Aronson, 1996.

4. *Panic Disorder: Critical Issues in Treatment* 1996;60(Suppl A).

5. *Panic Disorder: Different Clinical Populations* 1997;61(Suppl A).

References

Allgulander C, Lavori PW: Excess mortality among 3,302 patients with "pure" anxiety neurosis. *Arch Gen Psychiatry* 1991;48:599–602.

Ballenger JC: Toward an integrated model of panic disorder. *Am J Orthopsychiatry* 1989;59:284–293.

Ballenger JC: Panic disorder in the medical setting. *J Clin Psychiatry* 1997;58(Suppl 2):13–17.

Balter MB, Levin L, Manheimer DI: Cross-national study of the extent of anti-anxiety/sedative drug use. *N Engl J Med* 1974;290:769–774.

Barlow DH: *Anxiety and Its Disorders: The Nature and Treatment of Anxiety and Panic*. New York, Guilford, 1988.

Barlow DH: Cognitive-behavioral approaches to panic disorder and social phobia. *Bull Menninger Clin* 1992;56(Suppl A):A14–A28.

Barlow DH: Comorbidity in social phobia: implications for cognitive-behavioral treatment. *Bull Menninger Clin* 1994;58(Suppl A):A43–A57.

Baum C, Kennedy DL, Knapp DE, et al.: Prescription drug use in 1984 and changes over time. *Med Care* 1988;26:105–114.

Bemis J, Barrada A: *Embracing the Fear: Learning to Manage Anxiety and Panic Attacks*. Center City, MN, Hazelden, 1994.

Bergin AE, Garfield SL (eds.): *Handbook of Psychotherapy and Behavior Change*, 4th ed. New York, Wiley, 1994.

Boulenger JP, Lavallee YJ: Mixed anxiety and depression: diagnostic issues. *J Clin Psychiatry* 1993;54(suppl):3–8.

Bowlby J: *Attachment and Loss*, vol 1: *Attachment*. New York, Basic Books, 1969.

Bowlby J: *Attachment and Loss*, vol 3: *Loss: Sadness and Depression*. New York, Basic Books, 1980.

Brawman-Mintzer O, Lydiard RB: Generalized anxiety disorder: issues in epidemiology. *J Clin Psychiatry* 1996;57(Suppl 7):3–8.

Brown TA, Barlow DH, Liebowitz MR: The empirical basis of generalized anxiety disorder. *Am J Psychiatry* 1994;151:1272–1280.

Brown TA, O'Leary TA, Barlow DH: Generalized anxiety disorders. In: Barlow DH (ed.): *Clinical Handbook of Psychological Disorders: A Step-By-Step Treatment Manual*, 2nd ed., pp. 137–188. New York, Guilford, 1993.

Catalan J, Garth D: Benzodiazepines in general practice: a time for decision. *Br Med J* 1985;290:1374–1376.

Clark NM, Janz NK, Dodge J, et. al.: Managing heart disease: A study of experiences of older women. *J Am Med Wom Assoc* 1994;49(6):202–206.

Cohen LS, Heller VL, Rosenbaum JF: Treatment guidelines for psychotropic drug use in pregnancy. *Psychosomatics* 1989;30:25–33.

Craig KD, Dobson KS (eds.): *Anxiety and Depression in Adults and Children*. Thousand Oaks, CA, Sage, 1995.

Craighead LW, Craighead WE, Kazdin AE, et al. (eds.): *Cognitive and Behavioral Interventions: An Empirical Approach to Mental Health Problems*. Boston, Allyn & Bacon, 1994.

Craske MG, Meadows EA, Barlow DH: *Therapist's Guide for the Mastery of Your Anxiety and Panic II and Agoraphobia Supplement*. Albany, NY, Graywind Publications, 1994.

Davidson JRT: Use of benzodiazepines in panic disorder. *J Clin Psychiatry* 1997;58(Suppl 2):26–28.

Davidson JRT, van der Kolk BA: The psychopharmacological treatment of posttraumatic stress disorder. In: van der Kolk BA, McFarlane AC, Weisaeth L (eds.): *Traumatic Stress: The Effects of Overwhelming Experience on Mind, Body and Society*, pp. 510–524. New York, Guilford, 1996.

DuPont RL: Anxiety and addiction: a clinical perspective on comorbidity. *Bull Menninger Clin* 1995;59(Suppl A):A53–A72.

DuPont RL: Panic disorder and addiction: the clinical issues of comorbidity. *Bull Menninger Clin* 1997;61(Suppl A):A54–A65.

DuPont RL, DuPont CM, DuPont Spencer E: Anxiety disorders in the elderly. *Directions in Psychiatry* 1996a;16:3–11.

DuPont RL, Rice DP, Miller LS, et al.: Economic costs of anxiety disorders. *Anxiety* 1996b;2:167–172.

Fornazzari X, Freire M: Women as victims of torture. *Acta Psychiatr Scand* 1990;82:257–260.

Furey JA: Women Vietnam veterans: a comparison of studies. *J Psychosoc Nurs Ment Health Serv* 1991;29:11–13.

Gabbard GO: Psychodynamics of panic disorder and social phobia. *Bull Menninger Clin* 1992;56(Suppl A):A3–A13.

Gold MS: *The Good News about Panic, Anxiety, and Phobias: Cures, Treatments, and Solutions in the New Age of Biopsychiatry*. New York, Bantam, 1990.

Goldenberg IM, White K, Yonkers K, et al.: The infrequency of "pure culture" diagnoses among the anxiety disorders. *J Clin Psychiatry* 1996;57:528–533.

Greist JH: Anxiety disorders: the role of serotonin. *J Clin Psychiatry* 1996;57(Suppl 6):3–4.

Herbst PKR: From helpless victim to empowered survivor: oral history as a treatment for survivors of torture. *Women and Therapy* 1992;13:141–154.

Higgins ES: Obsessive-compulsive spectrum disorders in primary care: the possibilities and the pitfalls. *J Clin Psychiatry* 1996;57(Suppl 8):7–10.

Hirschfeld RM: The impact of health care reform on social phobia. *J Clin Psychiatry* 1995;56(Suppl 5):13–17.

Jefferson JW: Social phobia: everyone's disorder? *J Clin Psychiatry* 1996;57(Suppl 6):28–32.

Jefferson JW: Antidepressants in panic disorder. *J Clin Psychiatry* 1997;58(Suppl 2):20–25.

Johnson J, Weissman MM: Panic disorder, co-morbidity, and suicide attempts. *Arch Gen Psychiatry* 1990;47:805–808.

Judelson DR: Coronary heart disease in women: risk factors and prevention. *J Am Med Wom Assoc* 1994;49(6):186–191.

Katon W: Panic disorder: relationship to high medical utilization, unexplained physical symptoms, and medical costs. *J Clin Psychiatry* 1996;57(Suppl 10):11–22.

Katon W, Kleinman AM: Doctor-patient negotiation and other social science strategies in patient care. In: Eisenberg L, Kleinman AM (eds.): *The Relevance of Social Science for Medicine*, pp. 253–249. Datrecht, Holland, D Reisel, 1980.

Keller MB, Hanks DL: Anxiety symptom relief in depression treatment outcomes. *J Clin Psychiatry* 1995;56(Suppl 6):22–29.

Kendler KS: Twin studies of psychiatric illness: current status and future directions. *Arch Gen Psychiatry* 1993;50:905–915.

Kendler KS, Neale MC, Kessler RC, et al.: Generalized anxiety disorder in women: a population-based twin study. *Arch Gen Psychiatry* 1992;49:267–272.

Kendler KS, Neale MC, Kessler RC, et al.: Panic disorder in women: a population-based twin study. *Psychol Med* 1993;23:397–406.

Kennerley H: The prevention of anxiety disorders. In: Kendrick T, Tyler A, Freeling P (eds.): *The Prevention of Mental Illness in Primary Care*, pp. 188–206. Cambridge, Cambridge University Press, 1996.

Klein DF: Panic disorder and agoraphobia: hypothesis hothouse. *J Clin Psychiatry* 1996;57(Suppl 6):21–27.

Lieberman JA III: Compliance issues in primary care. *J Clin Psychiatry* 1996;57(Suppl 7):76–82.

Liebowitz MR: Mixed anxiety and depression: should it be included in DSM-IV? *J Clin Psychiatry* 1993;54(5, suppl):4–7.

Lucki I: Serotonin receptor specificity in anxiety disorders. *J Clin Psychiatry* 1996;57(Suppl 6):5–10.

Marshall JR: The psychopharmacology of social phobia. *Bull Menninger Clin* 1992;56(Suppl A):A42–A49.

Marshall JR: *Social Phobia: From Shyness to Stage Fright*. New York, Basic Books, 1994.

Marshall JR: Comorbidity and its effect on panic disorder. *Bull Menninger Clin* 1996;60(Suppl A):A39–A53.

Menninger WW (ed.): *Fear of Humiliation: Integrated Treatment of Social Phobia and Comorbid Conditions*. Northvale, NJ, Aronson, 1995.

Milrod BL, Busch FN, Cooper AM, et al.: *Manual of Panic-Focused Psychodynamic Psychotherapy*. Washington, DC, American Psychiatric Press, 1997.

Milrod B, Busch FN, Hollander E, et al.: A 23-year-old woman with panic disorder treated with psychodynamic psychotherapy. *Am J Psychiatry* 1996;153:698–703.

Murrey GJ, Bolen J, Miller N, et al.: History of childhood sexual abuse in women and depressive and anxiety disorders: a comparative study. *J Sex Educ Ther* 1993;19:13–19.

Petty F, Davis LL, Kabel D, et al.: Serotonin dysfunction disorders: a behavioral neurochemistry perspective. *J Clin Psychiatry* 1996;57(Suppl 8):11–16.

Pigott TA: OCD: where the serotonin selectivity story begins. *J Clin Psychiatry* 1996;57(Suppl 6):11–20.

Pollack MH: Treatment and outcome in anxiety disorders. *Currents* 1993;12:5–15.

Quadrio C: Families of agoraphobic women. *Aust N Z J Psychiatry* 1984;18:164–170.

Regier DA, Boyd JH, Burke JD, et al.: One-month prevalence of mental disorders in the United States: based on five Epidemiologic Catchment Area sites. *Arch Gen Psychiatry* 1988;45:977–986.

Regier DA, Myers JK, Kramer M, et al.: The NIMH Epidemiologic Catchment Area program: historical context, major objectives, and study population characteristics. *Arch Gen Psychiatry* 1984;41:934–941.

Renik O: The patient's anxiety, the therapist's anxiety, and the therapeutic process. In: Roose SP, Glick RA (eds.): *Anxiety as Symptom and Signal*, pp. 121–130. Hillsdale, NJ, Analytic Press, 1995.

Rosenbaum JF: Evaluation and management of the treatment-resistant anxiety disorder patient. *Bull Menninger Clin* 1992;56(Suppl A):A50–A60.

Rosenbaum JF: Treatment-resistant panic disorder. *J Clin Psychiatry* 1997;58(Suppl 2):66–67.

Rosenbaum JF, Pollock RA: The psychopharmacology of social phobia and comorbid disorders. *Bull Menninger Clin* 1994;58(Suppl A):A67–A83.

Rosenbaum JF, Pollock RA, Jordan SK, et al.: The pharmacotherapy of panic disorder. *Bull Menninger Clin* 1996;60(Suppl A):A54–A75.

Rosenbaum JF, Pollock RA, Otto MW, et al.: Integrated treatment of panic disorder. *Bull Menninger Clin* 1995;59(Suppl A):A4–A26.

Ross J: *Triumph over Fear: A Book of Help and Hope for People with Anxiety, Panic Attacks, and Phobias.* New York, Bantam, 1994.

Roy-Bryne PP: Generalized anxiety and mixed anxiety-depression: association with disability and health care utilization. *J Clin Psychiatry* 1996;57(Suppl 7):86–95.

Sable P: Attachment, anxiety, and agoraphobia. *Women and Therapy* 1991;11:55–69.

Shear MK, Cooper AM, Klerman GL, et al.: A psychodynamic model of panic disorder. *Am J Psychiatry* 1993;150:859–866.

Shear MK, Mammen O: Anxiety disorders in primary care: a life-span perspective. *Bull Menninger Clin* 1997;61(Suppl A):A37–A53.

Shear MK, Weiner K: Psychotherapy for panic disorder. *J Clin Psychiatry* 1997;58(Suppl 2):38–43.

Sichel DA, Cohen, LS, Dimmock JA, et al.: Postpartum obsessive compulsive disorder: a case series. *J Clin Psychiatry* 1993a;54:156–159.

Sichel DA, Cohen LS, Rosenbaum JF, et al.: Postpartum onset of obsessive-compulsive disorder. *Psychosomatics* 1993b;34:277–279.

Stahl SM: Mixed anxiety and depression: clinical implications. *J Clin Psychiatry* 1993;54(suppl):33–38.

Stokes PE: A primary care perspective on management of acute and long-term depression. *J Clin Psychiatry* 1993;54(Suppl 8):74–84.

Stoudemire A: Epidemiology and psychopharmacology of anxiety in medical patients. *J Clin Psychiatry* 1996;57(Suppl 7):64–72.

Street LL, Barlow DH: Anxiety disorders. In: Craighead LW, Craighead WE, Kazdin AE, et al. (eds.): *Cognitive and Behavioral Interventions: An Empirical Approach to Mental Health Problems,* pp. 71–88. Boston, Allyn & Bacon, 1994.

Wagner KD, Berenson AB: Norplant-associated major depression and panic disorder. *J Clin Psychiatry* 1994;55:478–480.

Wenger NK: Coronary heart disease in women: gender differences in diagnostic evaluation. *J Am Med Wom Assoc* 1994;49:181–185, 197.

Winnicott DW: *The Family and Individual Development.* London, Tavistock, 1965.

Wise MG, Griffies WS: A combined treatment approach to anxiety in the medically ill. *J Clin Psychiatry* 1995;56(Suppl 2):14–19.

Yonkers KA, Ellison JM: Anxiety disorders in women and their pharmacological treatment. In: Jensvold MF, Halbreich U, Hamilton JA (eds.): *Psychopharmacology and Women: Sex, Gender, and Hormones,* pp. 261–285. Washington, DC, American Psychiatric Press, 1996.

Yonkers KA, Gurguis G: Gender differences in the prevalence and expression of anxiety disorders. In: Seeman MV (ed.): *Gender and Psychopathology,* pp. 113–130. Washington, DC, American Psychiatric Press, 1995.

Zerbe KJ: Through the storm: psychoanalytic theory in the psychotherapy of the anxiety disorders. *Bull Menninger Clin* 1990;54:171–183.

Zerbe KJ: Anxiety disorders in women. *Bull Menninger Clin* 1995;59(Suppl A):A38–A52.

Chapter 2

Depression

Depression is a major mental health concern for women. Occurring two to three times more commonly in women than in men, the spectrum of mild-to-severe forms takes an enormous toll on family life and productivity. Unipolar depression and seasonal affective disorder (SAD), or winter depression, which is related to a change in daylight hours, predominate in females. In recent generations, there apparently have been earlier onset and increased incidence of depression in younger age groups. The postpartum period is the most likely time for a woman to become depressed (see Chapter 11).

Although major strides have been made over the past 25 years in diagnosing and treating affective disorders, the stigma of having an emotional problem impedes many people from seeking help early. One national poll found that 54% of the United States population view depression as a personal weakness and that 62% do not view depression as the health problem it truly is. Strikingly, 13% of those interviewed saw themselves as "really depressed" (National Mental Health Association, 1996). As these public opinion findings demonstrate, there are literally millions of people who fail to seek treatment because of shame, embarrassment, and limited understanding of the illness. Even in primary care, one half of all patients with depression remain unrecognized (Tylee, 1996) and hence untreated. It is estimated that 10% of patients in primary care have major depression, and that 20% to 30% of all those seen in this setting have depressive symptoms (Klerman and Weissman, 1992; Wells et al., 1992).

Both the varying definitions of the disorder and the standard measurement instruments that can be helpful in primary care as well as psychiatric practice (e.g., Beck Depression Inventory, Hamilton Rating Scale for Depression, Zung Self-Rating Depression Scale) may fail to gauge the depth of suffering of many patients who are inadequately treated. The diagnosis, treatment, and synthesis of relevant literature on depression are therefore more difficult than they appear.

First introduced in 1972, the term "major depression" continues in use today, although it is relatively nonspecific and means different things to different professionals (Parker, 1993). The majority of patients presenting to general medical practitioners do not meet the full diagnostic criteria listed in the fourth edition of the American Psychiatric Association's *Diagnostic and Statistical Manual of Mental Disorders* (1994), yet the adverse outcome for so-called subthreshold or subclinical depression is as high or higher than for major depression (Olfson et al., 1996). Morbidity in both groups is comparable: One fourth of patients make suicide attempts, about 20% lose at least 1 week of work per year, 15% use minor tranquilizers, and many subjectively report having had "the worst depression of my life" (Johnson et al., 1992; Olfson et al., 1996).

Two thirds of the estimated 6 million women with major depression or dysthymia remain undiagnosed. The annual cost in the United States is more than $25 billion, of which half results from reduced productivity and excessive absenteeism (Greenberg et al., 1993). The mean annual health care cost of primary care patients with depression is $4,246, almost double that for those without depression ($2,371). Only one fifth of the cost for patients with depression is related to mental health care; the remainder is for general medical care (Simon et al., 1995).

In the RAND Corporation analysis of outcome data, it was ascertained that depression is still underdiagnosed, although primary care providers treat 60% of those who are severely depressed (Sturm and Wells, 1995) and have access to more accurate ways of identifying the illness. Other problems associated with treatment of depression include poor medication choice and treatment focus and lack of patient counseling. For example, anxiolytics are overprescribed to depressed patients, whereas antidepressants are underutilized. Many patients refuse antidepressants because they inaccurately believe them to be addictive. Too little psychotherapy and patient education is provided, mainly because the average visit to the primary care physician is only 8 minutes long. More favorable depression outcomes result when clinicians are trained to provide increased patient education, brief cognitive-behavioral therapy, and adequate dosage and duration of pharmacotherapy, and when they integrate the help of care extenders such as nurse counselors (Katon et al., 1996; Schulberg et al., 1996).

Secondary prevention of depression is enhanced when primary care clinicians or care extenders ask open-ended questions, show empathy, and teach patients how to make behavioral and lifestyle changes (Table 2–1). Acute- and continuation-phase treatments of specific dosage and duration, in conjunction with greater recognition of subthreshold symptoms that tend to be dismissed, help address the needs of the millions of men and women whose social, family, and work functions are impaired by affective illness (Olfson et al., 1996; Schulberg et al., 1996). The first step, however, is enhancing one's diagnostic acumen with respect to depression, making sure that even the most subtle signs do not go unnoticed or unaddressed.

Patient Presentation

What is the "typical" presentation of depression in primary care? The hallmark features of dysphoric mood—feeling sad, blue, discouraged, hopeless, and "not caring about things any more"—usually are recognized by even an unseasoned practitioner (Table 2–2). However, actual cases are not often as neat as the clinical examples in textbooks and academic lectures. The symptoms that are most valuable in pointing to depression are persistent and pervasive lowering of mood, and loss of motivation, interest, and drive. The primary care clinicians must be alert to the patient who complains of a change in her activity level and lessened involvement in those chores, hobbies, or interests that once gave her pleasure (Table 2–3). At work, for example, the patient may note that she is putting off making decisions; she may describe how she moves more slowly through tasks, watching her work accumulate.

The observations of family members can reveal much about the patient's change in mood. Partners or children may casually mention that the patient has lost interest in activities that she enjoyed and that she has stopped cooking, cleaning, or participating in hobbies or family events.

Table 2–1. **Initial Assessment of the Patient with Depression**

Enhance caring attitude by an open demeanor
1. Show interest and concern. Ask about home, work, and family.
2. Address the patient's hidden concerns (e.g., embarrassment or shame about coming in for treatment or trouble functioning at home or at work; change in sexual desire; change in weight; decreased confidence in mental ability).
3. Challenge the stigma that accompanies emotional disorders. Some patients believe they lack "backbone" if they acknowledge their low self-worth, sadness, fatigue, or other symptoms of depression.
4. Be aware of verbal and nonverbal cues—not only in the patient but also in yourself.
5. Remember that women are more likely than men to discuss symptoms but avoid doing so unless they are given sufficient time.
6. Whenever possible, ask family members about their observations.

Educate patients about pharmacotherapy
1. Challenge notions about antidepressants. Many people mistakenly believe that these medications are addictive.

Check for somatic mimics of depression
1. Suspect depression in patients who present with a plethora of physical complaints, a lack of willingness to consider psychological explanations for their problems, or cues of emotional disturbance that surface late in the interview.

Develop interviewing skills
1. Make more eye contact. Listen patiently without interruption. Ask about feelings.
2. Ask open-ended questions. To convey that you are listening carefully and attentively, briefly summarize what the patient has told you.
3. Make empathic comments (e.g., "It must be very hard to get up and go to work in the morning, feeling like you do"; "You must be very worried about yourself, and your family, because you aren't able to maintain the pace you previously did").

Because of the comorbid anxiety that frequently accompanies depression, the patient may also complain of a continual state of apprehension. The somatic aspects of anxiety—palpitations, sweating, headache, and indigestion—lead to expensive medical workups that can be avoided if the commonly encountered mixed anxiety-depression syndrome is considered first.

Table 2–2. **When to Suspect Depression—Classic Presentation**

Persistent sad, anxious, or unhappy mood
Feelings of guilt, worthlessness, and helplessness
Feelings of emptiness, malcontent, and despair
Fatigue or decreased energy
Marked changes in sleep pattern
Appetite or weight loss—or, conversely, overeating and weight gain
Lack of desire or interest in sex
Poor self-esteem or lack of contentment with self

Table 2–3. **When to Suspect Depression—Other Common Indicators**

Symptom	Examples
Irritable mood or magnified behaviors	The patient is often moody or easily upset. "I find myself brooding about what my boss and assistants think about me all the time." "I always think my husband is mad at me, and I cry easily."
Any change in behavior	An ambitious female executive suddenly loses interest in her work and falls behind in her tasks. She may stay at home worrying or complain of fitful sleep. She also takes sick days and appears "lazy" to coworkers and friends. "I just don't care about my job or how my house looks anymore."
Sudden silences	A previously talkative and outgoing person withdraws, saying she wants to be alone all the time. The patient's significant other tells you that she "never talks to me anymore. She goes off and stares blankly at the fireplace."
Forgetfulness	The patient tells you she thinks she is developing Alzheimer's disease because she can't remember her best friend's phone number, always has to double-check appointments, and was humiliated when she forgot her child at the day care center. "I think I'm losing my mind."
Indecisiveness	A formerly assertive woman begins to have trouble making even small decisions, forgetting her menus, or deciding what to wear. The patient's partner tells you, "I have to decide every little thing now. She used to even tell me what to wear."
Poor grooming	A previously fastidious, fashionable dresser begins to look unkempt, reflecting a loss of interest or pleasure in self-care. The patient says, "I don't care how I look anymore. I don't have the energy or interest to style my hair."
Complaint of aches and pains despite negative workup	A patient without a history of somatization and in good physical health makes numerous visits to your office—always with a new physical complaint. She says her body is "falling apart" because she has backache and stomach pain, feels fatigued, and so on. She is frustrated because several physicians who have done "full medical workups never found anything wrong."

Certain obvious cognitive problems herald depression. Patients typically complain of an inability to concentrate or pay attention. Cognitive symptoms may initially lead the primary care clinician to suspect organic brain disease, but depression is the most common cause of decreased capacity to think clearly and learn new facts. These symptoms can be tested objectively in the office by asking the patient to do a few simple mathematical problems or by questioning her about some recent local or national events. Women usually brighten when asked about their families. But the patient who seems not to care about herself or others, who exerts enormous energy to answer questions, and who complains of fatigue and feelings of low self-worth is a prime candidate for a diagnosis of depression.

What to Listen for

The best diagnostic tool is still the clinician's ear. Make a mental note to assess each of these areas of potential distress in the patient: sleep, mood, activity level, loss of sexual interest, and suicide risk. Your own feeling state around the patient should be evaluated also.

Sleep. Although early morning awakening has long been considered the preeminent sleep disturbance with depression, the most common complaint is inability to fall asleep. Despite exerting enormous energy to "keep going" during the day, at night the patient may lie awake and worry. Rare but still characteristic symptoms include night awakening, feeling despondent or even suicidal, and weepiness. More typically, patients report that they feel unrefreshed after sleep. Like depression itself, sleep disturbances occur on a continuum, with the classic symptom of early morning awakening typically connoting a more severe depression.

Mood. As depression progresses, the patient's feelings devolve from a sense of "flatness" or "dullness" to a near-total "loss of feeling." Verbal individuals may describe their depression as a "black cloud hanging over me" or "feeling like I'm in a dark cave." Less sophisticated, more concrete-thinking patients do not have words to describe their emotions. They tend to somatize and emphasize physical complaints. Rarely do these complaints center on just one body system; rather, they tend to span a wide range—from headache, to stomach pain, to dyspepsia, to arthralgia, to backache. Continued physical complaints and costly workups that do not yield a specific bona fide diagnosis can be emotionally draining on the practitioner and can shroud recognition of the depression.

Those patients who are capable of expressing themselves in words report that their mood is not just normal sadness but something characteristically different. On occasion, the patient may report bursting into tears for no reason. However, with increasing severity, the patient becomes incapable of weeping. This ominous sign is a hallmark of severe depression—the sense that one is now becoming "beyond tears."

Activity Level and Loss of Sexual Interest. Early in the course of depression, a woman may be able to forget her physical or emotional state in the company of others; a highly attuned spouse or significant other may note a change that is not recognized by a friend or coworker. However, as the depression progresses, the patient feels weighed down by her misery and avoids opportunities to participate in outings or take on tasks that were once personally meaningful. She tends to avoid her friends. Women who once enjoyed sex or who were, at least, quite willing partners may lose interest and desire. But they often will not reveal this information, divulging it only when asked repeatedly by the physician.

Your Own Feeling State. In the presence of a depressed person, clinicians, like many friends and family members, are prone to take on the role of "cheerleading the patient." You may unwittingly find yourself saying to the patient, "Can't you see the bright side of things? Look at how much you have going for you. So many people care. You've got to stay active and keep moving." Depressed patients feel worse after such seemingly well-intentioned comments and are not reassured by compliments. Instead, they see the gloomy side of everything. Despite notable past achievements, they view themselves as failures; productive work and activities seem trivial. In the most severe cases, they describe themselves as hopeless and having no future, despite being told by their caregivers that their depression is eminently treatable.

Recognition and treatment of depression are both enhanced by the practice of verbal and nonverbal communication skills that demonstrate empathy, openness, interest, and concern (Howie et al., 1991; Tylee, 1996) (see Table 2–1). Clinicians sometimes feel depressed or sad themselves when interviewing a depressed patient. This state of "emotional contagion" (picking up on the patient's feelings) reflects the patient's capacity to successfully deposit raw emotions into a sensitive, receptive human being. Attunement to what one experiences with the patient, in terms of one's own mood, is frequently a clue to successful diagnosis and treatment.

Suicide Risk. The risk for suicide is greatest when the patient is preoccupied with thoughts of death and feels that life is not worth living. If the patient has made a previous suicide attempt and acknowledges having a suicide plan that might be used, the risk goes up substantially. However, *even persons with mild depression may try to kill themselves without warning*, so it is important for the physician and care extenders to ask frequently about thoughts of death, storing up prescribed or nonprescribed medications, or other ways that the patient may be planning to hurt herself. It is virtually impossible to predict suicide, but anguish and a sense of hopelessness are among the most immediate motives. This despair may result from the humiliation that follows after a catastrophic personal loss or an injury to self-esteem and self-confidence (Jack, 1987; Lewis, 1987). Illness, the loss of a job, the collapse of a marriage, the mortification about the actions of one's spouse or children, and the death of a family member are all precipitants the perceptive caregiver must attempt to recognize and address.

Clinical Example 2–1

A 50-year-old surgeon was convinced she would be sued for malpractice because of a small, residual scar that occurred after she sutured the lacerated thumb of an adolescent convict. Reassurances by colleagues, including her primary physician, failed to alleviate her feelings of guilt and self-reproach. She ruminated about her "mistake" and had to push herself to go to work. She lost 30 pounds and paced the floor at night; her husband

and children begged her to seek psychiatric support, but she refused. Her depression worsened, and her guilty preoccupation turned into a frank delusion. She believed that her action had deformed the patient, whose "symptoms are all my fault," that he would seek retribution by publicly maligning her, and that her career would be "totally ruined." Finally, she sought psychiatric help. In the initial interview, she denied wanting to kill herself, but then she stored up 2 weeks' worth of her prescribed antidepressant medication, impulsively swallowed it, and subsequently crashed her car into the wall of the hospital admissions office.

What to Watch for in the Clinical Setting

Neurovegetative Symptoms. Frequently encountered neurovegetative symptoms of depression—significant weight loss, decreased libido, poor appetite, terminal insomnia—indicate a profound depressive episode. A useful clinical tool is to ask the patient about a "loss of pleasure" in usual activities, such as eating, sleeping, or making love. Often, a depressed woman responds affirmatively when these empathic questions penetrate her defensive facade of "keeping up a good appearance and working hard." She may then be able to confirm her diminished energy, emotional lability, decreased vitality, and pessimism. Prime candidates may be those patients who report being (or *who you sense* are) more *irritable*, *labile*, or *fearful* than usual. Primary care clinicians who are aware of these subtle shifts in the patient's visage or activity level are in the best position to detect an early, more easily treated clinical depression.

Apprehension and Anxiety. In the past decade, research has also identified the high occurrence of "mixed states" of anxiety and depression (Klerman, 1990; Leibowitz, 1993; Parker, 1993). This frequently encountered comorbidity (sometimes as high as 50%) points the way toward specific diagnosis and more effective treatment. More women than men complain of the agitation (or restlessness) that accompanies depression. The anxious, depressed patient fidgets in the examining room chair, crosses and uncrosses her legs, plays with her jewelry, or tears tissues into little bits; while tousling her hair, she may frenetically stop to examine her fingers.

In more rural settings, a patient may not seek medical attention because of limited access to care, lack of knowledge, and resolute desire "to see the doctor only if something is really wrong with me." Such circumstances keep many who could be effectively treated early from getting adequate evaluation and treatment. A severe, agitated depression or melancholic state then evolves over a period of many months. The patient typically enters the examination room, ceaselessly pacing up and down. When the patient wrings her hands, tears at her hair, moans pleadingly, or expresses certainty that a calamity is about to occur, the diagnostic question is raised of an agitated depression versus a mixed bipolar illness. Because either condition is amenable to electroconvulsive therapy (ECT) or may be treated with aggressive pharmacotherapy, psychiatric consultation should be obtained whenever possible. This is particularly true if the primary care clinician is uncertain of the diagnosis (which can sometimes be made only after sufficient time and a longitudinal profile of the illness) or of the most expeditious route of treatment.

THE LONG-TERM NATURE OF DEPRESSION

Depressive disorders traditionally were viewed as time-limited episodes lasting 6 to 9 months; full recovery was expected even without treatment. This view has radically shifted over the past 20 years. Longitudinal studies of patients with one episode of depression have determined that most have other episodes and need long-term follow-up treatment. Depression is currently best understood as a chronic, albeit treatable, emotional illness (Hirschfeld, 1997; Kocsis et al., 1996; Kupfer et al., 1992; Mintz et al., 1992; Mueller et al., 1996; Rush, 1996; Wells et al., 1992).

Depressed persons have numerous interepisodic manifestations, including emotional lability, general anxiety, irritability, decreased vitality, hypochondriasis, pessimism, insomnia, and loss of affective resilience. Psychiatric research has demonstrated that treatment should be longer and sustained. Despite lengthy periods of illness, patients continue to recover (Mueller et al., 1996), although it is as yet impossible to distinguish those who will recover from those who will not.

Patients with dysthymia who receive adequate doses of medication can have a full remission of symptoms (Thase et al., 1996), and long-term maintenance appears to be effective in preventing relapse (Blacker, 1996; Kocsis et al., 1996). Maintenance medication is recommended for at least 2 years, but some patients may need it for decades (Rush, 1996). Most authorities concur that treatment should continue for an extended period after symptomatic improvement (Blacker, 1996; Kupfer et al., 1996). The physician should make frequent assessments for changes in symptoms that might warrant a change in treatment strategies. For example, a woman whose condition does not improve (or does so only minimally) is likely to benefit from an adequate dosage of another agent (Quitkin et al., 1996). The physician must be tenacious and hopeful, building the therapeutic alliance by repeating to the patient, "If this does not work, we will continue to try other medications."

THE IMPORTANCE OF COMPLIANCE

The patient should be asked about any medication side effects. Many times depression improves with pharmacotherapy, but sleep disturbance will not be normalized and sexual dysfunction may occur (Shen and Hsu, 1995). These side effects can result in poor compliance and an impaired quality of life. Some antidepressants themselves negatively affect sexual functioning and sleep. Clinicians should ask specifically about these domains so that the patient can be given, if necessary, a medication with a different mechanism of action (e.g., from a selective serotonin reuptake inhibitor [SSRI] to nefazodone) (see Chapter 13).

Other important factors are drug interactions, weight gain, and daytime sleepiness. Long-term tolerance of the selected agent is crucial for patient acceptance; a growing body of evidence suggests that a combination of medication and psychotherapy has many potential advantages for chronically depressed patients (Fava et al., 1996). These treatments tend to enhance each other by as yet unknown mechanisms. Improvement in one's sense of self-worth and ability to cope with life's vicissitudes appears to be a crucial variable with a positive effect on symptom management.

Research on the long-term nature of depression is now prompting the prophylactic use of antidepressants, usually for years in persons who have had two or three episodes. Specific guidelines continue to be elucidated, although the value of long-term pharmacotherapy and psychotherapeutic follow-up is likely to stand the test of time (Fava et al., 1996). In some studies, adjunctive cognitive-behavioral or interpersonal psychotherapy has been recognized as augmenting the effect of medication.

The primary care clinician plays a major role by educating the patient about depression, encouraging compliance with medication and therapy, and countering the natural tendency to feel shame or embarrassment about receiving psychological care. Simply emphasizing to the patient that depression is an illness with biologic underpinnings can help offset the patient's tendency to view herself as impaired or marred by the illness. It is important also to stress that the most thorough scientific studies now argue for long-term maintenance pharmacotherapy, particularly in patients who have had severe and recurrent symptoms or episodes (Kupfer and Frank, 1996). The majority of patients who do not improve are noncompliant with treatment or are not receiving a high enough dose of medication. Efforts must therefore be made to keep the patient on an adequate dosage (see "Present Treatment Options"), to minimize side effects, and to stay involved in psychosocial treatment.

ATYPICAL DEPRESSION

Atypical depression occurs three to four times more commonly in women than in men. This syndrome (which in the 1970s and 1980s was referred to as "hysteroid dysphoria") is characterized by sensitivity to interpersonal rejection and the inverse of traditional neurovegetative signs of depression. In practice, the female patient with atypical depression complains of carbohydrate craving, psychomotor agitation or anxiety, oversleeping and fatigue, and overeating. Some subgroups of women describe a pervasive need to consume chocolate; others tend toward having panic attacks (Hamilton et al., 1996; Nolen-Hoeksema, 1995; Shaw et al., 1995).

Family history is positive for the depressive spectrum of illnesses—female relatives with depressive disorder and male relatives with alcoholism or antisocial personality. This group of patients tends to be selectively responsive to the monoamine oxidase inhibitors (MAOIs). Preliminary data also suggest superior efficacy of some of the SSRIs.

SEASONAL AFFECTIVE DISORDER

This subtype of unipolar and bipolar disorder affects more women than men, usually between the ages of 21 and 30 years. Atypical neurovegetative features (hyperphagia, hypersomnia, weight gain, and anergia) that are recurrent and associated with a winter or summer seasonal pattern suggest the diagnosis (Shaw et al., 1995). Like other mood disturbances, SAD occurs on a continuum; both subsyndromal SAD (also known as the "winter blues") and its more severe counterpart respond well to light therapy. Patients who use a 10,000-lux light fixture that is easily obtained commercially find that they can, with experience, adjust the amount of light needed. Although it is possible to induce mania and hypomania with light therapy, a collaborative relationship with the patient minimizes these untoward consequences (Rosenthal and Orem, 1995).

MEDICAL MIMICS OF DEPRESSION

A complete medical workup is essential, because many physical conditions manifest as depression (Cummings, 1994; Gadde and Krishnan, 1994, 1996; Hall et al., 1978; Mason et al., 1993; Pies, 1994; Prange et al., 1984). The list of possible medical causes provided in Table 2–4 is not intended to be all-inclusive but rather to trigger clinical thinking during the initial visits with a patient who experiences a change in mood, cognition, responsiveness, energy, or self-worth.

Patients who somatize can be the bane of the primary care clinician's existence, unwilling as they may be to hear that their condition has no concrete, discernible physical cause. But some persons deemphasize their physical problems and initially present feeling weighed down with their personal misery. These patients must be investigated carefully for depression. In particular, a medical cause should be suspected in any woman who presents after age 40 with depression for the first time. In this group, an occult carcinoma could be the culprit.

Moreover, despite the abundance of food in our society, a number of women have subclinical eating disorders or are frankly malnourished (see Chapters 5 and 14). Indeed, malnutrition itself is often the underlying cause of depression, particularly in the eating-disordered or elderly patient.

Table 2–4. Medical Mimics of Depression

Endocrine disorders	**Neurologic disorders**
Hyperthyroidism	Multiple sclerosis
Cushing's syndrome	Early Huntington's chorea
Adrenocortical insufficiency	Parkinson's disease
Hypothyroidism	Stroke
Collagen vascular disorders	Vascular disease
Rheumatoid arthritis	Tumor or aneurysm
Systemic lupus erythematosus	Wilson's disease, Lewy body disease (rare)
Giant cell arthritis	**Neoplastic disorders**
Hematologic disorders	Lung
Anemia	Pancreas
B_1 (thiamine) deficiency	Lymphoma
B_3 (niacin) deficiency	Brain
B_6 (pyridoxine) deficiency	Breast
B_{12} (cyanocobalamin) deficiency	**Substance abuse disorders**
Folate deficiency	Alcohol
Infectious diseases	Cocaine
Hepatitis	Opiates
Human immunodeficiency virus (HIV)	Cannabis (potentially)
infection	**Nutritional/metabolic disturbances**
Influenza	Hypokalemia/hyponatremia
Mononucleosis	Uremia
Lyme disease	Subclinical or overt eating disorder
	Malnutrition, particularly in elderly or
	eating-disordered patients

IATROGENICALLY INDUCED DEPRESSION

Medications from "virtually every class of drugs have been implicated in causing depression" (Metzger and Friedman, 1994) (Table 2–5). Sex differences related to drug-drug interactions may be a confounding variable that heightens the propensity of women to develop depression when taking certain medications. In addition, concurrent medication use may influence the course of an illness or alter pharmacokinetics (Hamilton et al., 1996).

As more and more agents become available without prescription, it is especially wise to take a thorough history of the patient's use of prescribed and over-the-counter medications. The history should note *all medications*, even those that the patient considers not important enough to mention (Metzger and Friedman, 1994). It is often difficult to distinguish among symptoms of depression, medication side effects that resemble depression, and a new physical condition heralded by dysphoria.

For example, consider the case of a 60-year-old woman who could not sleep because of acute "hip pain." After taking prescribed benzodiazepines and ibuprofen for a month, she felt increasingly disabled physically and worried about her deteriorating mood. A complete evaluation by her physician led to the eventual diagnosis of metastatic bronchogenic carcinoma; the precipitants of the evaluation were her mood, pain, and medication concerns, each of which could have been the primary cause of her complaint. Only a thorough workup provided the answer, but not every evaluation leads to such concrete results.

Table 2–5. **Medications Commonly Causing Depression**

Cardiovascular agents	**Cancer treatments**
Antihypertensives	Methotrexate
Rauwolfia alkaloids (e.g., reserpine)	L-Asparaginase
Beta-adrenergic blocking drugs (e.g., propranolol)	Procarbazine
propranolol)	Alkylating agents
Methyldopa; clonidine	Vinblastine
Calcium-channel blockers (nifedipine;	**Neurologic agents**
verapamil; captopril), by case report	Phenytoin
Antiarrhythmics	Phenobarbital
Digitalis	Felbamate
Procainamide; bretylium; disopyramide	Carbamazepine
(rare)	**Gynecologic preparations**
Anticholesterolemic agents	Oral contraceptives, by case report
Pravastatin	**Psychotropic agents**
Respiratory agents	Antipsychotics
Corticosteroids	Barbiturates
Antituberculosis drugs	Meprobamate
Isoniazid	Benzodiazepines
Cycloserine	
Gastrointestinal agents	
Cimetidine	
Ranitidine	
Famotidine	

In making a differential diagnosis, it is helpful to establish the chronology of depressive symptoms in relation to starting, discontinuing, or changing the dose of a medication and to note any symptomologic shifts in mental status. Alcohol abuse and the use of illicit substances are growing among women (Chapter 4). Some patients drink alcohol, in particular, to self-medicate. Psychosocial stressors must be carefully assessed in this population. Moreover, in a kind of a reverse gender bias, *clinicians tend to minimize the amount of alcohol or drugs their female patients take*. Because alcohol is a depressant, its chronic use may induce a depressive affective state.

When a patient presents intoxicated and suicidal at the hospital emergency room, her depressive symptoms and suicidal feelings may remit after withdrawal from alcohol. However, the suicide rate in this subgroup is high, and aggressive treatment for substance abuse clearly is warranted (see Chapter 4).

GUIDELINES FOR TREATMENT

Discuss the Difference Between Depression and the "Blues." French novelist and essayist André Malraux, while researching for one of his books, asked an old priest what he had learned about the human condition after hearing confessions for so many years. The priest sagaciously observed: "There are so many sad people in the world."

Remind your patient that depression, unlike sadness, is not the typical unhappiness associated with everyday life. With sadness, one's sense of self-worth is not diminished. In contrast, with depression, a patient may feel gloomy, impoverished, lonely, lacking in self-confidence, and without a sense of personal agency. In fact, acute loss (bereavement) can be differentiated from depression because, after a death, the mourner still has self-esteem and self-worth despite having lost someone very dear (Caplan, 1990). The attributes of self-esteem enable the individual to do the work of grief, often emerging with restored confidence and a sense that "I am stronger than I once believed I was."

Review the Clinical Course of Depression. With current available treatments, the majority of patients improve. However, millions of people still do not receive any treatment or receive inadequate treatment. About 15% to 20% of patients do not improve despite repeated medication trials. For these persons, ECT may be helpful. Psychotherapy also appears to increase the response rate and to provide a protective shield for some persons. In practice, patients should have an adequate dosage of medication and should take it as prescribed. Studies reveal, however, that many patients are not compliant with medication and receive too low a dose; when these problems are corrected, the depression responds. The therapeutic alliance, in concert with depression-specific psychotherapy, is a crucial adjunct for state-of-the-art care.

Empathize with the Toll Depression Takes on Vitality. Counsel the depressed patient with empathy about how bad she feels about life and herself. Tell her that she will need courage and forbearance to confront an illness still stigmatized in our society. Addressing both her pain and the difficulty she encounters in seeking help is a good way to involve the patient in her own self-care.

Be Hopeful About the Treatability of the Illness. Reassure the patient that you understand her affliction and are not just giving her a pat on the back. In some cases, it may also be constructive to remind her that depression is a major public health problem, affecting as many as 25% of women and 10% of men over the course of a lifetime. It is the second most common psychiatric illness—and one of the most painful. Address the sense of shame the patient feels in having the illness and gently confront her tendency to believe that she has "let others down" (e.g., those with whom she has significant attachments).

Present Treatment Options. Review with the patient the genetic, neuro-transmitter, and neuroendocrine hypotheses that underlie depression (Gunderson and Phillips, 1991; Kendler et al., 1996; Mueller et al., 1996; Wells et al., 1992). Assuming the patient is willing to try an antidepressant, choose an option based on your own comfort and experience with the drug. Be sure to titrate the medication to an effective dose. Some studies suggest that at least 50% of patients in primary care practice are inadequately treated because the physician does not prescribe the dose to therapeutic levels or does not keep the patient on the drug for an adequate trial period (4–6 weeks).

Should the depression prove refractory to several trials of antidepressants from different classes (Table 2–6), consider a course of ECT. Especially with patients whose depression is life-threatening (those with extreme suicidality or psychosis), ECT may be a lifesaving procedure. Improvements in administration and anesthesia have made ECT safe and effective, with no major side effects. Although short-term memory problems can occur, the horror stories of yesteryear have largely disappeared. Nevertheless, many patients need to be reassured about contemporary practice, because they have seen only the media depiction of ECT. Patient education usually leads to acceptance of this most valuable treatment modality. The primary care clinician who has the family's and the patient's trust is often pivotal in acceptance of ECT.

COUNSELING TECHNIQUES FOR OFFICE SETTINGS

In most busy practices, clinicians have neither the time nor the clinical expertise to provide formal psychotherapy. Still, there are some basic psychotherapeutic techniques that clinicians or their care extenders can use in the office to support women trying to overcome depression.

Help the Patient Question Underlying Assumptions and Beliefs. Addressing the ways in which the patient sees the world as harsh or punitive enables her to arrive at a more even-handed perspective on events (Beck, 1976; Hollon and Carter, 1994). Then she can systematically work through those questions and beliefs and consider alternative explanations to problems. These are initial steps to promote rationality and challenge guilty self-recrimination.

Table 2–6. **Antidepressants**

Drug Class/ Generic Name	Trade Name	Usual Daily Adult Dose Range (mg)*	Special Considerations
Tricyclic Antidepressants (TCAs)			
Amitriptyline	Elavil, Endep	75–300	Should be avoided in
Amoxapine	Asendin	150–400	rapid-cycling bipolar
Desipramine	Norpramin, Pertofrane	75–300	illness.
Doxepin	Adapin, Sinequan	75–300	Frequent
Imipramine	Tofranil	75–300	pharmacodynamic
Maprotiline	Ludiomil	75–225	interactions with other
Nortriptyline	Aventyl, Pamelor	50–150	drugs; beware
Protriptyline	Vivactil	15–60	polypharmacy.
Trimipramine	Zurmontil	50–300	Blood level monitoring helps avoid toxicity.
Monoamine Oxidase Inhibitors			
Phenelzine	Nardil	45–90	Particularly useful in
Tranylcypromine	Parnate	20–50	atypical or refractory depression; dietary restrictions require patients' compliance.
New Generation Antidepressants			
Selective Serotonin Reuptake Inhibitors (SSRIs)			
Fluoxetine	Prozac	20–80	May cause loss of desire
Fluvoxamine	Luvox	100–200	for sex or anorgasmia;
Paroxetine	Paxil	20–50	may cause frequent
Sertraline	Zoloft	50–200	awakenings, poor sleep patterns, weight gain. Considered safe in overdosage.
Selective Norepinephrine Reuptake Blocker			
Bupropion	Wellbutrin	225–450	May be especially useful in bipolar patients who become depressed.
Serotonin and Norepinephrine Reuptake Blocker			
Venlafaxine	Effexor	75–375	May be especially useful in refractory or late-life depression.
5HT$_2$ Antagonist and Serotonin Reuptake Blockers			
Nefazodone	Serzone	300–500	Improved quality of sleep in 1 week; less sexual dysfunction than SSRIs.
Trazodone	Desyrel	150–500	Frequently used as adjunct with SSRIs to potentiate sleep.

*Beginning dose in geriatric patients is usually one third to one half of that for other adults; upper range generally is used only for severely depressed, treatment-refractory patients.

Emphasize the Need for Mastery and Improved Self-esteem. Even when medication or ECT is effective in treating symptoms, women need to increase their self-esteem, become more assertive, and feel less guilt-ridden to prevent depressive relapse (McGrath et al., 1990). Increasing problem-solving and coping skills is "one antidote to depression in some women," because "women are usually not taught as broad a range of problem solving and coping skills as are men" (McGrath et al., 1990, p. 50). Active interpersonal involvement in groups reduces social isolation and decreases depression, in part through distraction and companionship. Exercise, running, and weight lifting may be of particular value for depressed women, because these activities improve self-concept and potentially shift the patient's neurochemical balance.

Advocate Work on Relationships. Women are prone to develop a sense of self-sacrifice and self-betrayal in their relationships, and they tend to deny feelings of anger as well as depression (Lerner, 1985, 1987, 1993). Although both sexes have strong affiliative needs, women view emotional connectedness as their premier raison d'être and so may deny personal ambitions, achievements, and goals in order to sacrifice for others. The forums of support groups, therapy, and active listening may enable a patient to address the balance and interplay of personal goals and relationship needs.

The primary care clinician who empathizes with the myriad tensions and stressors women face in making career commitments while maintaining obligations to their family of origin, spouse, children, friends, and society provides a real service to the patient. Practitioners may also champion the needs of women to partake of counseling, psychotherapy, and peer support in order to become more confident in their capacity to control their own destiny and achieve a creative balance between personal and professional aspirations (Jack, 1987; Jamison, 1993; O'Connell and Mayo, 1988).

Encourage the Acquisition of Problem-solving and Coping Skills. Although specific techniques or manuals can help a patient through an initial episode of depression, more thorough long-term treatment should focus on helping her attain social, family, and job skills. In its widest context, overcoming depression necessitates commitment to enhancing knowledge, talents, and abilities so as to participate more effectively in work and family life.

Remind the Patient of the "Loss of Perspective." Caregivers who actively engage patients and remind them that their negative self-concepts, feelings of shame and humiliation, and relationship impasses may be signs that "the depression is talking again" not only aid in identifying the major manifestations of the disorder but also undermine "the apparent 'morale impairment' (the state of mind that threatens relationships, work, and life)" (Shuchter et al., p. 87). In essence, the therapist helps the patient identify any apparent distortions while reconstructing a healthier, more hopeful attitude about the future and the patient's capacity to deal with problems that arise.

Call Attention to the Importance of a Physically Healthy Lifestyle. This suggestion seems so self-evident as to be trivial, but it is often overlooked in practice. Yet many authorities now believe that dysphoric affect can actually be overridden or modified by regular exercise and by drawing on spiritual and religious beliefs. For women, developing a sense of personal power or agency is a particularly important coping practice that can be brought to light by the primary care clinician (Hamilton and Jensvold, 1992; Jack, 1987; Lewis, 1987). By reviewing stressful events and defining strategies that reduce them, and at the same time by advising patients to augment life's simple pleasures, clinicians can reduce their patients' maladaptive distortions.

PATIENT GUIDELINES FOR COPING WITH DEPRESSION

1. Depression is a mood disorder—not a sign of personal weakness. The disorder makes people feel dejected, despairing, and gloomy. It is important to try to maintain your perspective and to know "when the depression is talking to you" (Shuchter et al., 1996, pp. 87–88). The best scientific evidence supports the notion that depression occurs in repeated episodes, usually interspersed with periods of relative wellness. Fortunately, excellent treatment is now available.
2. Women experience depression twice as often as men. Although events associated with normal female physiology (e.g., menarche, premenstrual stress, postpartum period) are not responsible for depressive illness, women appear to be more likely to succumb to depression at these times. Other biologic factors that may be relevant to depression in women are thyroid disease and the use of contraceptives with high steroid content (Gadde and Krishnan, 1994; Mason et al., 1993).
3. Substance abuse, which is on the rise in women, tends to be associated with depression. Women sometimes attempt to self-treat their low moods with alcohol or other substances that mask an underlying depression. This combination can provoke a suicidal crisis. Avoid alcohol, opioids, marijuana, and so on, particularly if you are prone to depression.
4. The major vulnerability for depressive illness is family history of a mood disturbance. That is, a genetic factor appears to play a role. If one of your parents has had a mood disorder, you have a three to four times greater risk for developing depression in your lifetime. If both of your parents have had mood disorders, the risk is increased 10-fold. Despite this biologic risk, environment plays an important modifier role. Taking good care of yourself, which includes getting adequate rest, exercising regularly, and participating in treatment when indicated, can help control depressive episodes.
5. Depression can occur at any time in the life cycle. Although it tends to strike in the most productive years (ages 20 to 50), it can also appear in children, adolescents, and the elderly. Depressive episodes become more frequent and more severe if left untreated.
6. A thorough medical workup to rule out physical causes of depression is a crucial first step in treatment. Be sure to tell your physician about any change in your physical status and about all the medications you are taking, including over-the-counter medications and birth control pills. Any class of medication can contribute to causing depression; discuss with your doctor

any known physical illnesses or medications that could be compromising your well-being.

7. The brain is intimately involved in the cause of depression. Even with medication, you will no doubt need courage, resolve, and effort to overcome the illness. Although scientific research has not yet documented the precise biochemistry of depression, there are clues as to what makes people vulnerable. The brain chemicals known as neurotransmitters—especially dopamine, norepinephrine, and serotonin—are involved in the regulatory mechanism that controls the "limbic" or feeling part of the brain. This center links with the higher brain centers to control and coordinate emotional expression, drives in activity, and daily biologic rhythms. Disruption in cortisol, melatonin, and sleep patterns also can trigger depression. The important point is that depression is an illness with biologic roots which, in the modern age, can usually be treated quite successfully if you follow recommendations and do not give way to the pessimism that is part of depression.

8. Follow through on taking medications regularly and at prescribed doses, but also participate in individual or group counseling, if possible. The best studies show that medication and counseling or psychotherapy work synergistically. In fact, there are new psychotherapeutic methods specifically aimed at the treatment of depression. Whenever possible, take advantage of psychotherapy.

9. Because not all depression is hereditary or biologic in origin, pay attention to psychological issues that may be part of your depression. In some women, loss and stress are critical determinants. Women often sacrifice for others and yet feel they are letting their loved ones down if they become ill or depressed. Individual or group psychotherapy and support groups have been shown to be quite effective in helping address some of these underlying concerns. All women are challenged to straddle the dual concerns of relationship and career, but depression may be one final pathway for the sense of self-sacrifice and self-betrayal associated with living first and foremost for others. Women must find creative ways to address their multiple roles and aspirations.

10. Become an expert on your own illness. If you do not get better quickly, ask your doctor about new medications. Face down the problem of stigma. Get involved in local support groups or seek out psychotherapy as an adjunct to medication treatment. Read as much as possible about your illness, particularly making use of some new workbooks that you can find at your local bookstore or library (see "Resources for the Patient"). These will help you begin to use positive health practices and new behavioral strategies. Read the autobiographies of others who have struggled with depression to see how they dealt with the illness and to reassure yourself that you are not alone.

11. Assert your sense of self-agency and personal power. About one third of all depressed persons do not seek treatment because they are worried about their lack of insurance or money as a barrier to treatment. Become an activist, and demand that this clinical condition be handled at the same level as other medical illnesses. If those who administer your policy (e.g., managed care representatives) deny you benefits, then write to your state insurance commissioner or talk directly with your employer or union.

12. Disavow the myth that depression is a sign of weakness or a "normal" part

of life. These myths only make you less likely to seek out and engage in treatment. By all means, familiarize yourself with the signs and symptoms of clinical depression and work closely with your doctor to confront the illness. At least 80% of patients recover, or improve significantly, if they take adequate doses of medication and participate in psychotherapy.

ADDITIONAL GUIDELINES FOR PRIMARY CARE CLINICIANS

1. Each class of antidepressants has been shown to be highly effective in treating women. The side effect profile varies widely; some patients can tolerate more of the anticholinergic effects of the tricyclic antidepressants than others. The new SSRIs are preferred in primary care because of their low potential for side effects and their safety in overdosage. However, because they usually are more expensive than the tricyclics and can cause difficulties with sleep, weight gain, or sexual functioning, it is useful to be familiar with other agents. In the treatment of patients with anxiety and depression (mixed anxious depression), an MAOI may be the drug of first choice.
2. Good clinical practice suggests becoming familiar with one or two medications from each class (rather than attempting to prescribe the entire repertoire of agents available). Consider referral to a psychiatrist for patients who do not respond to two or three trials of medication at adequate dosage (see Table 2–6). In severe depression that does not remit after adequate medication trials, or when the patient is imminently suicidal, ECT can be lifesaving. Its status is gaining favor, especially in view of its safety and ease of administration in contemporary psychiatry and the consequently shorter hospital stays.
3. The kindling phenomenon and behavioral sensitization models suggest that vulnerability to depression worsens over time. Changes in the central nervous system can result from electrophysiologic and neurochemical events, leading to insecurity, hypersensitivity, anxiety, and depression (Shuchter et al., 1996). This presentation involves a recurrent and progressive course of episodes that appears to be more pronounced in women than in men. Experiencing repeated episodes of untreated depression results in recurrences that are less responsive to treatment than the initial episode. Kindling therefore may trigger more severe and accelerated episodes of mood disorders. Early intervention is crucial to prophylactically interrupt and block behavioral sensitization. Patients who comply poorly with medication may be at risk for more severe depression in the future.
4. Antidepressants can take weeks to become fully effective. During this time, patients need additional emotional support, perhaps through the use of care extenders or through referral for psychotherapy. A significant number of patients who commit suicide have seen a physician shortly before their death. You therefore should urge patients to make use of *all* avenues of interpersonal support, to structure their lives and stay busy, and to have an action plan in place should a crisis arise. Any time there is a partial but not complete response to treatment (e.g., when the patient is feeling a bit more energetic), the patient may be at high risk for suicide.
5. Make sure the patient is compliant with treatment. Many patients think that

taking medication is a sign of weakness, or they dislike particular side effects. Educate them about the high rate of success with the right medication regimen. Insist on honesty, particularly with respect to any untoward side effects (because this is a primary cause of poor compliance).

6. In the treatment of depression, the first indications of improvement are improved sleep and reduced fatigue, not necessarily improved mood. Be sure to tell patients to keep taking their medications, because they sometimes view any improvement as a sign that they are totally well.

7. It has been suggested that oral contraceptive use has a depressogenic side effect in 30% to 50% of women. Symptoms include irritability and reduced energy. Pyridoxine therapy usually reverses this iatrogenic effect in about 2 months.

SUMMARY

Women predominate over men in the spectrum of depressive disorders by a ratio of 2:1 to 3:1. Although there continues to be debate about why depression occurs so much more frequently in women—such as sociocultural versus biologic (hormonal) causes—there is no doubt that this disorder remains unrecognized and undertreated. Because depression is associated with a high rate of relapse and a long duration of episodes, appropriate treatment could help the majority of those not receiving care.

The primary care clinician is in a unique position to reverse the underrecognition and undertreatment of depression (Hirschfeld et al., 1997). Depression occurs in women of all ages. A thorough medical workup, taking into account prescribed and nonprescribed medications that may be implicated in the disorder, is a critical first step in treatment. Also essential to good care are the steps of *making the correct diagnosis, using appropriate and adequate doses of pharmacotherapeutic agents, and suggesting psychosocial therapies.* Contemporary research shows that many patients are noncompliant with medications or are prescribed inadequate doses of antidepressants for an inadequate duration; these factors exacerbate the economic costs and personal toll on family life and professional productivity.

To treat the millions of depressed women who are not receiving adequate care, physicians must first enhance their diagnostic skills and act as advocates for their patients. The stigma that prevents so many from seeking help can be reduced with primary provider support, recognition, diagnosis, and treatment. Collaboration between primary care physicians, psychiatrists, and other mental health professionals is ideal. However, the primary care clinician who is able to form a strong alliance with the patient dispels the myth that psychiatric disorders are not "real" illnesses. Employing the dual approaches of pharmacotherapy and psychotherapy diminishes the personal suffering and enormous societal toll taken by depression.

To help overcome the high suicide rate, occupational impairment, and impoverished interpersonal and family relationships caused by depression, physicians must ensure that contemporary, safe, effective, and economical treatments are available. Although it is useful to stress that depression has both hereditary and biologic foundations, women must also be encouraged to address the psychological aspects. Interviewing skills that focus on the often shrouded areas of loss and stress and the interpersonal sacrifices women make for others serve to bring unspoken mental anguish to the fore. Addressing the woman from a comprehensive perspective that combines biologic, social, and psychological approaches remains essential for individualized patient care.

Resources for the Patient

Burns DD: *Feeling Good: The New Mood Therapy.* New York, William Morrow & Co, 1980. New York, Avon, 1992.

This classic self-help guide for the treatment of depression is packed with useful tools and effective methods based on clinical research. Topics include how to defeat hopelessness and suicide, constructively deal with the stress of everyday life such as hostility, and talk back to one's inner critic. It is easy to read and widely accessible and has been rewritten in workbook format (The Feeling Good Handbook), *which is another self-help program to improve outlook and to overcome depression.*

Copeland ME: *The Depression Workbook: A Guide for Living with Depression and Manic Depression.* Oak Bridge, CA, New Harbinger Press, 1992.

This workbook provides an excellent summary for general readers concerning the clinical presentation and biologic underpinnings of affective disorder. Presented in question-and-answer format, with plenty of space for writing down notes, this book offers suggestions to help the patient become an active agent in her own treatment. In addition to explaining the role of medication, psychological therapies, and support groups, this resource is an excellent adjunct to help the patient develop a sense of mastery over depression and to encourage her to structure her thoughts and activities during those times when she may be more reluctant to participate.

Manning M: *Undercurrents: A Life Beneath the Surface.* San Francisco, HarperCollins, 1994.

This remarkable journal by a female psychologist tells the story of her spiraling descent into and arduous emergence out of clinical depression. Full of humor and personal vignettes, it presents the author's multiple roles as mother, wife, daughter, and professional—all of which women will relate to. Also of interest is Dr. Manning's own treatment history. She openly reveals how multiple trials of medication failed to alleviate her depression, which was handled successfully by a course of ECT, along with psychotherapy. This book offers the inspiration of hope and wise encouragement for all patients but is particularly useful for those who have had several episodes of depressive illness.

Thorn J: *You Are Not Alone: Words of Experience and Hope for the Journey Through Depression.* San Francisco, HarperCollins, 1993.

In this marvelously accessible book, the author includes brief personal stories of a number of men and women who have struggled with the vicissitudes of depression. There is something for everyone in these first-person accounts, including suggestions and testimonials about what does and does not work in treatment. Implicit throughout is the sense that one can grow in the course of one's life journey and can positively benefit from the experience of treatment. Words of hope and comfort underscore the essential steps to take when seeking professional help and support groups.

Resources for the Clinician

Gut E: *Productive and Unproductive Depression: Success or Failure of a Vital Process.* New York, Basic Books, 1989.

For the health care clinician who wants to understand more about the psychology and psychodynamic issues underlying many cases of depression, this book provides a very readable yet thorough summary. Free of psychiatric jargon and leavened with many interesting clinical examples, it offers a perspective on how psychotherapeutic under-

standing can benefit patients when other treatments do not. Also presented are concrete suggestions on how to deal with depression more productively. Family and sociocultural influences are reviewed, as are suggestions for self-help and professional aid. This substantive primer should prove of use to clinicians who are interested in doing more counseling of the clinically depressed in their daily practice and to those who simply want to learn more about the human side of the illness.

McGrath E, Keita GP, Strickland BR, et al.: *Women and Depression: Risk Factors and Treatment Issues.* Final report of the American Psychological Association's National Task Force on Women and Depression. Washington, DC, American Psychological Association, 1990.

This finely detailed overview of risk factors, research issues, and treatment considerations is the final report of the American Psychological Association's National Task Force on Women and Depression. It will no doubt serve as a special reference manual for primary care clinicians who treat a significant number of women in their practice. The final section on populations at risk (minorities, adolescents, the elderly, lesbians, the poor) is a unique supplement.

Shuchter SR, Downs N, Zisook S: *Biologically Informed Psychotherapy for Depression.* New York, Guilford, 1996.

A state-of-the-art office reference for the mental health professional or primary care practitioner who treats depressive disorders, this comprehensive overview beautifully summarizes the biologic and psychological models of depression. Particularly useful are the sections on "biologically informed psychotherapy," which is essentially a series of supportive techniques for implementation in daily office practice. Highly comprehensive, yet utterly pragmatic, this text will be a standard reference on the treatment of depression for some years to come.

Styron W: *Darkness Visible: A Memoir of Madness.* New York, Random House, 1990.

In only 84 pages, this Pulitzer Prize–winning author brings to the public eye one of the finest clinical portraits of depression ever written. Styron clearly documents his descent into his own private hell and demonstrates the personal cost of depression in his personal and professional life, but he also offers insight into what constitutes successful treatment. This narrative memoir conveys the patient's perspective on what having severe depression is like; it helps even seasoned professionals to put themselves into the patient's shoes and can also be used as a patient resource.

References

American Psychiatric Association: *Diagnostic and Statistical Manual of Mental Disorders,* 4th ed. Washington, DC, American Psychiatric Association, 1994.

Beck AT: *Cognitive Therapy and the Emotional Disorders.* New York, International Universities Press, 1976.

Blacker D: Maintenance treatment of major depression: A review of the literature. *Harv Rev Psychiatry* 1996;4:1–9.

Caplan G: Loss, stress, and mental health. *Community Ment Health J* 1990;26:27–48.

Copeland ME: *The Depression Workbook: A Guide for Living with Depression and Manic Depression.* Oak Bridge, CA, New Harbinger Press, 1992.

Cummings JL: Depression in neurologic diseases. *Psychiatr Ann* 1994;24:525–531.

Fava GA, Grandi S, Zielezny M, et al.: Four-year outcome for cognitive behavioral treatment of residual symptoms in major depression. *Am J Psychiatry* 1996;153:945–947.

Gadde KM, Krishnan KRR: Endocrine factors in depression. *Psychiatr Ann* 1994;24:521–524.

Gadde KM, Krishnan KRR: Depression in endocrine disorders. *Directions in Psychiatry* 1996;16:1–7.

Greenberg PE, Stiglin LE, Finkelstein SN, et al.: The economic burden of depression in 1990. *J Clin Psychiatry* 1993;54:405–418.

Gunderson JG, Phillips KA: A current view of the interface between borderline personality disorder and depression. *Am J Psychiatry* 1991;148:967–975.

Gut E: *Productive and Unproductive Depression: Success or Failure of a Vital Process.* New York, Basic Books, 1989.

Hall RCW, Popkin MK, Devaul RA, et al.: Physical illness presenting as psychiatric disease. *Arch Gen Psychiatry* 1978;35:1315–1320.

Hamilton JA, Grant M, Jensvold MF: Sex and treatment of depressions: When does it matter? In: Jensvold MF, Halbreich U, Hamilton JA (eds.): *Psychopharmacology and Women: Sex, Gender, and Hormones,* pp. 241–260. Washington, DC, American Psychiatric Press, 1996.

Hamilton JA, Jensvold M: Personality, psychopathology, and depressions in women. In: Brown LS, Ballou M (eds.): *Personality and Psychopathology: Feminist Reappraisals,* pp. 116–143. New York, Guilford, 1992.

Hirschfeld RMA: The long-term nature of depression. *Psychiatr Ann* 1997;26:313–314.

Hirschfeld RMA, Keller MB, Panico S, et al.: The National Depressive and Manic-Depressive Association consensus statement on the undertreatment of depression. *JAMA* 1997;277:333–340.

Hollon SD, Carter MM: Depression in adults. In: Craighead LW, Craighead WE, Kazdin AE, et al. (eds.): *Cognitive and Behavioral Interventions: An Empirical Approach to Mental Health Problems,* pp. 89–104. Boston, Allyn & Bacon, 1994.

Howie JGR, Porter AMD, Heaney DJ, et al.: Long to short consultation ratio: A proxy measure of quality of care for general practice. *Br J Gen Pract* 1991;41:48–54.

Jack D: Silencing the self: The power of social imperatives in female depression. In: Formanek R, Gurian A (eds.): *Women and Depression: A Lifespan Perspective,* pp. 161–181. New York, Springer, 1987.

Jamison KR: *Touched with Fire: Manic-depressive Illness and the Artistic Temperament.* New York, Free Press, 1993.

Johnson J, Weissman MM, Klerman GL: Service utilization and social morbidity associated with depressive symptoms in the community. *JAMA* 1992;267:1478–1483.

Katon W, Robinson P, Von Korff M, et al.: A multifaceted intervention to improve treatment of depression in primary care. *Arch Gen Psychiatry* 1996;53:924–932.

Kendler KS, Eaves LJ, Walters EE, et al.: The identification and validation of distinct depressive syndromes in a population-based sample of female twins. *Arch Gen Psychiatry* 1996;53:391–399.

Klerman G: Depression and panic anxiety: The effect of depressive co-morbidity on response to drug treatment of patients with panic disorder and agoraphobia. *J Psychiatr Res* 1990;24(suppl 2):27–41.

Klerman GL, Weissman MM: The course, morbidity, and costs of depression. *Arch Gen Psychiatry* 1992;49:831–834.

Kocsis JH, Friedman RA, Markowitz JC, et al.: Maintenance therapy for chronic depression: A controlled clinical trial of desipramine. *Arch Gen Psychiatry* 1996;53:769–774.

Kupfer DJ, Frank E: Maintenance therapy for chronic depression: A controlled clinical trial of desipramine [commentary]. *Arch Gen Psychiatry* 1996;53:775–776.

Kupfer DJ, Frank E, Perel JM, et al.: Five-year outcome for maintenance therapies in recurrent depression. *Arch Gen Psychiatry* 1992;49:769–773.

Lerner HG: *The Dance of Anger: A Woman's Guide to Changing the Patterns of Intimate Relationships.* New York, Harper and Row, 1985.

Lerner HG: Female depression: Self-sacrifice and self-betrayal in relationships. In: Formanek R, Gurian A (eds.): *Women and Depression: A Lifespan Perspective,* pp. 200–221. New York, Springer, 1987.

Lerner HG: *The Dance of Deception: Pretending and Truth-Telling in Women's Lives.* New York, HarperCollins, 1993.

Leibowitz MR: Mixed anxiety and depression: Should it be included in *DSM-IV*? *J Clin Psychiatry* 1993;54(suppl 5):4–7.

Lewis HB: The role of shame in depression in women. In: Formanek R, Gurian A (eds.): *Women and Depression: A Lifespan Perspective,* pp. 182–199. New York, Springer, 1987.

Manning M: *Undercurrents: A Life Beneath the Surface.* San Francisco, HarperCollins, 1994.

Mason GA, Walker CH, Prange AJ: L-Triiodothyromine: Is this peripheral hormone a central neurotransmitter? *Neuropsychopharmacology* 1993;8:253–258.

McGrath E, Keita GP, Strickland BR, et al.: *Women and Depression: Risk Factors and Treatment Issues.* Final Report of the American Psychological Association's National Task Force on Women and Depression. American Psychological Association, Washington, DC, 1990.

Metzger ED, Friedman RS: Treatment-related depression. *Psychiatr Ann* 1994;24:540–544.

Mintz J, Mintz LI, Arruda MJ, et al.: Treatments of depression and the functional capacity to work. *Arch Gen Psychiatry* 1992;49:761–768.

Mueller TI, Keller MB, Leon AC, et al.: Recovery after 5 years of unremitting major depressive disorder. *Arch Gen Psychiatry* 1996;53:794–799.

National Mental Health Association: "Breaking out of the box": A national survey conducted January 19–26, 1996 (sponsored by Eli Lilly Co.). *Neuroscience News* 1996;1(1):3.

Nolen-Hoeksema S: Epidemiology and theories of gender differences in unipolar depression. In: Seeman MV (ed.): *Gender and Psychopathology*, pp. 63–87. Washington, DC, American Psychiatric Press, 1995.

O'Connell RA, Mayo JA: The role of social factors in affective disorders: A review. *Hosp Community Psychiatry* 1988;39:842–851.

Olfson M., Broadhead E, Weissman MM, et al.: Subthreshold psychiatric symptoms in a primary care group practice. *Arch Gen Psychiatry* 1996;53:880–886.

Parker G: Presentation and course of affective disorders. *Current Opinion in Psychiatry* 1993;6:1,4–9.

Pies RW: Medical "mimics of depression." *Psychiatr Ann* 1994;24:519–520.

Prange AJ, Loosen PT, Wilson IC, et al.: The therapeutic use of hormones of the thyroid axis in depression. In: Post RM, Ballenger JC (eds.): *Frontiers of Clinical Neuroscience*, vol 1: *Neurobiology of Mood Disorders*, pp. 311–322. Baltimore, Williams & Wilkins, 1984.

Quitkin FM, McGrath PJ, Stewart JW, et al.: Chronological milestones to guide drug change: When should clinicians switch antidepressants? *Arch Gen Psychiatry* 1996;53:785–792.

Rosenthal NE, Oren DA: Light therapy. In: Gabbard GO (ed.): *Treatments of Psychiatric Disorders*, 2nd ed., pp 1263–1273. Washington, DC, American Psychiatric Press, 1995.

Rush AJ: Ongoing needs in depression. World Congress of Psychiatry, August, 1996, Madrid, Spain.

Schulberg HC, Block MR, Madonia MJ, et al.: Treating major depression in primary care practice: Eight-month clinical outcomes. *Arch Gen Psychiatry* 1996;53:913–919.

Shaw J, Kennedy S, Joffe RT: Gender differences in mood disorders: A clinical focus. In: Seeman MV (ed.): *Gender and Psychopathology*, pp. 89–111. Washington, DC, American Psychiatric Press, 1995.

Shen W, Hsu J: Female sexual side effects associated with selective serotonin reuptake inhibitors: A descriptive clinical study of 33 patients. *Int J Psychiatry Med* 1995;25:239–248.

Shuchter SR, Downs N, Zisook S: *Biologically Informed Psychotherapy for Depression*. New York, Guilford, 1996.

Simon G, Ormel J, Von Korff M, et al.: Health care costs associated with depressive and anxiety disorders in primary care. *Am J Psychiatry* 1995;152:352–357.

Sturm R, Wells KB: How can care for depression become more cost-effective? *JAMA* 1995;273:51–58.

Styron W: *Darkness Visible: A Memoir of Madness*. New York, Random House, 1990.

Thase ME, Fava M, Halbreich U, et al.: A placebo-controlled, randomized clinical trial comparing sertraline and imipramine for the treatment of dysthymia. *Arch Gen Psychiatry* 1996;53:777–784.

Thorn J: *You Are Not Alone: Words of Experience and Hope for the Journey Through Depression*. San Francisco, HarperCollins, 1993.

Tylee A: Secondary prevention of depression. In: Kendrick T, Tylee A, Freeling P (eds.): *The Prevention of Mental Illness in Primary Care*, pp. 167–187, London: Cambridge, 1996.

Wells KB, Burnam MA, Rogers W, et al.: The course of depression in adult outpatients: Results from the Medical Outcomes Study. *Arch Gen Psychiatry* 1992;49:788–794.

Chapter 3

Bipolar Disorder

Bipolar disorder, also known as manic-depressive illness, is one of the most severe psychiatric illnesses. It adversely affects the patient's mood, activity, and thought processes. (See Table 3–1 for a more definitive list of historical symptoms.) Characterized by one or more manic episodes and typically by one or more depressive episodes, the disorder manifests by an elevated, expansive, irritable mood and a host of behavioral symptoms. Because persons with mania are dangerous to themselves and to others, this disorder is considered one of the few emergencies in psychiatry (Bowden, 1996a).

Affecting 1% to 1.6% of both men and women, bipolar disorder occurs at about the same frequency in either gender, and without regard to national origin (Leibenluft, 1996; Weissman et al., 1996). Although gender differences have only begun to receive systematic study, there appear to be significant gender-related issues regarding the course of this illness and response to treatment. For women, pregnancy and the postpartum period are times of special risk for onset and recurrence. In addition, all the effective mood-stabilizing agents pose special risks during pregnancy.

Women have a higher rate of "rapid-cycling" and "mixed-state" forms of bipolar disorder. What constitutes diagnostic verifiability for each of these forms is still a matter of some controversy. Bipolar women appear to be at higher risk than bipolar men for development of depressive episodes. Although bipolar illness is inherently treatable (Bowden, 1996a, 1996b; Bowden et al., 1996; Bowden and McElroy, 1995; Cohen et al., 1995; Dunner, 1993; Keck et al., 1996a; Kupfer

---

Table 3–1. **Historical Symptoms of Bipolar Spectrum**

Mood	Poor social boundaries
Inappropriate humor or euphoria	Sexually overactive and provocative
Irritation or anger	Frequent interrupting; boastfulness
Disinhibition	Uncontrolled spending
Heightened sensory experiences (e.g., "That's the bluest tie I've ever seen!")	**Thought**
	Poor judgment
Activity	Distractibility
Increased energy	Litigiousness
Poor impulse control	Denial
Decreased need for sleep	Flight of ideas
Pressure of speech	Grandiose ideas and delusions
Increased social contact	Recurrent psychosis
	Recurrent thought disorder; depression

and Frank, 1997; Sachs, 1996; Schou, 1997; Tohen et al., 1996), those forms that preferentially affect women are particularly challenging to control clinically. As a result, it is important to address this disorder in regard to women's health (Leibenluft, 1996).

Despite commonly held notions that bipolar illness carries a good prognosis, current data indicate otherwise. At least 10% of patients have a chronic course, with a significant number failing to recover even from the initial episode (Gershon and Soares, 1997; Schou, 1997; Solomon et al., 1995). The rate of suicide attempts is 19% to 25%; over a 30-year time span, almost 1 of every 10 bipolar patients dies from suicide. Despite well-defined criteria, the illness is commonly underdiagnosed because it has many different presentations. Any *recurrent* affective or psychotic disturbance should prompt the clinician to suspect bipolar disorder. For identification and treatment purposes, consultation with a psychiatrist is often required.

Some studies suggest that many people with mood disorders do not receive effective treatment despite its availability and efficacy. As many as two thirds of patients with bipolar illness who could receive help do not get it, often because they fail to recognize that they have a treatable illness (Keck et al., 1996a, 1996b). In 1979, the U.S. Department of Health, Education, and Welfare estimated that a woman who develops bipolar disorder at age 25 can be expected to lose 9 years of life expectancy overall, with a 14-year loss in productivity during her lifetime. This pronounced risk is largely a result of suicide among these patients. With treatment, however, many of the hazards associated with the illness can be eliminated, leading to increased life expectancy, enhanced productivity, diminished risk of suicide, and improved quality of life (Blazer, 1996; Gitlin et al., 1995; Gitlin and Altshuler, 1997; Keck et al., 1996b; McElroy et al., 1996; Tohen et al., 1996).

Bipolar disorder is often complicated by other psychiatric problems, most notably substance abuse (Brady and Sonne, 1995). All persons with bipolar disorder should be counseled to avoid intoxicants, because they can lead to treatment failure. Patients with bipolar disorder may attempt to self-medicate—with alcohol or street drugs—their irritability, agitation, sudden mood or behavior changes, and depression. The increased use of psychoactive substances (particularly cocaine and hallucinogens) has resulted in greater recognition and treatment when both bipolar disorder and substance abuse occur simultaneously. Patients with a substance abuse history may complain of manic, hypomanic, depressive, or mixed affective symptoms, leading some authorities to suspect a causal relationship.

An Unquiet Mind, the popular autobiography by psychologist and researcher Kay Jamison (1995), has raised awareness about the clinical presentations and personal toll of this malady. Both professionals and the lay public have developed a working knowledge of the disorder through popular accounts of the lives of artists and writers (Jamison, 1993; Middlebrook, 1991). The widely acclaimed book *Touched with Fire: Manic-depressive Illness and the Artist's Temperament* (Jamison, 1993) charted the spiraling downhill course, punctuated by intensely hyperactive periods of productivity and creativity, of Sylvia Plath, Anne Sexton, Ernest Hemingway, Ezra Pound, Vincent van Gogh, Paul Gauguin, Virginia Woolf, Georgia O'Keeffe, Mark Twain, and Tennessee Williams, to name only a few. Jamison cited the ability of these artists to function on only a few hours of sleep, their proclivity to work intensely and relentlessly, and their capacity to experience and to express profoundly deep and varied emotions, thus illuminating—for both the professional and the layperson—the cost of human suffering inherent to mania and hypomania. But what becomes apparent in the study is that not all the sequelae of this illness are necessarily negative. Increased energy, increased speed of thought, decreased need for sleep, and grandiosity may be conducive to artistic flair and originality. The enormous productivity and élan of manic-depressive individuals not infrequently stirs resentment in bystanders who are unaware of the price those afflicted must pay.

Jamison's (1995) harrowing description of her own struggle with manic-depressive illness is a powerful, gripping, and brutally honest portrait that has spurred others affected by the disorder to ask questions and seek treatment. In the daily practice of primary care, it is increasingly common to find patients who are sophisticated consumers familiar with the "addictive euphoric manias" (restlessness and irritability) and the "wildly agitated, paranoid, and physically violent" crises that Jamison describes so vividly. This author's courage to go public with her illness has made it possible for others with a similar personal history and incapacitating symptoms to seek help, with the requisite courage to counter the stigma and sense of personal isolation and humiliation that accompany mental illnesses more than physical disorders.

RECOGNIZING BIPOLAR ILLNESS

The full-blown symptoms of mania are not difficult to recognize (Table 3–2). Because both bipolar I and bipolar II disorders tend to "breed true," it is important to look closely at family history. Bipolar I patients more often have relatives with bipolar I illness, and the same holds true for bipolar II disorder. Bipolar II patients are more likely to have seasonal depression (i.e., patients become more depressed in winter than in summer) and have more suicide attempts. Bipolar illness runs a different course than unipolar depression; it affects younger persons, produces more episodes of illness, and requires more frequent hospitalizations.

During their training, many clinicians have known someone who appeared to

---

Table 3–2. Manifestations of Bipolar I and Bipolar II Disorder

Bipolar I Disorder	Bipolar II Disorder
Psychosis	Personality disturbance or disorder of temperament (borderline-like)
Paranoia	Seasonal depression
Rapid mood cycling	Alcohol and/or substance abuse
Recurrent schizophrenia-like symptoms	Rapid mood cycling
Recurrent depression	Premenstrual dysphoria; premenstrual mood disturbance
Mania	Impulse difficulties
Bizarre behavior	Interpersonal sensitivity
Substance abuse and/or self-medication	Recurrent depression
	Mood instability

have unlimited energy for work, speed in thinking and in accomplishing tasks, and a diminished need for sleep. These talented, ambitious persons arouse envy, if not suspicion, in their ability to get work done—often despite the chaos they create, usually at the expense of others. One such person during my own medical school training was a gifted surgical resident with expertise beyond her years in teaching, writing, and clinical acumen. It was not uncommon for her to rouse her students and give a lecture at 3 a.m., after she had worked a 36-hour shift. Her boastfulness, demandingness, frequent irritability, and provocative sexual flirtatiousness—with both men and women—alienated this otherwise brilliant woman from the attending staff and junior colleagues.

As in many patients whose premorbid personality may be an attenuated expression of affective illness (Akiskal, 1994; Akiskal et al., 1985), this resident went on to develop a full-blown manic episode requiring pharmacologic and hospital treatment after many years of a seemingly temperamental "personality" disturbance (Kopacz and Janicak, 1996; Peselow et al., 1995). Personality disorders can mimic affective disorders; some patients with cyclothymic personalities may develop a variant of bipolar disorder, but some simply have normal mood swings. Many patients have episodic depression and mania (or hypomania) for years but with insufficient severity, duration, and symptoms to meet the full criteria for bipolar disorder (Swann, 1995). They may manifest a prolonged period of poor social judgment, increased energy and activity, and excessive irritability. Rarely, a bipolar II patient develops full-blown mania. However, studies demonstrate that many patients respond positively to the antimanic agents that ameliorate these "hyperthermic" mood swings (Jacobsen, 1993; Johnson and McFarland, 1996).

Sometimes mania comes "out of the blue," but most often there are prodromal symptoms that can alert the clinician early. Consider incipient bipolar illness in the patient who is a compulsive talker and constantly interrupts others. Family members may complain of this and other behavioral control problems, such as spending too much money, being irritable, and showing poor judgment. Boastful, extroverted, impatient individuals have the hyperthermic temperament characteristic of manic-depressive (particularly bipolar II) illness. Others are more petulant and driven, sometimes living between compulsive investment in their activities and explosive temper outbursts that are alienating in their work and family life. Denial of illness during a manic high is very common.

SECONDARY MANIAS

Primary care clinicians are called on to rule out physical disease as a cause of bipolar disorder in the psychiatric population. Concomitantly, in primary care practice, organic factors that cause mania must always be considered in the differential diagnosis, especially in the patient who presents initially with mania or hypomania without a family history. Some of these illnesses tend to affect women more than men. Although correction of the underlying organic (toxic, metabolic, infectious) factors may reverse the manic presentation, many organic factors (trauma, stroke, aging, human immunodeficiency virus [HIV] infection, neoplasia) are not reversible (Evans et al., 1995; Krauthammer and Klerman, 1978). In fact, secondary manias can be especially difficult to treat. The primary care clinician should work in concert with a psychiatrist for titration of psychotropic drugs and initiation of psychosocial interventions.

Many of the available data concerning secondary manias are derived from single case reports, small case series, and anecdotal accounts. The classic retrospective review (Krauthammer and Klerman, 1978) found that prescribed medications and drugs of abuse, infections, neoplasms, epilepsy, and various metabolic disturbances can cause the same hyperactive, sexually indiscreet, agitated, and grandiose symptomatology that is often found in bipolar patients. Closed head injury, mental retardation, and HIV infection also have been associated with mania.

Of particular note is late-onset mania, a geriatric condition that is becoming more prevalent as our elderly population increases (Evans et al., 1995). This heterogeneous group of disorders runs the gamut from classic bipolar disorder to organic states; neurologic conditions are a frequent cause. Be alert to any underlying organic impairment, negative family history for affective disorder, or dominant irritable mood with persecutory delusions. These patients also tend to be resistant to the usual antimanic agents.

In female patients, particular attention should be paid to iatrogenic causes of secondary mania. For example, antidepressants, which are more commonly prescribed to women than to men, tend to induce rapid cycling and the organic manic state (Owley and Sharma, 1996). Calcium supplementation, increasingly used in menopausal women, has also been implicated in some cases of secondary mania. (See Table 3–3 for a list of organic causes of secondary mania.)

With respect to treatment, although lithium carbonate may be effective in some patients with secondary mania, it is no longer the drug of choice. Adverse side effects seem to limit its usefulness in this subgroup. To stabilize mood in patients with secondary mania, anticonvulsants, particularly divalproex sodium (Keck et al., 1996c) and carbamazepine, have been shown to be effective and

Table 3–3. **Common Organic Causes of Mania (Secondary Manias)**

Infectious disease	**Prescribed and over-the-counter medications**
Benign herpes simplex	Amphetamines
Influenza	Decongestants
Neurosyphilis	Bronchodilators
HIV infection	Corticosteroids
Encephalitis or equine fever	Antidepressants (particularly tricyclics)
Neurologic disease	Isoniazid
Tumor	L-Dopa
Cerebrovascular disease	Calcium replacement therapy (occasional)
Aneurysm	Oral contraceptives (possible)
Multiple sclerosis	**Drugs of abuse**
Closed head injury	Amphetamines
Mental retardation or developmental delay	Cocaine
Metabolic disturbances	Cannabis (questionable)
Thyrotoxicosis	**Other**
Renal dialysis	Caffeinated beverages
Postoperative states	
Anemia	
Vitamin B_{12} deficiency	

well tolerated. Most importantly, any underlying medical disturbance or etiologic factors should be corrected first. Treatable causes, such as vitamin B_{12} deficiency, caffeinism, and misuse of over-the-counter medications, are easily overlooked (Owley and Sharma, 1996). Inadequate monitoring of thyroid replacement therapy for hypothyroidism may be an unsuspected cause of organic mania.

It is virtually impossible to know at the outset whether the syndrome will remit with correction of the organic cause alone or whether antimanic pharmacotherapy will be a necessary adjunct. Most practitioners aggressively treat the secondary mania with pharmacotherapy because of the syndrome's physical and psychosocial morbidity, particularly in patients with irreversible neurologic disorders associated with trauma, stroke, and acquired immunodeficiency syndrome.

EFFECTS OF THE FEMALE REPRODUCTIVE SYSTEM ON BIPOLAR ILLNESS

Menstruation

Whether the phases of the menstrual cycle affect the course or symptoms of bipolar illness is a matter of debate. No systematic studies have yet been carried out, and those case reports that are available lack long-term follow-up to document whether a particular phase of the cycle is consistently associated with relapse. Some reports (Leibenluft, 1996) do link severe premenstrual tension with rapid-cycling bipolar disorder. But other studies (Shaw et al., 1995) suggest that social incapacitation due to menstrually related mood symptoms is no more common among bipolar women than among normal women. Psychosocial support, particularly individual or group therapy, may be useful in reducing the stress that augments menstrual disorders.

Pregnancy

When a patient with known bipolar illness becomes pregnant, the clinician and patient are presented with difficult decisions. Untreated bipolar illness poses special risks to both mother and baby, but every mood-stabilizing agent can cause teratogenic effects. The main fetal risks for lithium carbonate are cardiac defects (e.g., Ebstein's anomaly), polyhydramnios, premature labor, neonatal hypothyroidism, and neonatal toxicity. Neonatal toxicity results in the transient problems of abnormal respiratory patterns, cyanosis, hypotonia, decreased suckling and motor reflexes, hypoglycemia, and poor myocardial contractility. Carbamazepine and sodium valproate (e.g., divalproex) increase the risk of neonatal hemorrhage, which can be prevented by administering vitamin K to the mother during the last 1 to 2 months of pregnancy and to the infant at birth. A rare but fatal complication of sodium valproate is acute liver failure in the infant. The congenital risks of lithium are not as great as originally thought, and many experts are recommending ongoing prophylaxis for women who are at risk for puerperal instability (e.g., bipolar disorder, puerperal psychosis).

The decision as to whether to continue mood-stabilizing agents during pregnancy requires collaboration between doctor and patient. The risk of recurrence of bipolar illness in the mother must be balanced against the physical risk to the fetus. Although discontinuation of antimanic agents has, until rather recently, been a standard practice, prospective studies (Cohen et al., 1995; Finnerty et al., 1996) have found no difference in overall teratogenesis between pregnant women taking lithium and matched control subjects not exposed to this medication. Consequently, some patients have continued on lithium throughout pregnancy, labor, and delivery. In at least one naturalistic study of 27 pregnant patients, those bipolar women who remained on lithium had a significantly lower rate of relapse (Cohen et al., 1995). The investigators concluded that, given "the potential impact of maternal psychiatric illness on child development, the value of aggressive treatment of women at risk for puerperal illness becomes more compelling" (Cohen et al., 1995, pp. 1643–1644).

Usually, exposure has already occurred in the first trimester, before the patient knows she is pregnant (Finnerty et al., 1996). If the patient has a good therapeutic alliance, excellent family support, and personal awareness about her illness, the decision may be made for a trial of medication discontinuance. However, if symptoms exacerbate, a resumption of medication, hospitalization, or ECT will be necessary. Because a pregnant woman with acute mania is prone to poor judgment and is unlikely to follow through with prenatal and postnatal care for herself or the baby, the risks and benefits of discontinuing mood stabilizers must be thoroughly explained in an informed consent process (Finnerty et al., 1996). If a manic relapse occurs, the patient may be more reluctant to seek help or to collaborate with treatment.

Neuroleptic and anxiolytic agents may be employed for acute stabilization, but these treatments are not optimal mood stabilizers, nor are they totally safe for the fetus. A host of psychological issues should also be reviewed, including the patient's fears of motherhood, her reactions to the baby and to her changing self-image and body image, and the potential for abandonment. Psychiatric consultation may be particularly useful in (1) rendering state-of-the-art medication management and (2) providing psychosocial support and therapy. Appropriate group, peer, and family support may be available in the community to help the patient navigate the major life change of childbirth and learn about the expectable life phase events of motherhood that may prove uniquely challenging.

The postpartum period is a time of high risk for the patient with bipolar disorder. The rate of relapse during the puerperium ranges between 20% and 50%, although prophylactic treatment with lithium reduces that rate to about 10% (Cohen et al., 1995). The primary care clinician should be aware that a postpartum depression that first appears to be unipolar may evolve into a full-blown bipolar illness. Women with a history of both a bipolar episode unrelated to childbirth and a puerperal episode have a greater than 50% risk of an affective episode after a subsequent delivery. This risk has led most experts to conclude that "there is no other time in life of a male or female bipolar patient when the risk of an episode is higher than it is for a female bipolar patient in the postpartum period, especially if she has had a previous puerperal episode" (Leibenluft, 1996, p. 166). The primary care clinician must emphasize these findings in counseling the bipolar patient who wishes to have another child. In these complex cases, the psychosocial and pharmacologic recommendations must be tailored to the individual patient.

Menopause

The effects of menopause on bipolar illness have not been well studied. As the adult population ages, more case reports and naturalistic studies may clarify the extant reports in the literature. These current contradictory case studies describe a worsening or a lessening of the frequency of the manic-depressive cycle at the time of the female climacteric. Until studies confirm the most typical patterns and receive just attention in the literature, it is a wise course to listen for any changes in affective intensity or temperamental shifts and then to tailor the treatment to the individual patient.

Many women feel reassured by a clinician who honestly shares information on areas where science is still lacking. Underscoring the value of good self-care and of reducing episodes of emotional stress encourages a better prognosis. It is crucial to pay careful attention to issues of pharmacotherapy, especially with patients who are being treated with both a mood stabilizer and other medications for physical illnesses. Therapeutic levels of mood stabilizers should be obtained routinely, but especially in those patients whose use of other medications may affect the bioavailability of a particular mood stabilizer.

GUIDELINES FOR TREATMENT

Bipolar disorder is one of the most challenging psychiatric disorders to treat. Diagnosis is often complicated and difficult, compliance with medical and psychosocial interventions is poor, and suicide rate is high. Health care clinicians may find it particularly frustrating to work with patients who are reluctant to follow through on their advice, especially in the presence of a life-threatening illness. For this reason, it may be wise to involve a mental health professional, preferably a psychiatrist skilled both in psychotherapy and in pharmacotherapy, in the care of women with bipolar illness. The primary care clinician plays a pivotal role in making appropriate referral. This process involves considering bipolar illness in the differential diagnosis by ruling out secondary manias and treating the patient and helping the patient collaborate with treatment.

Clinical and research experiences demonstrate that bipolar patients benefit greatly from pharmacologic treatment and psychosocial intervention, but those whose illness is atypical (e.g., mixed-state, rapid-cycling) warrant intensive follow-up (Bowden, 1996b; Solomon et al., 1995; Swann, 1995). Women tend to have higher rates of these disorders. They may require frequent and regular titration of medications, including the periodic use of benzodiazepines or antipsychotics to curtail a manic swing. The unpredictability of the course of bipolar illness, in conjunction with the patient's impulsivity, may necessitate involvement with the court system to institute commitment and to counsel the patient's spouse and children.

General recommendations about the care of the bipolar patient in a primary care setting fall into the three domains of psychosocial intervention, pharmacotherapy, and special considerations of conception, pregnancy, and menopause. In regard to specific psychotherapeutic interventions, little research has been published on the techniques that are most effective with this population. However, becoming aware of psychosocial aspects of the disorder and interviewing patients with appropriate counseling maneuvers are essential for optimal care. Psychotherapy helps women recognize the indicators of the illness. For example, they may feel an intensification of sexual feelings and fantasies, or they may become more irritable in general, or they may find that their thinking is speeding up and their sleep patterns are shifting. Helping patients to become aware of these indicators enables the clinician to determine when best to increase the dosage of the mood-stabilizing agent.

Although mood stabilizers reduce the economic costs of prolonged hospitalization, usually bring the manic state under rapid control, and lessen the truly dangerous effects of the episodes, they are not panaceas. The social and personal costs of repeated episodes are high (Bowden, 1996b; Keck et al., 1996a). Awareness of psychosocial stressors and their particular meaning to the patient can help prevent relapse. In addition to the supportive counseling techniques of giving advice, empathetically validating the patient, affirming her courage in the face of adversity, and encouraging her treatment compliance, the primary care clinician may adapt the following guidelines for face-to-face office counseling. Giving the patient a handout of written instructions (such as the Patient Guidelines listed below) accentuates compliance with taking of medications and following through with psychosocial interventions.

In presenting guidelines for pharmacotherapy and those areas of special concern to women (e.g., pregnancy), an effort has been made to group the most salient aspects of general care as a starting point. In all likelihood, additional mood stabilizers will become available in the near future. Clinicians who routinely treat patients with bipolar disorder should refer to current periodicals, texts, or pharmacotherapy handbooks, because the medications, their dosages, and the requirements of therapeutic monitoring are in a rapid state of evolution (Bowden, 1996b). However, the following counseling principles and suggestions for self-care and compliance are likely to stand the test of time.

PATIENT GUIDELINES FOR COPING WITH BIPOLAR DISORDER

1. There are good weapons to treat bipolar disorder. With systematic trials, the medication that works best in stabilizing your moods can be found.
2. Report any signs of relapse or side effects of medication to your doctor. Become an expert on your illness, recognizing that recurrences can come "out of the blue." Nevertheless, there are many positive health practices you can use to manage your illness.
3. Beware of the use of alcohol, drugs of abuse, even small amounts of caffeine, and over-the-counter medications. Sometimes just a little of these substances can exacerbate bipolar disorder.
4. Learn techniques to manage stress at your job and at home. Be sure to take time out for leisure activities. Practice good sleeping habits and report any diminished need for sleep to your physician, because this is often an early warning sign of relapse.
5. Stick with the treatment. For a long period, you may suspect that the mood stabilizer is not doing you much good; but research shows that those people who keep taking their medication have fewer and less severe relapses (Blazer, 1996; Gitlin et al., 1995; Keck et al., 1996a; Solomon et al., 1995). If you do decide to stop the medication, consult with your doctor and taper the medication very slowly (Baldessarini et al., 1996).

6. Take advantage of individual and group psychotherapy. These treatments can help reduce the stress that triggers mania or depression and can help you deal with the loss of self-esteem that accompanies long-term illness. Local community support groups can also be an invaluable part of treatment.

7. It may seem unfair that you cannot do what is "normal" for others, and this legitimately causes anger. Talk about such feelings with a trusted friend or counselor, or in a support group.

8. Feelings of self-destructiveness or suicide may come "out of the blue." Discuss with family members ahead of time how to deal with this and other life crises that can be a byproduct of your illness. If you become suicidal, call your doctor immediately. Try to remember that suicidal thinking is a symptom of your illness, not a sign of personal or moral failure. The crisis will pass even though it feels hopeless at times.

9. Build your self-esteem. Emotional problems are associated with stigma and the irrational sense that we cause our own problems. Working on your own sense of personal power, relationships, and career will help you to feel that you are doing all you can to care for yourself. Moreover, there is evidence that increased feelings of self-worth actually lessen the proclivity toward depression.

10. Remember that self-sacrifice and self-betrayal have deep roots in our culture (Lerner, 1985, 1987, 1993) and can lead to feelings of demoralization. While developing and nurturing strong ties to others (children, partner, parents, friends), do not neglect yourself, as women are sometimes prone to do. Try to concentrate on your own growth, too. This can buffer you in times of loss or stress. A reservoir of self-efficacy and competency enables you to nurture. Recognize that the achievements of others for whom one cares and the maturation of children can arouse feelings of competition and conflict. Deal with rivalrous feelings as openly and straightforwardly as possible.

ADDITIONAL GUIDELINES FOR PRIMARY CARE CLINICIANS

The following goals and strategies are recommended as ways to facilitate better treatment of bipolar patients.

Make an Accurate Diagnosis

Accurate diagnosis of bipolar illness is the first step toward proper treatment.

1. As many as 66% of treatable patients never receive the care they need because the diagnosis is missed. Consider bipolar illness in any woman with recurrent psychosis or depression, irritability, boastfulness, and poor impulse control (see Table 3–2). Patients usually see three or four doctors before receiving the correct diagnosis. Often, bipolar I patients who are psychotic are misdiagnosed as having schizophrenia.

2. Bipolar disorder is a lifetime illness in which "the number of atypical cases challenges those that are 'typical'. . . . Regardless of the patient's age, the clinician should expect the unexpected" (Blazer, 1996, p. 102). Help the patient and her family to learn as much about the illness as they can. Be

sure to give support and hope to family members, who often can become discouraged.

3. The mechanisms underlying the increased incidence of rapid cycling in bipolar women are poorly understood. Women may be exposed to more antidepressant medications than men because they tend to suffer from more depressive episodes. They are also treated for depression more aggressively than men are, and they seek treatment more often. These differences may result in part from gender role stereotyping or stigma.

4. The prevalence of rapid cycling in women could be a result of iatrogenic illness induced by the tricyclic class of antidepressants. In general, *avoid the use of tricyclics for depressed bipolar patients*. Still, these patients frequently need medication. Bupropion is now considered a safer choice for women in the depressed phase who need medication.

Make Appropriate Psychosocial Interventions with Patient and Family

A growing body of literature suggests that life events trigger relapses of bipolar disorder, even in those patients who are treated with mood stabilizers (Gitlin and Altshuler, 1997).

1. Bipolar illness can be particularly hard to bear for family members who find it difficult to live with unpredictability and mood swings. Counsel family members on ways to reduce daily stress and emotional reactivity as much as possible.

2. Counsel family members to understand and accept that treatment will be needed beyond immediate control to long-term with one of the mood-stabilizing agents such as lithium, divalproex sodium, carbamazepine, gabapentin, or lamotrigine.

3. Psychosocial impairment is high in the bipolar patient. State-of-the-art treatment necessitates providing patients with strategies for dealing with the work, interpersonal, and family problems that will arise.

4. There are insufficient studies available to argue for one preferred mode of psychotherapy over others in bipolar disorder (in contrast to pure depressive disorders). Still, some of the cognitive-behavioral and interpersonal strategies deemed effective for the treatment of unipolar illness are likely also to help patients with bipolar illness. Individual therapy helps patients develop needed skills to prevent relapse. Gaining insight and increasing one's repertoire of coping skills in interpersonal or cognitive-behavioral therapy can have long-lasting benefits and can empower the patient to become an expert in the illness and its treatment. Decreased rates of hospitalization and improved socioeconomic functioning have been reported in those persons who have been part of successful group therapy.

5. Psychosocial therapies may also improve outcome by providing social support during trials of pharmacologic agents, by improving compliance, by reducing functional morbidity, and by serving as preventive agents in their own right. Because manic-depressive illness is a heterogeneous disorder, some subtypes may respond preferentially to the addition of particular psychotherapeutic interventions, but this research question requires further study.

6. Women in particular may respond to specific psychotherapeutic techniques

or modalities that enhance self-esteem and their ability to exert personal control in their lives. It is therefore important to encourage activities that enhance the patient's sense of self-worth.

7. Be aware of the disruption of circadian rhythm in bipolar patients. Urge patients to follow good sleep hygiene. The prodrome of a manic episode is often typified by lack of sleep. In some cases, mania may be averted by the use of sleeping medications such as temazepam (Restoril).

8. As a preventive measure, tell patients not to let themselves become overly tired, hungry, or angry. These states appear to precipitate relapse of the affective disorder. The primary care clinician should spend time counseling patients on how to regulate their lifestyle, sleep patterns, and exercise routines to serve as secondary preventive strategies.

9. Patients with bipolar illness should be taught that alcohol and caffeine and substance abuse can have adverse effects on the long-term course of their illness. Conservative treatment is aided by a substance-free lifestyle for the bipolar patient.

10. After the disease is under good pharmacologic control and the patient has established a good working relationship with caregivers, review with her the hereditary nature of bipolar disorder.

11. To enhance compliance, remind patients that medication prophylaxis reduces mortality (Gershon and Soares, 1997; Schou, 1997). This occurs via decreases in suicidality and the emotional distress and physical risks associated with the disease.

Stabilize Moods with Appropriate Pharmacotherapy

Because 90% of all bipolar patients have multiple episodes, long-range treatment should be offered to prevent relapse. In addition to psychosocial support, patients should be prescribed a mood stabilizer. The best predictor of poor prognosis is a lack of compliance with pharmacologic treatment.

There are now three effective agents to treat acute mania: lithium, divalproex sodium (Bowden, 1996b; Johnson and McFarland, 1996; Keck et al., 1996c), and carbamazepine. These may be taken alone, together, or in conjunction with antipsychotics or benzodiazepines. Two new anticonvulsants, lamotrigine and gabapentin, have been found in open-label studies, case reports, and case series to also be effective. These novel agents should be considered when primary and adjunctive therapies are ineffective. Specialty consultation is advised until further research defines specific indications in bipolar illness.

Lithium. It is well established that manic symptoms will resolve, usually within 1 to 2 weeks, if a patient taking lithium can obtain a blood level of 0.8 to 1.2 mEq/L. An oral loading dose is discouraged because of significant gastrointestinal side effects. Long-term prophylaxis with levels of 0.5 to 0.8 mmol/L is effective and reduces side effects. Routine and regular determinations of serum lithium levels are a safeguard against underdosage or overdosage. Kidney damage caused by lithium, feared two decades ago, has not been borne out with clinical and research data (Kupfer and Frank, 1997; Schou, 1997).

About 20% to 40% of patients obtain no relief from lithium. Failure of lithium prophylaxis is associated with a high frequency of prior mood episodes, rapid cycling, mixed mania, and personality disturbance. Rapid-cycling or mixed states (which tend to occur more often in women) respond well to anticonvulsants such as divalproex or carbamazepine.

Lithium treatment causes hypothyroidism in both men and women, but women appear to be more sensitive to lithium's thyrotoxic effect. Studies of people taking lithium (Leibenluft, 1996; Prange et al., 1984; Shaw et al., 1995) suggest a higher percentage of hypothyroidism in women than in men. Because hypothyroidism is associated with secondary affective symptoms and other morbidities, thyroid status should be assessed at least semiannually in the female patient.

Divalproex Sodium and Carbamazepine. Although both divalproex sodium and carbamazepine are effective for maintenance treatment (Sachs, 1996; Solomon et al., 1995; Swann et al., 1997), sodium valproate is being used increasingly as a first-line drug for bipolar illness. In counseling the female patient, however, clinicians should be aware that high rates of menstrual disturbance, polycystic ovaries, and hyperandrogenism have been demonstrated in those taking valproate for epilepsy. Valproate has also been implicated in congenital abnormalities in the offspring of women patients.

Also called sodium valproate (Depakote), divalproex sodium should produce an antimanic response within 1 to 4 days, with 1 to 2 weeks needed for a full response. An oral loading dose is well tolerated (20 mg/kg per day); a serum level of 45 to 125 µg/mL is correlated with a good antimanic response. Depressive symptoms during manic episodes appear to respond preferentially to divalproex (Swann et al., 1997).

The maximum effect of carbamazepine on mania occurs at 7 to 14 days and on depression at 14 to 21 days. Clinical response is correlated with dosages of 600 to 1,200 mg/day; therapeutic levels may be used but are not always correlated with a clear response.

Risks During Pregnancy and Menopause

Lithium has revolutionized the treatment of bipolar disorder and significantly reduced the rate of relapse and recurrence. However, case reports have indicated that lithium treatment during pregnancy increases the likelihood of Ebstein's abnormality in the baby. Some reviews (Finnerty et al., 1996; Leibenluft, 1996) indicate that the risk of congenital anomalies in offspring of lithium-treated women is considerably lower than previously reported. Still, lithium use during pregnancy should be minimized. If a decision is made to discontinue, the primary care clinician will need to work in concert with the patient's family and mental health team to offer increased psychosocial support.

A modest but consistent body of literature supports the notion that the risk for a new episode of bipolar illness is lower for pregnant than for nonpregnant women. Increased progesterone has been posited as part of the mechanism that accounts for the reduced frequency of bipolar episodes during pregnancy. Still, manic episodes do occur during pregnancy.

In some women with known bipolar illness, medication may be decreased cautiously during pregnancy, but doing so is controversial. However, during the postpartum period, the likelihood of a new manic episode is increased significantly.

Except for pregnancy, little attention has been focused on the implications of bipolar illness for a woman's reproductive status. Serum lithium levels may vary systematically throughout the menstrual cycle, but in most women oral contraceptives do not appear to affect lithium levels significantly.

If the bipolar patient is taking carbamazepine and an oral contraceptive, it is important to consider the interaction between the two medications. Because carbamazepine increases hormone clearance, women taking it need a higher dose of oral contraceptives to obtain adequate protection. This is particularly important because carbamazepine has been associated with neonatal hepatic dysfunction and hemorrhage.

The effects of exogenous estrogens and progesterones on the course of bipolar illness have not been explored. As a result, the particular impact of hormone supplementation in menopausal bipolar women remains unknown.

Psychopharmacologic treatment with lithium during pregnancy is becoming more common; risks and benefits must be weighed in each individual case. Because there is substantial morbidity from bipolar illness for both mother and baby, women with bipolar disorder appear to benefit from puerperal prophylaxis with mood stabilizers (Cohen et al., 1995). Although it is best to avoid treatment during the first trimester, there are times when it cannot be avoided. As Finnerty and associates (1996) wisely commented, "As physicians, we are naturally inclined to avoid risks that we *create* (e.g., by prescribing a drug), but it is important to weigh the magnitude of those risks against the risks of the untreated illness" (p. 262). In addition, as pregnancy progresses, lithium requirements increase because of the increased glomerular filtration rate.

For the acutely manic patient presenting in the emergency room, the benzodiazepines lorazepam (Ativan) and clonazepam (Klonopin) are currently the first line of treatment. Both perform well to bring acute symptoms of mania under control and are reasonably safe to the fetus.

SUMMARY

Bipolar disorder is a major public health problem, affecting 1% to 1.6% of the adult population. About 50% of these patients are women. Although major strides have been made in the diagnosis of the spectrum of bipolar-related disorders, it is estimated that 30% to 60% of those who could benefit from medication do not receive it. Clinicians should suspect bipolar disorder in a patient with any recurrent affective or psychotic illness and should become attuned to the subtle, subclinical presentations of this malady.

In the female workforce alone, the estimated cost of diminished productivity (impaired work performance) caused by affective symptoms from bipolar disorder is $9 billion. This figure does not include the mortality costs due to suicide, the enormous emotional costs and suffering of the patient and her family members, and the high utilization of nonpsychiatric medical care. Lithium carbonate and the anticonvulsants divalproex sodium and carbamazepine have been shown to be highly cost-effective in both the acute and maintenance phases of the disorder. However, patient compliance with medication regimens is sporadic. Efforts must be made to enhance compliance among patients taking mood stabilizers, which tend to prevent relapse in a significant number of cases.

Although the availability of lithium, divalproex sodium, and carbamazepine has expanded the number of available therapeutic options, these agents differ in their onset of action, side effects, and clinical features. Primary care clinicians play an essential role in recognizing bipolar disorder and encouraging patients to take advantage of pharmacologic and psychosocial interventions. Before initiating therapy, the clinician must distinguish bipolar disorder from secondary manias, those medical conditions that "mask" a more functional disturbance.

Pregnancy and the puerperium present special challenges in the treatment of bipolar disorder. Because women patients seem to have a greater incidence of the "rapid-cycling" form of bipolar illness, bupropion may be a better medication choice during the depressed phase of the illness, particularly if there is not full control with a mood-stabilizing agent. Comorbidity is high with other psychiatric illnesses, particularly alcoholism and substance abuse. Specific treatment for the comorbid condition may be necessary.

Because of the complexity of presentation, the high morbidity, and the suicide rate associated with bipolar disorder, treatment by a specialist is highly recommended. However, the primary care clinician can be instrumental in the management of this disorder by encouraging the patient to comply with treatment, by supporting the patient and family members during times of crisis, and by offering suggestions about positive health practices that can attenuate the illness.

As with other disorders, the primary care clinicians must encourage the bipolar patient to become an expert on her own illness to ensure she gets the treatment she needs. Managed care systems have not always been supportive of patients with severe mental disorders. The primary care clinician and the patient must join forces, therefore, with mental health practitioners to educate case managers about cost offset, employers about productivity, and political representatives about the value and effectiveness of treatment. Aggressive pharmacologic maintenance treatment, patient and family education, psychotherapy, and rehabilitation are necessary to facilitate a high quality of care for this severe, relapsing, and costly illness.

Resources for the Patient

Jamison KR: *An Unquiet Mind: A Memoir of Moods and Madness.* New York, Alfred A. Knopf, 1995.
   The author's personal torment with bipolar illness is described in this poignant, accessible autobiography. The reader emerges with a sense of what it is like to be manic-depressive. This book will help the patient not only to understand her illness better but also to realize that very successful people who are affected by it can go on to lead fulfilling lives. The benefits of both psychotherapy and pharmacotherapy are described, as is the toll of denying or keeping the illness secret because of stigma.
Duke P, Hochman G: *A Brilliant Madness: Living with Manic-depressive Illness.* New York, Bantam Books, 1993.
   This popular celebrity's autobiography is a heart-wrenching tale of her struggle to overcome bipolar illness and lead a creative, fulfilling life. Patty Duke's admission of her illness and her recounting of her recovery provide a unique perspective and perform a real service for patients and professionals alike. She explains the course of her illness and treatment experiences and the personal cost in terms of failed opportunities and relationships. She also offers speculation about the disease's connection to creativity. Detail is provided about the hereditary and biologic bases for the illness, treatment modalities, and the impact of the illness on family and friends. Numerous interviews by experts in the field provide state-of-the-art information about causes, medication, and psychotherapy, underscoring the need for patients to involve them-

selves in healing by complying with medications and using support groups whenever possible. A list of resources and references for mentally ill patients and their families is included at the end. A section addressing the suffering of family members who must come to grips with the disorder in a loved one may be suggested for the patient, her spouse, and children.

Duke P, Turan K: *Call Me Anna: The Autobiography of Patty Duke.* New York, Bantam Books, 1987.

Although this book provides less detailed clinical information than Ms. Duke's later book, her moving story about living with bipolar illness is thorough and persuasive. An interesting read for the general reader as well as for the clinician, this text benefits from the author's honesty, which will no doubt inspire in others the courage, determination, and commitment to stick with treatment. Her successful rehabilitation with a combination of psychotherapy and medication, along with her vivid description of the impact of the disorder on her life, provides a view of the illness not possible from mere clinical texts alone.

Resources for the Clinician

Jamison KR: *Touched with Fire: Manic-depressive Illness and the Artistic Temperament.* New York, Free Press, 1993.

The relationship between manic-depressive illness and creative accomplishment is reviewed. These biographic sketches teach much about the experience of mania and hypomania. Although the author's purpose is to delineate the similarities and differences between mood disorders and creativity, readers will also learn much about the various directions the illness may take, its painful and fluctuating course, and new pathways for research.

Leibenluft E: Women with bipolar illness: Clinical and research issues. *Am J Psychiatry* 1996;153:163–173.

An articulate, comprehensive overview about gender differences in bipolar illness and the effects of the female reproductive system on the course of the illness and its treatment.

Frances A, Doherty JP, Kahn DA: The expert consensus guidelines series: Treatment of bipolar disorder. *J Clin Psychiatry* 1996;57(Suppl 12A):5–88.

This supplement to the Journal of Clinical Psychiatry *offers a comprehensive set of treatment guidelines for the generalist and the specialist alike. Almost any clinical question that could come up in the care of the bipolar patient is addressed from the perspective of an expert panel. Treatment pathways, specific recommendations, and treatment options are reviewed. Following the patient from the initial presentation to follow-up, the authors offer guidelines and algorithms to address all phases of treatment and, in particular, to suggest what to do after complications arise or when therapy proves inadequate. The handout section at the end of the supplement for patients and their families is a useful adjunct for those who monitor the treatment of many bipolar patients in their practice.*

References

Akiskal HS, Chen SE, Davis GC, et al.: Borderline: An adjective in search of a noun. *J Clin Psychiatry* 1985;46:41–48.

Akiskal HS: The temperamental borders of affective disorders. *Acta Psychiatr Scand* 1994;89(suppl):32–37.

Baldessarini RJ, Tondo L, Faedda GL, et al.: Effects of the rate of discontinuing lithium maintenance treatment in bipolar disorders. *J Clin Psychiatry* 1996;57:441–448.

Blazer DG: Lifetime perturbations of bipolar disorder. *Am J Psychiatry* 1996;153:100–102.

Bowden CL: The efficacy of divalproex sodium and lithium in the treatment of acute mania. *Directions in Psychiatry* 1996a;16:i–vi.

Bowden CL: Dosing strategies and time course of response to antimanic drugs. *J Clin Psychiatry* 1996b;57(suppl 13):4–9.

Bowden CL, Janicak PG, Orsulak P, et al.: Relation of serum valproate concentration to response in mania. *Am J Psychiatry* 1996;153:765–770.

Bowden CL, McElroy SL: History of the development of valproate for treatment of bipolar disorder. *J Clin Psychiatry* 1995;56(suppl 3):3–5.

Brady KT, Sonne SC: The relationship between substance abuse and bipolar disorder. *J Clin Psychiatry* 1995;56(suppl 3):19–24.

Cohen LS, Sichel DA, Robertson LM, et al.: Postpartum prophylaxis for women with bipolar disorder. *Am J Psychiatry* 1995;152:1641–1645.

Duke P, Hochman G: *A Brilliant Madness: Living with Manic-depressive Illness.* New York, Bantam Books, 1993.

Duke P, Turan K: *Call Me Anna: The Autobiography of Patty Duke.* New York, Bantam Books, 1987.

Dunner DL: Diagnosing and treating bipolar II disorder. *Directions in Psychiatry* 1993;13:1–6.

Evans DL, Byerly MJ, Greer, RA: Secondary mania: Diagnosis and treatment. *J Clin Psychiatry* 1995;56(suppl 3):31–37.

Finnerty M, Levin Z, Miller LJ: Acute manic episodes in pregnancy. *Am J Psychiatry* 1996;153:261–263.

Frances A, Doherty JP, Kahn DA: The expert consensus guideline series: Treatment of bipolar disorder. *J Clin Psychiatry* 1996;57(suppl 12A):5–88.

Gershon S, Soares JC: Commentary: Current therapeutic profile of lithium. *Arch Gen Psychiatry* 1997;54:16–20.

Gitlin MJ, Altshuler LL: Unanswered questions, unknown future for one of our oldest medications. *Arch Gen Psychiatry* 1997;54:21–23.

Gitlin MJ, Swendsen J, Heller TL, et al.: Relapse and impairment in bipolar disorder. *Am J Psychiatry* 1995;152:1635–1640.

Jacobsen FM: Low-dose valproate: A new treatment for cyclothymia, mild rapid cycling disorders, and premenstrual syndrome. *J Clin Psychiatry* 1993;54:229–234.

Jamison KR: *An Unquiet Mind: A Memoir of Moods and Madness.* New York, Alfred A. Knopf, 1995.

Jamison KR: *Touched with Fire: Manic-depressive Illness and the Artistic Temperament.* New York, Free Press, 1993.

Johnson RE, McFarland BH: Lithium use and discontinuation in a health maintenance organization. *Am J Psychiatry* 1996;153:993–1000.

Keck PE, McElroy SL, Bennett JA: Health-economic implications of the onset of action of antimanic agents. *J Clin Psychiatry* 1996a;57(suppl 13):13–18.

Keck PE, McElroy SL, Stanton SP, et al.: Pharmacoeconomic aspects of the treatment of bipolar disorder. *Psychiatr Ann* 1996b;26(suppl 7):S449–S453.

Keck, PE, Nabulsi AA, Taylor JL, et al.: A pharmacoeconomic model of divalproex vs. lithium in the acute and prophylactic treatment of bipolar disorder. *J Clin Psychiatry* 1996c;57:213–222.

Kopacz DR, Janicak PG: The relationship between bipolar disorder and personality. *Psychiatr Ann* 1996;26:644–650.

Krauthammer C, Klerman GL: Secondary mania: Manic syndromes associated with antecedent physical illness or drugs. *Arch Gen Psychiatry* 1978;35:1333–1339.

Kupfer DJ; Frank E: Commentary: Forty years of lithium treatment. *Arch Gen Psychiatry* 1997;54:14–15.

Leibenluft E: Women with bipolar illness: Clinical and research issues. *Am J Psychiatry* 1996;153:163–173.

Lerner HG: *The Dance of Anger: A Woman's Guide to Changing the Patterns of Intimate Relationships.* New York, Harper & Row, 1985.

Lerner HG: Female depression: Self-sacrifice and self-betrayal in relationships. In: Formanek R, Gurian A (eds.): *Women and Depression: A Lifespan Perspective,* pp. 200–221. New York, Springer, 1987.

Lerner HG: *The Dance of Deception: Pretending and Truth-Telling in Women's Lives.* New York, HarperCollins, 1993.

McElroy SL, Keck PE, Stanton SP, et al.: A randomized comparison of divalproex oral loading versus haloperidol in the initial treatment of acute psychotic mania. *J Clin Psychiatry* 1996;57:142–146.

Middlebrook DW: *Anne Sexton: A Biography.* Boston, Houghton Mifflin, 1991.

Owley T, Sharma R: Drug-induced mania: A critical review. *Psychiatr Ann* 1996;26:659–664.

Peselow ED, Sanfilipo MP, Fieve RR: Relationship between hypomania and personality disorders before and after successful treatment. *Am J Psychiatry* 1995;152:232–238.

Prange AL, Loosen PT, Wilson IC, et al.: The therapeutic use of hormones of the thyroid axis. In: Post RM, Ballenger JC (eds.): *Depression in Neurobiology of Mood Disorders,* pp. 311–322. Baltimore, Williams & Wilkins, 1984.

Sachs G: Is divalproex sodium an appropriate initial treatment for bipolar depression? *Psychiatr Ann* 1996;26(suppl 7):S454–S459.

Schou, M: Forty years of lithium treatment. *Arch Gen Psychiatry* 1997;54:9–13.

Shaw J, Kennedy SH, Joffe RT: Gender differences in mood disorders: A clinical focus. In: Seeman MV (ed.): *Gender and Psychotherapy,* pp. 89–111. Washington, DC, American Psychiatric Press, 1995.

Solomon DA, Keitner GI, Miller IW, et al.: Course of illness and maintenance treatments for patients with bipolar disorder. *J Clin Psychiatry* 1995;56:5–13.

Swann AC: Mixed or dysphoric manic states: Psychopathology and treatment. *J Clin Psychiatry* 1995;56(suppl 3):6–10.

Swann AC, Bowden CL, Morris D, et al.: Depression during mania: Treatment response to lithium or divalproex. *Arch Gen Psychiatry* 1997;54:37–42.

Tohen M, Zarate CA, Zarate SB, et al.: The McLean/Harvard First-Episode Mania Project: Pharmacologic treatment and outcome. *Psychiatr Ann* 1996;26:S444–S448.

Weissman MM, Bland RC, Canino G, et al.: Cross-national epidemiology of major depression and bipolar disorder. *JAMA* 1996;276:293–299.

Chapter 4

Misuse of Substances

The misuse of substances by women (e.g., alcoholism, abuse of illicit and prescription drugs, nicotine dependence) has dramatically increased in the past 50 years. In this chapter, special attention is paid to the two most common addictions in women—alcoholism and nicotine dependence—but most of the core concepts apply to the diagnosis and treatment of all cases of substance misuse. Special issues related to misuse of prescription drugs are explored in Chapter 1 (Anxiety Disorders), Chapter 7 (Insomnia), and Chapter 8 (Somatization and Hypochondriasis).

Startling facts about the impact of substance abuse must inform not only the clinician's practice but also the national health agenda: Alcohol and drug dependence are among the most prevalent illnesses. Deaths from addictive disorders account for one fourth to one third of all deaths in the United States (Hurt et al., 1996). It is estimated that alcoholism alone contributes to 100,000 deaths annually and costs the country $99 billion, about 37% of which is attributed to lost productivity. Addiction expert Robert DuPont (1997a) gives a broader context for these statistics:

> More than 30 million Americans alive today will experience addiction to alcohol and other drugs in their lifetime. Sixteen percent, or about 1 in 6, will themselves suffer from addiction to alcohol and other drugs. Four out of 10 American families are directly affected by addiction . . . the number one preventable health problem in the United States and throughout the developing nations of the world . . . . No part of the nation and few extended families have been spared the deadly, overwhelming, and confusing grip of addiction (pp. 3–4).

Many of the facts clinicians rely on to care for women with addictions are based on studies of men. But notable differences between men and women have been identified regarding patterns of use, epidemiology, medical and social consequences, and treatment (Blume, 1986; Blume et al., 1992; Lex, 1991). Research has attempted to close this gender gap, shifting attention over the past 25 years to the special problems and therapeutic needs affecting female patients who abuse substances.

WOMEN AT RISK

Women who have problematic substance use are increasingly found in all settings (Table 4–1). As women have entered the workplace and gained greater economic independence, their misuse of substances has been exacerbated. In the past, many more men than women had substance use problems and suffered the consequences of addiction; this gender gap appears to be closing. Almost 10% of women younger than 30 years of age are estimated to have an alcohol

---

Table 4–1. **Risk Factors for Misuse of Substances by Women**

Depression
Anxiety
Eating disorder
One or both parents with a history of substance abuse
Stressful life events
Avoidant coping style
Partner who drinks or abuses substances
Physical and sexual victimization in childhood
Sexual dysfunction and/or high-risk sexual behavior
Sexual orientation (possible)

---

use disorder. One of three alcoholics in the United States is female. Women's health is impaired by the direct toxic effects of substances on the body, the sapping of psychological stability, and the long-term, unrelenting havoc rendered on relationships, livelihood, and overall quality of life.

Substance-abusing women report an amalgam of family and marital problems. In addition to being prone to being victims of violence and abuse, they report a high degree of marital and family strife and feelings of inadequacy and loneliness. They engage in frequent suicide attempts. Their lives are riddled with upheaval. They may divorce but continue to function well at work; they may be fired from countless jobs but share a substance-abusing life with a partner. Whenever these women become isolated, they tend to leave their adult responsibilities to their children.

Children reared in substance-abusing families are at higher risk for a range of developmental and emotional problems. They commonly exhibit the emotional symptoms of low self-esteem, harbor feelings of shame and hopelessness, engage in deviant and high-risk behavior, and are hampered by poor social and learning skills. These children are prone to later drug use themselves, in part because of genetic predisposition but also because of neglect and poor role modeling in their family of origin.

The failure of physicians to bring up the topic of substance abuse and to be frank about the toll it takes on the lives of men and women is a major gap in our national health care agenda (Crits-Cristoph and Sigueland, 1996; Gordis, 1996; Wesson and Ling, 1996). As DuPont (1997a) comments:

> Every major social and community institution has been hit by addiction, although many continue to ignore it, treating it as if it were an uncommon problem experienced only by a small number of troubled people. Addiction affects people of all ages and in all walks of life and is an equal opportunity destroyer (p. 4).

A Patient's Perspective

As useful as these facts may be regarding the global and societal costs of addiction, few medical texts or lists of problems tell the tale as starkly and trenchantly as the words of an actual patient. In recounting her near-demise from alcoholism, journalist Caroline Knapp (1996) reveals how her addiction "made the confusion go away; it provided an easy way out, an escape from my internal life" (p. 67). She shares the insight of a friend who called alcoholism

" 'the disease of more,' a reference to the greediness so many of us tend to feel around liquor, the grabbiness, the sense of impending deprivation, and the certainty that we will never have enough" (p. 53). The questions clinicians ask their patients, although professionally apt, sound surprisingly sterile, even mundane, when compared with the "real questions" Knapp asks herself (and which can easily be applied to most other addictions):

> When someone pours you a glass from that bottle, do you take careful note of the level of liquid in the glass, and measure it secretly against the level of liquid in other glasses, and hold your breath for just a second until you are sure you have enough? Do you establish an edgy feeling of relationship with that glass, that wine bottle; do you worry over it, care about it, covet it, want all of it yourself? Can you bear the thought that it might run out, that you might be left sitting there without it, alone and unprotected? (pp. 52–53).

But the loss of control—and the multiple tolls—resulting from addiction go even further. Countering the notion that addiction is simply a biologic matter, Knapp realizes, in her recovery, that she drank to avoid conflict, to manage strong feelings, and to eschew compelling psychological hunger. In essence, she comes to understand in treatment that

> You drink to avoid those painful choices as you wake up in the morning, and all those choices are still with you, still unfaced; all those unresolved problems are hanging around your neck like pieces of lead, weighing you down, keeping you from moving forward. Humiliating. And terrifying, because I can't see an end to it. . . . My life could go on and on and on like that, just as my father's had (p. 217).

These "late-onset," subjective consequences are not included in the kinds of epidemiologic statistics ("hard data") cited previously. In fact, substance abuse is perceived as such a staggering problem that many clinicians give up before addressing it on an individual basis. Frustration with treating the illness runs high, in part because primary clinicians rarely feel that they are in a key position to have a positive impact. But nothing could be further from the truth. The following sections examine why so many patients don't get help and then consider some straightforward strategies for recognizing these women in medical practice.

WHY FEW WOMEN SEEK HELP

Lack of Recognition

The primary care clinician is increasingly being called on to recognize and care for the singly or multiply addicted patient. As managed health care reshapes the practice of medicine, addiction treatment that previously was provided by psychiatrists or addiction specialists, or in residential drug abuse treatment programs, is shifting to outpatient care by generalists.

To enhance opportunities for recovery, medical clinics overseen by family practitioners, internists, gynecologists, and their care extenders (e.g., Advanced Registered Nurse Practitioners) must be equipped to recognize substance misuse in women patients, to suggest avenues of intervention, and to teach coping skills (Table 4–2) (Fleming et al., 1997; Miller and Swift, 1997; Wesson

---

Table 4–2. **Initial Assessment of the Patient with "Potential"
Substance Misuse**

---

1. Consider substance abuse or multiple substance use in the diagnosis.
2. Discuss health consequences, especially those related to women's more rapid development of cardiovascular, gastrointestinal, and liver diseases ("telescoping").
3. Address the "relational context" of substance use (e.g., partner with substance abuse problem, history of physical abuse or violence).
4. Ask the woman's partner or adult children to get a more objective perspective on the extent of use; involve them in treatment.
5. Recommend that the patient visit a 12-step group, and remind her that these are free. Have available the phone numbers of local Alcoholics Anonymous (AA), Narcotics Anonymous (NA), and Women for Sobriety (WFS) groups.
6. Consider residential or structured day treatment if abuse is severe or long-standing.
7. Empathize with and help address practical issues of employment, housing, physical health, legal issues, and childcare.
8. Be aware of community resources and chemical dependency experts and counselors.
9. Consider interaction between substance use and any complaint of impaired sexual functioning.
10. Educate about gender roles, gender socialization, and the tendency of women to self-blame for substance abuse.

---

and Ling, 1996). Treatment guidelines, including counseling techniques and pharmacotherapy suggestions, are included at the end of this chapter.

Limited Access to Services

The challenge of increasing access to services for addictive disorders begins when the patient opens the front door of the primary clinician's office. Many inpatient treatment centers for addictions have closed, and the 28-day inpatient stay is no longer considered the "gold standard" of care. This added marketplace pressure places a greater burden on primary care clinicians to manage these life-threatening illnesses. Fortunately, a majority of addicted patients can be helped by a range of outpatient approaches (Miller and Swift, 1997).

Because addicts are often motivated to seek drug abuse treatment only during a crisis (Wesson and Ling, 1996), the barriers and delays of managed care in accessing treatment are likely to result in the failure of millions of patients to receive the help they need so desperately. This will not be the case if the primary care clinician is vigilant and persistent in diagnosing the problem, has readily available some effective techniques for intervention, and knows how to seek out additional specialty support. Although addiction to alcohol or drugs is clearly life-threatening, many women can benefit from new pharmacotherapies, outpatient psychotherapy, highly structured day or residential treatment, and 12-step fellowships.

Physician Preferences

Physicians avoid treating both male and female addicts, but the woman with a substance abuse problem has been additionally disparaged by the misperception that she is weak-willed, promiscuous, sexually aggressive, or frankly antisocial. To render effective care, clinicians must confront their tendency to hold onto these stereotypes. Of course such patients can be humbling to physicians, because they can tenaciously thwart one's best efforts (DuPont, 1997b; Vaillant, 1983). But outcome studies reveal that the majority of even the most refractory patients can and do improve. Being interested in the person, maintaining a sense of purpose and helpfulness, and having confidence about one's skills in treating addictions all help promote long-term recovery.

Unrecognized Costs to Society

The costs to society in days lost at work, accidents, disrupted family life, and poor quality of life are difficult to quantify objectively. Clearly, alcohol and drug abuse inflate the cost of general medical care. As Wesson and Ling (1996) state, "Enlightened self-interest will dictate that health maintenance organizations and other capitated health care providers provide effective drug abuse treatment services" (p. 1792). An additional onus on the primary care clinician is the securing of benefits, including specialty care, for the patient with a complicated problem or multiple addictions.

Family Attitudes

A major obstacle for the woman who needs treatment is denial and obfuscation on the part of friends, significant others, and family members. They avoid recognizing that the woman actually has a substance abuse problem, and sometimes they actively oppose her efforts to get help. On other occasions, stigma itself may be the primary impediment (e.g., shame or embarrassment when acknowledging that one's wife, daughter, or mother is an alcoholic).

Family responsibilities also contribute. Primary care clinicians understand that some women live in dire economic circumstances or are preoccupied with caring for children. When these women do begin to take time for themselves, they may experience guilt about diverting necessary family resources for their own needs. To successfully engage and retain female patients, some creative treatment programs now offer childcare. Your role is to underscore that effective parenting means taking care of oneself, and that addicted persons not only place their loved ones at special risk but also cannot be fully "present" for their care.

Some experts suspect that women do not seek treatment for substance abuse because they worry about being declared unfit mothers and losing custody of their children. In some jurisdictions, the high treatability of women substance abusers has been emphasized to counter public concern and minimize legal action. Here the primary clinician may also play an essential role by providing education about contemporary treatment. Ultimately, this approach has a positive impact on the family and the social systems to encourage more acceptance of the addicted woman. It concomitantly reinforces to the patient that positive strides can be made. Life-affirming goals can be met so that recovery can enhance—not derail—family life.

Psychiatric Comorbidity

Female substance abusers are highly comorbid for other psychiatric illnesses. Untreated, they ultimately face an increased mortality rate. Common but frightening is the alcoholic patient who presents in the emergency room as depressed, suicidal, and intoxicated. Once sober, she may find that her depression remits. However, at least 30% of these patients have a primary diagnosis of both depression and alcoholism (Hesselbrock and Hesselbrock, 1993; Woody et al., 1995a). When sober, such patients respond to antidepressants (e.g., tricyclics, selective serotonin reuptake inhibitors [SSRIs]) that have a positive effect on their moods and dependence problems.

Other dual diagnoses commonly encountered include the anxiety disorders, eating disorders, and antisocial and borderline personality disorders. Concomitant use of alcohol and sedative drugs is a commonly recognized pattern of mixed dependency. Sometimes a well-meaning clinician prescribes benzodiazepines for a physical or emotional problem (see Chapter 7). Although this strategy can be useful with nonaddicted patients (particularly when use is brief and crisis-focused), rapid tolerance develops in those prone to substance abuse. Prescribing a benzodiazepine is tantamount to prescribing poison (Greenfield, 1996; Lex, 1991, 1995).

Be wary also about the use of tobacco by these patients. Tobacco addiction is highly correlated with alcoholism and other drug dependencies. In the past, tobacco use was not discouraged. In part, the oral gratification of smoking and the camaraderie with others who smoke appeared to have a soothing and sustaining effect on persons attempting to abstain from "hard" drugs. Because cumulative mortality has been found to be extremely high, nicotine dependence treatment is now viewed as imperative in the multiaddicted patient (Hurt et al., 1996).

ALCOHOLISM IN WOMEN: A COMMON, COMPLICATED CONCERN

Women who abuse alcohol now number about 6 million in the United States alone. These women typically develop problem drinking later than men. Although less apt to drink daily and continually or to engage in binges, women progress much more rapidly from the onset of a drinking problem to the later stages of alcoholism—a phenomenon termed "telescoping" (Blume, 1992; Lex, 1991, 1995; North, 1996). A number of factors account for this rapid progression (e.g., social stigma, medical complications, family patterns, and response to loss).

Keeping Secrets

A woman alcoholic appears to face greater social stigma than a man in admitting her problem. She may discern that peers and professionals alike view her as an evil or a promiscuous "fallen woman." Experience often confirms her worst fears. Thus arises a clinical conundrum in diagnosing the female alcoholic: How does the primary care clinician address the possibility of substance misuse, knowing that the woman is more likely to keep her drinking secret and solitary? *Few patients of either gender readily identify alcohol abuse as their chief complaint* (Table 4–3) (Miller, 1997; North, 1996; Wilsnack and Beckman, 1980).

Medical Complications

Female alcoholics have a death rate 50% to 100% higher than that of their male counterparts; they lose an average of 15 years of life expectancy as a

Table 4–3. **Evaluation of the Female Alcoholic**

Physical clues
  Weight loss
  Hoarse voice
  Hypertension (mild)
  Puffy, edematous face; engorgement of conjunctival vessels
  Bruises, cuts, or scratches (indicating physical trauma or accidents)
  Tremors, sweating, spider nevi, alcohol on breath (these signs appear late)
Laboratory clues
  Elevated gamma-glutamyl transpeptidase (GGT)
  Increased mean corpuscular volume (MCV)
  Elevated aspartate aminotransferase (AST) relative to alanine aminotransferase (ALT)
  Low serum potassium
  Elevated fasting triglyceride
Assessment clues
  Multiple addictions, including tobacco
  Deterioration in physical and/or mental health, family life, work, and finances (legal
    problems are common)
  Drinking when alone
  History of depression
  Complaints about sexual dysfunction, low energy, and/or trouble sleeping (e.g.,
    rebound awakening followed by self-medication with alcohol)

result of cirrhosis, circulatory disorders, suicide, homicide, and alcohol-related accidents. Women rapidly develop the serious cardiovascular, gastrointestinal, and liver complications of alcoholism, another aspect of the telescoping phenomenon (Lex, 1995). When women and men consume comparable amounts of alcohol, women have higher blood levels even when size differences are taken into account. The increased bioavailability of alcohol results from decreased gastric oxidation. This contributes to the acute and chronic complications of alcoholism in women (Frezza et al., 1990). The incidence of cirrhosis in women is rapidly increasing, as is the number of women arrested for driving while intoxicated. Drinking has also been linked to an increased risk of breast cancer. Other less lethal but serious consequences are the high prevalence of amenorrhea, anorgasmia, dysmenorrhea, infertility, and early menopause (Lex, 1991; North, 1996; Wilsnack, 1995; Wilsnack and Beckman, 1980).

Medical consequences are the same for women as for men; they include peptic ulcer disease, liver function abnormalities, hypertension, acquired immunodeficiency syndrome and other sexually transmitted diseases, and a history of occupational or automobile accidents. Other psychological sequelae that may alert you or your care extender to problems with chemical dependency are anxiety (Chapter 1), depression and thoughts of suicide (Chapter 2), domestic violence and/or a history of sexual abuse (Chapter 6), psychosomatic complaints (Chapter 8), and sexual dysfunction and marital disruption (Chapter 13).

Family Patterns

Women are likely to have a family history of alcoholism or to have a spouse with alcohol use problems. Although men appear to do their heaviest drinking in young adulthood (ages 21 to 34), the rate of drinking among women continues to climb into midlife (ages 50 to 64). Alcoholism in older women is also on the rise, particularly among those who live alone, have few social supports, or have lost a significant relationship (Goldstein et al., 1996). In this group, alcoholism is most prominent among divorced, separated, and unemployed women and those whose children do not live with them.

Family members may not tell you in the office about the deteriorating problems at home that can only be surmised. But they may quietly take your advice after they leave. More than one woman has been encouraged to obtain treatment after seeing the films *The Days of Wine and Roses, A Woman Under the Influence,* and *When a Man Loves a Woman.* Likewise, the powerful reminiscence by former Senator George McGovern (1995) of his daughter's death by alcoholism authoritatively acknowledges the pain—and the love—of family members have the addicted person. This book is highly recommended as a first step for families struggling with addiction (see "Resources for Patients").

Significant Loss

Like so many other psychological disorders, risk for alcoholism is linked to sustaining a *significant loss*—either in one's adult role or in a relationship. Risk factors associated with alcoholism in the younger adult group (ages 21 to 34) are unemployment, childlessness, and being single; these women are unable to assume their expected adult roles (Cirillo, 1995, 1996; Wilsnack and Beckman, 1980). Risk among older women is linked to the loss of a significant relationship or job, lack of employment outside the home, and even the "empty nest" syndrome.

MAKING THE DIAGNOSIS

Questions to Avoid

Because substance abuse transcends age, race, and socioeconomic background—and is often *denied* by the patient—diagnosis can be difficult. Clinicians are taught that asking the patient how much she drinks or uses rarely proves useful. So often she may minimize or even be unaware of the amount. If she is aware, she will find ways to dodge your well-intentioned queries because she believes she must have the substance to *survive.* As Caroline Knapp (1996) further describes her own compulsion to keep drinking despite numerous, dangerous consequences:

> The need is more than merely physical: it's psychic and visceral and multilayered.
> There's a dark fear to the feeling of wanting that wine, that vodka, that bourbon:
> a hungry, abiding fear of being without, being exposed, without your armor (p. 54).

Moreover, as in male patients, there is no pathognomonic sign to aid detection (Mello, 1980; North, 1996). Some recommend having female patients fill out a health questionnaire that focuses on issues of emotional stress and chemical dependency. These questionnaires, although useful, tend to pick up only late-stage disease. The clinician also must rely on the patient's veracity.

Questions to Ask

The alcoholic patient usually is more willing to answer questions that center on the physical sequelae of alcoholism, such as gastric distress, anxiety, low energy, sexual dysfunction, insomnia, disrupted sleep, and infertility. It is careful attention to these physical complaints that alerts most primary care clinicians to the patient's alcoholism (Fleming et al., 1997; Miller and Swift, 1997).

The *CAGE* mnemonic is widely employed as an evaluation tool to substantiate the diagnosis of alcohol-related problems. It is easy and takes less than 1 minute of your time (Barnes and Bor, 1996; Blume et al., 1992; Ewing, 1984). To get a more objective reading of alcohol use, ask the patient the following four questions: (1) Have you ever *C*ut down on your drinking? (2) Have you ever been *A*nnoyed by criticism of your drinking? (3) Have you ever felt *G*uilty about your drinking? (4) Have you felt the need for an *E*ye opener? Addiction specialists believe that a single "yes" to any of these four questions strongly suggests a serious alcohol problem. Two or more positive responses increases the likelihood to about 90%.*

When such detective work pays off and the patient acknowledges a problem, the clinician must confront his or her own tendency to shy away from challenging the patient's denial of the extent of her problem. The physician may turn away from the patient, or from the sordid details of her substance history. Listening to this painful material can be difficult. Physicians may feel the heavy onus of responsibility. They may be reminded of an alcohol or a substance problem in their own family of origin and so may be unexpectedly confronted with visceral memories of personal anguish long since past.

Clinicians may also be angry or frustrated when hearing about how an innocent person was psychologically or physically injured by the patient. Most clinicians also have had to endure insults from, and to maintain composure in the face of, intoxicated patients, some of whom have not survived their addiction. Thus clinicians may feel a sense of defeat or intolerance before they begin. Any or all of these factors are likely to contribute to difficulty in responding to the patient with a substance problem and in maintaining equanimity, patience, and a desire to be helpful (Vaillant, 1983).

ADDITIONAL FACTORS TO ASSESS IN THE HISTORY

Multiple Substance Use

Because women who abuse one substance are often addicted to others, the clinician must always inquire about other drug use in a comprehensive examination (Hall, 1994; Lex, 1995; Wilsnack, 1995). Be wary of the negative answer.

---

*Research found that the *TWEAK* questionnaires may be more specific for diagnosing alcoholism in women (Bradley et al., 1998). The *TWEAK* mnemonic in your practice involves asking the woman (1) How many drinks can you hold? Three or more indicates *T*olerance. (2) Have relatives or friends *W*orried about you in the past year? (3) Do you need to take a drink (*E*ye opener) to get started in the morning? (4) Has a friend or family member told you that you said or did something you cannot remember? (*A*mnesia.) (5) Have you tried to cut down your drinking? (i.e., *K*ut down.) (See Bradley et al., 1998.)

The patient may attempt to cover up these ancillary addictions. She may even have changed her drug or alcoholic beverage of choice in the hope of controlling her intake (Stammer, 1991). Keep the issue of potential multiple addictions at the forefront of your thinking to avoid being surprised when you learn about these concealed behaviors.

Other Emotional Problems

Women who misuse substances typically present to their primary care clinicians as depressed or suffering from a series of physical ailments—the so-called psychosomatic complaints. These problems often do require medical attention, and the physician may appropriately prescribe medication. However, the substance abuse problem is often overlooked (Lisansky Gomberg and Nirenberg, 1993; McCrady and Langenbucher, 1996; Miller and Swift, 1997).

For example, a well-meaning clinician may be responsible for an iatrogenic addiction. In attempting to deal with the patient's manifest symptoms of depression or anxiety, the clinician may inappropriately prescribe a benzodiazepine. The real issue of substance abuse, particularly alcoholism, then gets overlooked. As the authors of *Women and Drugs* (Peluso and Peluso, 1988) point out, some women who are "diagnosed as using too much alcohol" are given benzodiazepines instead, "a procedure that one doctor likens to treating lung cancer with cigarettes. 'Your patients don't get better,' another doctor has said, 'They just smell better'" (p. 36).

Family History

If a spouse, partner, or adult child is available for questioning, ask the patient for permission to speak with that person. This interaction promotes collaboration and provides objective details. However, significant others may also feel reluctant to acknowledge the depth of the problem and may unwittingly tend to perpetuate it (the so-called codependency issue).

This problem is all the more reason to involve loved ones in the treatment whenever possible and to urge them to also seek help (e.g., Al-Anon/Alateen). Know the support networks in your community, and review the long-term medical and psychological risks. Empathize with the family members' distress and point out the heartbreak of losing a loved one to addiction. This approach prompts them to muster the courage to confront the tendency to avoid the problem or to give in to the patient's denial. Substance abuse is a family problem, and all members suffer from its consequences (McGovern, 1995).

Alcoholism in women appears to be strongly correlated with a family history of alcohol problems. There is growing evidence that both heredity and environment play etiologic roles. One form of alcoholism may be more environmentally determined and another more genetically mediated (Hill, 1995); how much variance is explained by inheritance and how much is moderated by personal factors remains at issue. Clearly, a genetic diathesis is important, but several studies now demonstrate the ways in which environment modifies these hereditary attributes. For example, living with a partner or spouse who uses substances greatly exacerbates a woman's tendency to do so (Bepko, 1991; Toneatto et al., 1992; Wilsnack, 1995). These facts may aid in counseling the patient and in maintaining the high degree of vigilance necessary for initial interventions in the primary care setting (Anthony et al., 1995; Fleming et al., 1997; Hall, 1994).

The reasons women use substances differ from those of men. Family histories of women reveal a background of abandonment, divorce, or death of a loved one in childhood. Female alcoholics are also more likely than males to have grown up with an alcoholic father perceived as caring but inconsistent. These women may turn to alcohol or drugs as a way to make interpersonal connections or to identify with their father. Moreover, their use of alcohol is an attempt to deal with feelings of inadequacy, lack of nurturance, emotional or physical abuse, abandonment, and painful memories of childhood (Wallace, 1992; Windle et al., 1995).

What precisely gets inherited to cause addiction is not yet known. Quite possibly, these hereditary factors may not be specific to a particular substance. Differences in temperament, variations in sensitivity to the rewarding or adverse qualities of a substance, idiosyncratic capacities to tolerate repeated exposure, nonidentical rates of metabolism, distinct taste preferences, and individual abilities to relate memories of drinking experiences to their consequences are inherited characteristics that lead to unique phenotypic expression (Anthony et al., 1996; Gordis, 1996).

Blum and colleagues (1996), working in 14 independent laboratories, have associated the A1 allele of the dopamine D2 receptor gene with a number of addictive-impulsive-compulsive disorders they call the "reward deficiency syndrome." Although these investigators have not proven that the A1 allele is the only cause of severe alcoholism, they have linked it as a factor in several forms of the disease. Persons who carry this allele have a 47% chance of developing one of the disorders of the reward deficiency syndrome (i.e., alcoholism, drug abuse, compulsive gambling, bingeing, or attention deficit disorder).

Patients may be reminded that the discovery of neurochemicals such as dopamine and the D2 receptor is the first step toward finding new pharmacologic agents. These agents may be very helpful adjuncts in long-term sobriety. For example, craving and anxiety are demonstrably reduced when A1 carriers are treated with the D2 agonist bromocriptine (Lawford et al., 1995). In the future, genetic markers may be used for early identification and treatment of alcohol and drug abuse, thereby arresting, if not preventing, the devastating course of addiction. As Blum and colleagues (1996) summarize,

> Identifying individuals with the A1 allele offers the possibility of helping individuals before alcoholism or substance abuse affects their lives. We foresee the possibility for better treatment, new forms of prevention, and the removal of the social stigma attached, not only to alcoholism, but also to related "reward seeking" behavior comprising the reward deficiency syndrome (p. 144).

Although many patients glean knowledge and hope about their disorder by learning some of the nuances of the emerging neuroscience of substance abuse, most benefit more from their primary clinician's straightforward emphasis on the mixture of genetic and environmental contributions in causing substance misuse. *Despite genetic proclivity, one still must use the substance to suffer the consequences. This clarification helps women take responsibility for those aspects of the problem they can control,* such as the environment they are exposed to every day and the jeopardy they place themselves in when loved ones engage in high-risk behaviors (Rivara et al., 1997).

Overemphasis on biologic vulnerability can become a convenient scapegoat, depriving the woman of taking on the far weightier—but essential—task of self-confrontation by making a spiritual inventory and enlisting resources for personal growth. After reviewing the hereditary influence on expression of these illnesses, you should call attention to how a return to health can occur only when both clinician and patient embrace the view that the patient must be accountable for herself.

> The most fundamental aspect of the disease of addiction is dishonesty, and the most fundamental value needed to get well is honesty. I have come to the conclusion that *honesty* is the one-word antidote for all forms of addiction . . . . Recovery often comes when it is least expected. Getting well from addiction is, in any event, an inside job, one that only the addicted person can do.
>
> (DuPont, 1997b, p. 375)

Sexual Abuse and Family Violence

Inquire about any history of physical abuse, sexual abuse, or family violence (Windle et al., 1995). When your patient is both a mother and a substance abuser, it can be assumed that her children are assuming primary caretaking roles in the family, especially for the care of younger siblings. The children of substance-abusing mothers are at high risk for developmental, physical, and emotional problems. Sexual abuse often occurs within the family nexus of a mother who is unable to fulfill her adult roles. Children, with natural desire to emulate adults, tend to turn to early substance use themselves.

Children raised in homes where one or both parents abuse substances are prone to exhibit low self-esteem, shame, and hopelessness; they engage in high-risk behavior; and they fail to learn and socialize appropriately for their age. To avoid being at home, some attempt to excel in another area of life (e.g., school, athletics). These efforts are aimed toward coping with complicated, noxious family problems. They take their toll on the emotional health and psychological development of the child (Knapp, 1996; Stammer, 1991; Unumb, 1992).

In effect, children of substance abusers suffer from having to grow up too soon, to fend for themselves instead of being fended for. Research confirms the commonsense perception that the prospects for healthy adjustment and maturation of children are poor when they witness years of a troubled marital relationship, endure verbal barrages or physical violence, receive inconsistent discipline and caregiving, and suffer the effects of financial strain and social isolation.

Another common and important problem for primary clinicians to acknowledge and address is the battered husband syndrome. Although women who physically injure often go unreported owing to the man's shame, evidence suggests that this problem is on the rise in our society. As a whole, however, women tend to verbally abuse more often than to physically attack (Cirillo, 1995). Verbal violence is especially prone to occur when the woman is under the influence of substances.

You may experience verbal belligerence yourself, or you may witness one of your support staff or a patient's family member being the unwelcome recipient of a verbal barrage. This loss of ancillary ego control on the part of the patient leads even the most experienced, mellow professional to feel anger, frustration, and resentment (Toneatto et al., 1992). The understandable defense of "not wanting to treat" the addicted patient comes in part from memories and experiences with addicted persons who were ungrateful and demeaning. DuPont's advice is again balm for the wounded healer (Nouwen, 1972) who attempts to stay the course with the most recalcitrant patient:

> I have learned never to give up and that recovery from addiction is always possible, even in the most hopeless cases . . . . Respect, but do not fear, the disease of addiction, which is a powerful and pitiless teacher for patients and therapists alike.
>
> (DuPont, 1997b, p. 375)

Treatment steps are outlined in Table 4–4.

SUBSTANCE ABUSE IN SPECIAL POPULATIONS

The primary care clinician should be cognizant that special groups of women are at particular risk for alcoholism and other forms of chemical dependency. However, research on risks for women of different ethnic, religious, and cultural backgrounds is still incomplete. These broad generalizations are meant not to stereotype individuals but rather to heighten awareness when dealing with patients of particular backgrounds. Sensitivity to ethnic and cultural issues does aid diagnosis and treatment planning. Research in this area is likely to evolve quickly as the importance of addressing cultural nuances becomes more widely accepted as essential for rendering optimal medical care.

Table 4–4. **Steps in Treating the Substance-Abusing Female Patient**

1. Detoxify the patient.
2. Confront the patient's denial.
3. Enlist support of family members; confront any tendency on their part to disavow the problem.
4. Insist on abstinence.
5. Refer the patient to self-help groups, particularly AA, NA, or WFS.
6. Educate the patient about the combined role of genetics and environment.
7. Avoid medications that promote dependence.
8. Encourage participation in psychotherapy.
9. Stay involved in the patient's care, even if referral to a specialist is made.
10. Arrange residential treatment when appropriate, particularly for patients with multiple relapses.
11. Consider legally mandated treatment in severe cases.
12. Expect relapses.
13. Consider trials of pharmacotherapy (e.g., disulfiram or naltrexone to help prevent relapse in alcoholism; antidepressants for alcoholic or nicotine-dependent patients).
14. Educate the patient about physical and developmental effects in children (e.g., fetal alcohol syndrome, problems with school and social role performance).

Socioeconomic Status

Although lower socioeconomic status has been implicated in the development of substance abuse, research confirms that more alcohol is used among the affluent, who can afford it. Yet alcoholism and other substance abuse problems are prevalent among homeless women, and they occur in at least half the female criminal population.

Minorities

Minority women, who often are unable to fulfill their life's ambitions and goals, may be at particular risk for excessive drinking. Cultural factors must be taken into account in integrated treatment planning. For example, African-Americans tend to turn to extended family networks and church organizations in times of crisis. Distrusting institutional medicine, African-Americans who return to their church or who reaffirm spiritual values are likely to increase their chances of treatment success (Aponte, 1996; Harris-Offutt, 1992). African-Americans may be motivated to stop smoking to "free themselves of addiction encouraged by tobacco companies" (Manley, 1996, p. 172).

People of Hispanic heritage constitute the fastest growing minority group in the United States, representing approximately 9% of the population. As Hispanics have become more acculturated, their drinking patterns have shifted from complete abstinence or socially controlled drinking at celebrations to more prevalent, and potentially abusive, consumption. Hispanic women who drink to excess tend to be American-born, middle-aged, economically middle class, and better educated than prior generations. Frequently, those who suffer a loss of social support as their cultural roots are cut off become more frequent and heavier users (Liepman et al., 1993).

Substance abuse and its consequences constitute the foremost health problem facing Native Americans. Symptomatic of a myriad of social problems confronting these cultures, alcohol-associated mortality rates are higher among Native Americans than among the overall U.S. population. Patterns of substance use differ between male and female Native Americans, but drinking appears to be increasing among the younger generation in general.

Surveys indicate that a majority of Native American women drink socially but a significant minority are heavy drinkers. Native American women are particularly affected by husbands who drink heavily; they have fewer social and economic resources than other groups to deal effectively with the illness. Perhaps foreshadowing an increased pattern of substance abuse to come, some of the most frequently reported predictors of dependency and abuse are found in the Native American population. These include boredom, low self-esteem, economic deprivation, social discrimination, and political marginalization (Liepman et al., 1993).

The Elderly

Substance abuse and tobacco use frequently remain unrecognized and inadequately treated among the elderly, in whom they diminish the overall quality of life. Clinicians must inform patients that quitting smoking and cutting down on other addictive substances can increase both the length and quality of life. The initial interview should include routine questions about past and present tobacco, alcohol, and prescription drug use (Goldstein et al., 1996). Elderly patients rely on prescribed medications to cope with physical aches and pains. Older people receive a disproportionately large number of prescriptions for psychoactive drugs from their physicians, which contributes to their increased incidence of addiction. Potential problems include the risk of adverse effects among drugs, including alcohol. The increased sensitivity to drugs, changes in drug metabolism, and social consequences of living alone or within a society that frankly discriminates against the aged appear to place the older woman at a higher risk for a substance problem (Greenfield, 1996).

Alcohol abuse appears to be less common among the elderly than the general population, but the statistics may actually be deflated. Consequences of heavy drinking that bring younger women to the attention of professionals (e.g., car accidents, driving under the influence citations) are underreported in the elderly and may occur less frequently. Many elderly persons stop driving but are at greater risk for solitary drinking because they are more isolated. Drinking alone is particularly dangerous and is quite common in women as a group.

The elderly are also prone to take medications that interact. Even modest consumption of alcohol, benzodiazepines, or narcotic preparations can be hazardous for an older person with impaired metabolism, diminished excretion, or chronic illness (Hall, 1994). Hospitalization for detoxification is usually indicated, because elderly persons have longer and more severe withdrawal reactions (Goldstein et al., 1996). To engage the patient in the long term, clinicians must address denial within the context of a supportive environment.

Athletes

As female athletes have enjoyed greater recognition and success, they have faced added pressures to achieve. Substance misuse has increased among athletes who attempt to compete despite an injury with the help of pain killers. Continual use of prescription narcotics for pain leads to addiction. Women athletes are also requesting more prescriptions of exogenous steroids to aid in body building. Physicians must discourage athletes, their coaches, and their trainers from these destructive practices. Athletes, like young women in general, may also turn to drugs for recreational purposes or to relax after competitions.

The clinician must be alert to the special concerns of athletes who may request stimulants to enhance performance, to aid in weight loss, or to participate in an event despite substantial pain. Good clinical care demands that unhealthy use of these drugs be discouraged. Remind the patient that ultimately her performance will be compromised. These patients benefit from sound clinical advice and positive role modeling from non-substance-using athletes.

Lesbians

Early studies reported a higher prevalence (30%) of alcohol abuse among homosexual than among heterosexual women (Wilsnack, 1995). An objective basis for this discrepancy has not been borne out in the scientific literature; empiric information about any increased substance abuse is contradictory. Although some studies indicate a twofold increase among lesbians, other research reveals no difference in the pattern of substance use between homosexual and heterosexual women. Nevertheless, the clinician should be alert to those risk factors in the homosexual patient that may increase her tendency to misuse substances (see Chapter 13). These include low self-esteem, depression, a history of physical or sexual abuse or violence, and a partner with a substance abuse problem (Wilsnack, 1995).

LONG-TERM SOCIAL CONSEQUENCES OF ADDICTION

Women with addictive disorders have a high mortality rate. Fifteen percent of women who attempt suicide have an alcohol-related problem. Alcoholic liver disease, accident, injury, and trauma are the usual causes of death; tobacco use significantly increases mortality in the substance-using population (Hurt et al., 1996). The most frequently reported social problems are driving while intoxicated, violence toward a spouse, household disruption, and inability to parent properly. Chronic substance use appears to be associated with an increased risk of violent death; the risk of homicide is increased for non-substance-abusing persons living in households where someone actively abuses alcohol or drugs (Rivara et al., 1997)

One of the "hidden costs" of long-term alcohol abuse that is hard to measure in concrete economic terms is its impact on children. The parent who is unable to consistently care for her children presents society with a formidable problem: These children often are left with awesome responsibilities that they cannot adequately handle and lack of the family or social supports that are necessary to produce healthy adults.

SPECIAL ISSUES IN THE CHILDBEARING POPULATION

The childbearing population includes women who are not yet pregnant, pregnant women, and women who have recently delivered. Although prenatal addiction to drugs (especially cocaine) has received inordinate media attention, use of any psychoactive substance during pregnancy is cause for concern because safety has not been established (Raskin, 1997).

The teratogenic potential of all drugs—including cigarettes, alcohol, and cocaine—must be explained to women of childbearing age as a primary preventive measure. Review with your patient in a general way the known cognitive, emotional, and behavioral problems of infants exposed prenatally to low or moderate doses of psychoactive substances. Encourage abstinence if the woman wants to become pregnant.

Clinicians who emphasize the biologic risks of perinatal addiction may err by neglecting the psychosocial factors and psychiatric morbidities that affect the woman and her baby. Pregnancy provides a unique, potentially positive time to involve an addicted woman in treatment, and many patients do avoid using substances "to care for the baby." Do not neglect the special vulnerabilities of the postpartum period. Relapse is highest when psychosocial stress is high;

sometimes providing support to the woman's spouse or partner during pregnancy or in the postpartum period is essential (Raskin, 1997). The partner then can nurture the woman, minimizing those stressors that fuel addiction.

As a general rule, clinicians are advised to discuss the benefits of abstinence for the woman—not just for her child or children. In the rush to be helpful to children, the clinician may identify with concerns for the children and may appear solely concerned about their welfare. The woman may then feel neglected, irritated, or narcissistically wounded. Suggest how she can take steps forward for her own growth by involving herself in treatment. This approach enables her to feel cared for as an individual and fosters her chances of achieving abstinence. In essence, you are telling the woman that her needs matter. This approach is one that is probably neglected by others in her life, including her own parents or support system. Treatment that focuses on having a healthy baby is "incomplete"—and likely to fail—because it

> carries two risks: disenfranchisement of the mother . . . and high relapse rates after childbirth . . . . Clinicians must be aware of the almost universal socialization regarding maternal sacrifice and the idealization of motherhood that we share with our addicted pregnant patients. We must challenge our patients to develop genuine internal motivation for recovery.
>
> (Raskin, 1997, p. 301)

Fetal Alcohol Syndrome

Alcoholism is the cause of multiple birth defects. It has been associated with mental retardation, Down's syndrome, and spina bifida. Alcohol causes reduced somatic growth, morphologic abnormalities (including the characteristic facial dysmorphology), and generalized central nervous system impairment (Little and Wendt, 1993). Fortunately, the full fetal alcohol syndrome (FAS) is rare and results only after very heavy drinking by the mother.

Still, women tend to feel very guilty and blame themselves for any problem affecting their child. Reassurance from the caregiver is essential, lest the patient sabotage her chances for sobriety out of guilt.

While stressing the sequelae of alcoholism and drugs of abuse to your patient, emphasize that research demonstrates that effects are greatest when chemicals are used in the first trimester or in the weeks before delivery. It is not yet known whether women can drink safely at all during pregnancy, but conservative practice indicates abstinence should the patient wish to conceive.

The ways in which alcohol affects the fetus may be influenced by race or ethnic origin and socioeconomic status. Native Americans have the highest rate of FAS. African-Americans have a rate six times higher than that of Caucasians. These discrepant rates have only lately been noted in the scientific literature; the reason for them is unknown. However, the children of poor women do appear to be at higher risk of fetal alcohol effects than those of middle-class women, indicating that socioeconomic status plays a significant role in expression.

NICOTINE ADDICTION

The number of women smokers has undergone a steep upward climb over the past two decades. Adolescent females are the fastest growing group of new smokers, and women smokers may soon outnumber men smokers. A higher percentage of African-American than Caucasian women smoke, and they tend to experience greater health consequences, including higher rates of cardiovascular disease, pregnancy complications, infant mortality, and low birth weight.

Just as in the other addictions, women often have less knowledge than men about the consequences of smoking. Health care practitioners must place greater emphasis on educating women about these risks. Even though more people are aware that they are endangering their health, surveys show that the clinician's advice is the main reason people stop smoking (Hajik, 1996; Manley, 1996). Don't underestimate your potential to help by monitoring progress and encouraging the patient to quit. But be aware that the foe is a formidable one. Heavy users of heroin and cocaine report that it is easier to give up those drugs than to stop smoking.

On average, men tend to smoke more cigarettes than women, but nicotine is more rapidly cleared by a man's kidneys. Therefore, men and women receive approximately equivalent amounts of nicotine despite the heavier smoking by men (Mermelstein and Borrelli, 1995).

Nicotine has significant effects on food consumption and body weight (Manley, 1996; Ockene and Kristeller, 1995). Smokers weigh 6 to 8 pounds less than nonsmokers. Women who want to stop smoking are sensitive to the possibility of gaining weight in our body-conscious society (see Chapter 5), and weight gained after the cessation of smoking has a greater effect on them than it does on men. Many women anecdotally tell of gaining much more than the average 8 pounds. Little wonder, then, that women smokers frequently cite the possibility of weight gain as a major deterrent to stopping smoking.

When nicotine is withdrawn, other gender differences become apparent. Women are more likely to experience craving for cigarettes than men, but men suffer from more physical side effects. The menstrual cycle appears to bear on the success of withdrawal and continued abstinence. Women who have premenstrual dysphoria experience more severe nicotine withdrawal (Greenfield, 1996).

Smoking affects the metabolism of drugs in women (Greenfield, 1996); they respond preferentially to certain pharmacologic agents in stopping smoking. Whereas nicotine gum has been shown to have a more beneficial effect in men, clonidine (Catapres) appears to be more beneficial in women.

Women appear to benefit from social supports and the encouragement of their significant others when they attempt to quit. Interventions that target the prevention of depression and have a standard smoking cessation component are more likely to succeed in the woman patient with a mood disorder (Hajik, 1996; Hall et al., 1994).

Women, Depression, and Nicotine Addiction

Women have a harder time quitting smoking because of their higher rate of depression. Eighty percent of women with a history of major depression are or have been tobacco addicts. Sometimes depression leads to nicotine dependence as a kind of self-medication for early mood changes. But depression and nicotine dependence also appear to be linked genetically. Twin studies suggest that a high rate of either depression or nicotine use predicts a high rate of the other

(Borrelli et al., 1996; Ferguson et al., 1996; Mermelstein and Borrelli, 1995; Stage et al., 1996).

Considerations for Treatment of Nicotine Dependence

1. Refrain from taking a "one size fits all" (DuPont, 1995) approach to the woman who is nicotine addicted. As in the treatment of all addictions, research has shown that physicians play a crucial role in helping patients to stop smoking simply by mentioning its negative health consequences (Fleming et al., 1997; Mermelstein and Borrelli, 1995). To quit, all some women need is your prompting and inducement. A follow-up visit or call from you or your care extender may be a positive motivating force.
2. Assess the patient for any history of depression. Depressed patients require more physician involvement. Your ongoing support and encouragement cannot be overestimated in helping a woman deal with the dual problem of nicotine addiction and mood disorder.
3. Direct the patient to seek more adequate coping methods and life-affirming activities in dealing with life's inevitable imperfections and problems. Of all types of treatment, cognitive-behavioral methods to stop smoking have been tested and found to work best. The most successful quitters appear to have the greatest number of strategies and relapse prevention skills to influence them during times when they are tempted to start smoking again (Farquhar and Spillar, 1990; Ockene and Kristeller, 1995).
4. Remember that women worry about gaining weight if they stop smoking. Research bears out that these fears are warranted. Suggest ways of reducing tension that also aid weight control. For example, increasing the amount of exercise to three 30- to 40-minute periods per week counters the metabolic effects of stopping smoking while promoting overall well-being. The tendency to gain weight after quitting is minimized.

   In reality, it is difficult to reassure a woman that any weight gain is acceptable in our appearance-conscious, externally focused society. Still, efforts can be made to help the patient counter stereotypic social norms regarding appearance. Remind her that smoking is a much greater risk to health than is the gaining of a few extra pounds.
5. Suggest ways of meeting oral needs (e.g., chewing gum) that do not include eating more food. One professional woman kept a pack of cloves available whenever she was tempted to light up. This noncaloric spice replaced her craving for menthol. She also bought a pair of "oriental clanging balls" that she clasped in her hands while making calls to her clients. She joked with her physician that these "power tools" helped her deal with obstreperous customers. Previously, she would have relied on a cigarette.
6. Offer pharmacologic support. Nicotine replacement therapy relieves withdrawal symptoms and cravings while the patient learns cognitive and behavioral techniques to help her stop smoking. Compared with cigarettes, the nicotine delivery system offers a lower, slower rate of dispersal. The four available modalities (gum, skin patch, nasal spray, and inhaler) can be purchased over the counter at a price about equal to the cost of cigarettes (Manley, 1996; Ockene and Kristeller, 1995).

The antihypertensive clonidine is used to ease several kinds of drug withdrawal. It has been found to be effective in promoting cessation of smoking in women (Greenfield, 1996). Serotonin-enhancing substances (e.g., fluoxetine, tryptophan) may also be selectively beneficial because of their ability to help prevent depressed mood and weight gain (Mermelstein and Borrelli, 1995). Bupropion (Wellbutrin SR sustained-release formula; Zyban) has been approved by the U.S. Food and Drug Administration as an adjunct therapy in smoking cessation. It is reported to reduce withdrawal symptoms and decrease the urge to smoke.

7. Address the need for inner soothing that smokers must confront if they want to stop. Treatment with an antidepressant may be considered for the woman with a history of depression or current depression. More research must be done to support the links among smoking, depression, and stress reduction; in the meantime, discuss with patients how they may be using smoking as a coping strategy. If you choose to prescribe Zyban, be sure that the patient is *not* taking another antidepressant. Toxicity could result.

8. Be sensitive to the fact that changes reported during phases of the patient's menstrual cycle are real, not signs of malingering or hysteria. When a woman has significant premenstrual symptoms, nicotine withdrawal symptoms may become more intense (Greenfield, 1996; Mello et al., 1989; Mermelstein and Borrelli, 1995). At this time, she may need more pharmacologic support to manage her withdrawal. Advise women to try to stop smoking early in their cycle. They are then less likely to experience the discomfort, malaise, and irritability of their premenstrual symptomatology.

9. Most importantly, educate female patients from adolescence to maturity about the risks of nicotine addiction, stressing its effects on the smoker's lifetime health and on the health of each family member. Review bona fide risks to the fetus in a mother who smokes (e.g., miscarriage, low birth weight). Stress that newborns of women who smoke have a slightly delayed development, a higher rate of attention deficit disorder, and an increased likelihood of developing asthma and other respiratory problems.

10. Underscore that *smoking is responsible for many more deaths than all forms of drug abuse combined* and that smoking diminishes one's overall quality of life.

PATIENT GUIDELINES FOR COPING WITH SUBSTANCE USE PROBLEMS

Acknowledge Your Addiction

1. Denial and dishonesty are hallmarks of addiction. Denial affects not only you but also all those around you. Addiction does not cure itself. It will worsen until it is treated, taking a heavy toll on you and those you love.

2. Remember that patterns of substance abuse are complicated and individually variable. Negative consequences often go unrecognized because not all women who misuse substances do so uncontrollably or all the time. Yet the problem is still real. If you find that you are concealing, rationalizing, or blaming others for your problem, the time to get help is *now*.

3. Learn all you can about addiction. Some of the books recommended at the end of this chapter will teach you how others have mastered their addiction problems. By reading and learning, you are networking with other men and women who have traveled similar paths and can provide excellent feedback and insight to support you in overcoming addiction. In essence, their testimonials say, "It *can* be done, and *you* can do it."

4. Recognize the considerable consequences of substance abuse. They include marital and relationship conflicts, legal problems, dangerous driving and accidents, job losses, emotional and physical illnesses, and family arguments and violence. Actual dependence involves additional symptoms, including drug tolerance and withdrawal reactions when you are away from your drug of choice. You may have made several attempts to cut down or stop; but you continue drinking or using substances despite their serious health effects. Gradually, preoccupation with the substance takes up so much of your time and life that nothing else seems to matter.

Look for Support in Numbers

1. The mutual aid groups of Alcoholics Anonymous (AA), Narcotics Anonymous (NA), and Women for Sobriety (WFS) are the most time tested and reliable ways to begin recovery from addiction to alcohol and other drugs (DuPont, 1997a; DuPont and McGovern, 1994; Kirkpatrick, 1977/1990; Knapp, 1996). Many people mistakenly believe that these groups are religious in orientation. Although you will be asked to admit that you are powerless over your drug of choice and need help from your Higher Power, and you will be urged to pray or meditate while taking a "full inventory" of yourself, such groups embrace no particular religious practice or faith. You will benefit greatly by being honest about your problems with others. You will also learn helpful skills and receive support from others who are recovering. These groups are free and are available in almost all communities, 7 days a week, 24 hours a day.

2. Recognize that you have special needs and issues as a woman that must be addressed in treatment. Some AA fellowships are for women only, as is WFS. Some women who must be hospitalized or must enter residential treatment prefer a program serving only recovering women.

   Although scientific evidence is lacking about the benefits and limitations of programs tailored just to women, some patients find them helpful because they focus on women's unique struggles in maintaining relationships and raising children; they offer opportunities for support and strength from other women. The need to affiliate with women can also be met by having women caregivers (e.g., chemical dependency counselor, psychotherapist, AA sponsor).

3. Seek positive role models, especially those who have overcome an addiction themselves. These individuals will be able to help you with any stigma you may face because of addiction, receiving treatment, or dealing with your multiple roles as a woman. The key point is to *find those groups or individuals who can help you to improve your self-worth and to create positive, life-affirming relationships. Growth of self-esteem is the foundation for solid recovery.*

Make Use of New, Available Medications

1. Seek your doctor's advice concerning medications to help recovering patients. Learn all you can about them. Pharmacists have excellent literature, or you can call your local library, mental health association, or women's treatment cooperative. This material is usually free.

   Disulfiram (Antabuse) helps protect against relapse by blocking the normal metabolism of alcohol. Naltrexone, used for years in the treatment of heroin addiction, was approved in 1995 to prevent alcohol relapse. Alcoholics who take naltrexone feel less craving, drink less, and are less likely to lose control of their drinking.

   Some studies have shown that tricyclic antidepressants and selective serotonin reuptake inhibitors help alcoholics to cut down on their alcohol intake and alleviate depression. These drugs can be helpful also to smokers who want to quit. Methadone is only one of a host of drugs now available to help during opiate withdrawal. Your physician can help you determine the most effective medication from this rapidly expanding group of new possibilities. The choice of medication depends on the particular substance or substances you have struggled with.

2. Although these medications can help you comply with substance abuse treatment, they are not "magic bullets." Research has shown that patients who receive psychotherapy, increase their coping skills, and put into place a relapse prevention program are the most likely to successfully recover from a serious addiction. To get well, you must change a dangerous habit that has become part of your identity. Determine those times when you are most vulnerable to stress, deal with your guilt and shame about abuse, and—by all means—work on your self-concept.

Develop a Relapse Prevention Program—But Keep It Simple

1. About 40% to 50% of patients with substance abuse problems have mild to moderate cognitive problems while actively using. These cognitive problems usually get better with long-term abstinence. However, at the beginning of treatment, you will want to keep your treatment plan simple because you are not "running on full power." Be sure to review instructions with your health care team. Use notebooks and write yourself memos.

2. Take advantage of cognitive-behavioral psychotherapy to increase coping skills. Probably everyone—not just patients with substance abuse problems—can benefit from social skills training and methods for handling stress. You will also benefit from practicing how to manage social situations without substances. What cognitive-behavioral therapy does is teach you how to refuse drinks politely and how to monitor and deal with your own feelings. You also learn a number of problem-solving strategies so that you can take charge of your life and weather its ups and downs.

3. Work with your counselor or psychotherapist on specific techniques you can use to develop an individual relapse prevention program. You may decide to keep a diary to identify those skills you now have and those you want to develop further. Write down what situations you find the most challenging.

4. Become a member of a relapse prevention group. These groups give you the opportunity to rehearse stressful situations. Rehearsal lets you anticipate conflictual situations and find ways to deal with whatever problems are likely to arise. These groups also provide role models (in the form of counselors and other recovering people) to help you make necessary life changes.
5. Learn what "drives" your addiction. Psychotherapy is one tool to help you effectively master the issues that perpetuate your turning to substances as a "friend" or coping mechanism. Recovering women need to deal with interpersonal issues (e.g., what constitutes a healthy, supportive relationship), social issues (e.g., domestic violence, history of childhood sexual abuse), and feelings of self-esteem. Addressing these psychosocial concerns must be part of both your ongoing treatment and any solid relapse prevention program.

Know the Risks Associated with Pregnancy and Parenting

1. Women with alcohol and drug problems have a higher risk of fetal abnormalities when they actively use during the first trimester. It is advisable to stop altogether, or at least reduce, your use of alcohol, tobacco, or any nonprescribed or illicit substance during pregnancy or when you are trying to become pregnant. Because most women worry about possible injury to their babies, many are able to cut down or even completely stop if they choose to have children.
2. If you decide to become pregnant, that may be a prime time to enter a formal treatment program. However, do it for yourself, not just "for the baby" (North, 1996).
3. Recognize that the postpartum period is a time of high risk of relapse for recovering substance abusers. Fatigue, "baby blues," and the time and energy required to care for a newborn all take their toll on a mother. Yet this time can also be gratifying and give your life a sense of meaning and purpose. Be sure to seek out extra support. Some treatment programs now offer childcare for recovering women. This resource can be an essential support and can help you to take advantage of your treatment program.
4. Remember, the best care you can give your child as a parent is to take care of yourself. Without renewed energy and complete sobriety, you will not be able to be the loving, mature parent you want to be.

Decide to Stay Abstinent

1. Most authorities believe that the most appropriate long-term goal for treatment of substance abuse is lifelong abstinence. With respect to problem drinking, this issue has generated a great deal of controversy (Vaillant, 1996). Although some problem drinkers are able to moderate their drinking, available evidence indicates that total abstinence is preferable. Most professionals consider controlled drinking possible only in milder cases of alcohol abuse (Valliant, 1996).
2. If you decide that you can cut back without abstaining, be sure to discuss the pros and cons of this decision with your health care team. Be honest with

them about your choice of direction. There are some cognitive-behavioral programs devoted to helping women reduce their drinking through short-term counseling. Referral to one of these programs may aid you in your decision regarding abstinence versus moderate drinking.

Never Give Up

1. Stay optimistic about the long-term results of treatment. In the beginning you may feel overwhelmed and defeated. This is your disease speaking, not the real you. As you get better, your self-worth improves and you gain more strength to take on the day-to-day battles.
2. Take solace in the number of research studies emerging in the medical literature that indicate good results for the treatment of addictions. However, improvement appears strongest with long-term treatment. So stay involved in your 12-step program, remain connected to your physician and health care team, and take advantage of psychotherapy. It, too, has been shown to be of real benefit for the recovering woman.

ADDITIONAL GUIDELINES FOR PRIMARY CARE CLINICIANS

Screen for Alcohol and Drug Abuse in Your Practice

1. Keep an open eye and an open ear for substance use problems, because they so frequently are unrecognized. Even brief interventions in primary medical settings have been shown to be surprisingly effective (Barnes and Bor, 1996; McCrady and Lagenbucher, 1996; Parish, 1997).
2. Talk to the patient's partner, spouse, and adult children. Be direct with your patient: "Do you have any objection if I speak with your spouse about your problem?" You may find that family members are themselves unaware (Blume et al., 1992; Wilsnack and Beckman, 1980) or deny the extent of the illness. Some spouses may be comfortable with the status quo (the so-called codependency problem). They may be reluctant to give up "the roller coaster ride of life with a female alcoholic" (Cirillo, 1996).
3. Confront denial. It is still the primary obstacle to receiving treatment. The primary care clinician who identifies the problem and empathically acknowledges it to the patient and her family is providing the crucial first step to recovery. Offer needed education and make treatment recommendations.

Refer Your Patient to Self-Help Fellowships

1. Encourage participation in 12-step fellowships such as AA, NA, and WFS. Overwhelming research shows that involvement in this kind of support group is the most effective tool in countering addiction. Although some people do get better without them, most do not do well without taking advantage of the advice and sponsorships offered by these free resources (DuPont and McGovern, 1994; McLellan et al., 1993).

2. Stay vigilant about the stressors on the family. There are groups such as Al-Anon for partners or Alateen for children and adolescents. Most professionals are not aware that Alateen is a fellowship of teenagers affected by a relative's alcoholism and not a group for adolescents seeking help for their own problems with alcohol (DuPont, 1997a; Miller, 1997). Don't stop encouraging participation in these supportive venues—even if the family member does not take your suggestion at first.
3. Attend several open meetings in your local community to fully understand how the 12-step fellowship process works. You will meet members of AA, NA, or WFS who are willing to serve as sponsors for patients. Providing names, telephone numbers, and access to a telephone in the office are concrete ways to introduce patients to these fellowships. Sometimes dialing the number yourself makes a powerful statement to the patient or family member. It also reinforces how serious you are about the problem and your willingness to be involved in treatment.

Support the Patient's Need to Learn from Other Women

1. Women appear to have a special need to affiliate with other women in treatment. Women-only AA and NA meetings have proliferated in some communities, WFS is also popular; this group offers additional tools for building self-esteem, a boon for many female patients entering a recovery process (Kirkpatrick, 1977/1990; Moyar, 1987; Stammer, 1991).

   WFS promotes the development of a positive identity without substances by suggesting self-affirmation, meditation, sound nutrition, and tools to increase self-confidence and self-responsibility. About 80% of WFS members also attend AA, but some women find the WFS sessions especially supportive, intimate, and life-enhancing (Kirkpatrick, 1977/1990).
2. Some women who misuse substances find it particularly helpful to work with a female therapist or female substance abuse counselor who is herself a recovering person. Female affiliations of this kind may offer women the healthy role modeling that is essential to an alcohol-free lifestyle (Moyar, 1987; Peluso and Peluso, 1988).

Recommend Family Therapy

1. Enhanced strategies for dealing with conflict in the patient's family are essential to recovery. Attaining and maintaining sobriety requires a shift in the entire family system. Skilled family therapy helps your patient's partner to provide much-needed support and to recognize his or her role in the addiction cycle (Bepko, 1991; Blume, 1986; Wilsnack, 1995).
2. Stress that *substance abuse is a disease the entire family must conquer.* Family members also need encouragement to face their own struggles, including those related to misuse of substances. Without addressing the salient family issues, the entire treatment process is likely to flounder.

Advocate Participation in an Individual Psychotherapy Process

1. Get to know those therapists in your community who have expertise in addiction treatment and enjoy working with this patient group. Although the specific role that psychotherapy plays with patients who abuse addictive substances has long been controversial, new data suggest that improvement is more robust when psychotherapy is also employed. Treatment that is longer term appears to be highly efficacious and cost-effective (Dodes, 1988; Khantzian, 1995; McLellan et al., 1993; Unumb, 1992; Woody et al., 1995; Wurmser, 1992).

2. There has also been great controversy about what constitutes appropriate, pragmatic psychotherapy. Psychotherapy helps the addicted patient by (1) identifying relationship problems, (2) finding alternative modes of problem solving, and (3) increasing comfort in discussing personal experiences and identifying feelings that foster intimate relationships (DuPont, 1997b; Levin, 1995). Remind third-party payers when you intercede for the patient that research has demonstrated the cost-effectiveness of psychotherapeutic approaches; this tactic helps ensure that your patient receives adequate compensated services (Anthony et al., 1995; Crits-Cristoph and Sigueland, 1996; Hall et al., 1994).

3. Educate your patient, her family, and third parties about the rationales for recommending therapy. Underscore that psychotherapy of the addicted person provides time, active interest and concern, and nonjudgmental positive regard. A therapeutic relationship is built to sustain the addicted person in times of despair. In order to give up their addiction and stay sober, people who use drugs as companions must develop a "capacity to be alone" (Levin, 1995; Winnicott, 1965).

   Although the chemical gives the illusion of being good company or of having a friend (see Knapp, 1996; Stammer, 1991), it actually precludes development of mature interpersonal relationships. Therapy explores why a particular person has difficulty being alone and how to build a sense of identity without turning to substances.

4. Remind your patients that working in psychotherapy is difficult. It takes time, energy, money, and commitment. Sometimes a person becomes depressed as she works on core issues. Those patients who are able to achieve sobriety must mourn the loss of the chemical as their primary companion, address the inner pain that the substance temporarily but inadequately anesthetized, and confront a magical fantasy that the substance gives them ultimate love, power, and the desires of the heart.

   A sense of failure is pervasive and must be overcome to counter the narcissistic insults of career setback, rejection, and humiliation. Psychotherapy works by replacing the drug with

   > something that does the job better—relationship . . . . The long-term goal must be the internalization of psychic structure, that is, acquiring the abilities to self-soothe, modulate and maintain a reasonably high level of self-esteem, tolerate affects, and feel securely cohesive, enduring, and capable of initiative (Levin, 1995, p. 206).

Clearly, goals of developing a firm sense of identity and becoming less vulnerable to aloneness and narcissistic injury cannot be achieved in one or two sessions.

5. Expect slips to occur. Keep an attitude of interest and belief that sobriety can be achieved as emotional pain becomes endurable (Levin, 1995). The patient will turn to you for encouragement. Tell her that, over the long run, sobriety will be easier and more rewarding because she will be living up to her ideals. This will build self-esteem and increase a sense of personal comfort. Remind the patient and third parties that those who receive psychotherapy have greater earning power, less income from welfare, and strikingly lower hospital admission rates than those who do not—all indications of the greater cost-effectiveness of psychotherapy. It benefits both the patient and society for the patient to stay involved in treatment (Crits-Cristoph and Sigueland, 1996; Lisansky Gomberg and Nirenberg, 1993).

6. Psychotherapy also helps addicted people cope with emotional needs that are separate from their addiction. One must understand that the disease of addiction is a disease of the entire self that has spiritual and existential dimensions. Addicted women can recover and can have "a good life, but to do so they must stay sober and have sound values based on humility, persistence, honesty, and resilience" (DuPont, 1997b, p. 374).

Use the New Pharmacologic Agents

There are now four primary categories of drugs used to control alcohol consumption: adversive agents, opioid antagonists, serotonergic agents, and TCAs. In general, pharmacologic therapeutic approaches have shifted from the primary use of adversive or deterrent agents, such as disulfiram, to that of opioid antagonists and groups of drugs employed in the treatment of depression (Meza and Kranzler, 1996).

1. Adversive Agents

   Although the research literature on the efficacy of disulfiram in women is not robust, it should be considered in the patient with severe alcoholism who has multiple relapses. The usual daily dose of Antabuse is 125 to 150 mg. Although it is never recommended as the sole treatment, it can be an important aspect of a comprehensive program for some women. If you employ this agent in your practice, be sure to remind your patient that even the small amounts of alcohol in perfume or mouthwash may precipitate adverse reactions (Frances and Franklin, 1989; Meza and Kranzler, 1996; Miller, 1997).

2. Opioid Antagonists

   Opioid antagonists reduce the risk of relapse to heavy drinking in alcohol-dependent patients (O'Malley, 1995; O'Malley et al., 1996). They modulate alcohol's positive reinforcing effect by blocking endogenous opioids in the nucleus accumbens region of the mesolimbic dopamine system. In essence, the clinical usefulness of the opioid antagonists comes from blocking the apparent "priming" effect of the initial drink, reducing alcohol craving, and reinforcing properties of the drug.

   Naltrexone (ReVia, oral dose 50 mg/day) reduces the rate of alcohol relapse by delaying the time of consumption of the first drink after detoxification.

This also reduces the reinforcing effects of alcohol (Volpicelli et al., 1995). It is of greatest benefit when combined with supportive therapy, relapse prevention skills training, and education to increase coping; drinking frequency appears to become attenuated with use (O'Malley et al., 1992; Volpicelli et al., 1992, 1995a,b).

Although naltrexone provides patients with a good start in their recovery, the optimum duration of treatment is unknown. Findings suggest that patients benefit from longer treatment than the 12-week duration employed in the initial research studies.

Possessing few side effects, naltrexone has been shown to be a safe drug in those groups in which it has been tested. Most studies have been done in male populations, so that direct application to female alcoholics remains unknown. According to some studies, the effects of naltrexone may last for several months, even after the patient stops taking it. Apparently, those patients who do take it regularly feel less craving, drink less, and are less likely to lose control if they take a drink (O'Malley et al., 1996). If you use it in your practice, be sure to stress to patients that studies indicate *better treatment outcomes when it is administered within the context of psychosocial interventions* (O'Malley, 1995; O'Malley et al., 1992; Volpicelli et al., 1992, 1995a,b).

3. Serotonergic Agents

Almost 800,000 women alcoholics suffer from clinical depression (Mason et al., 1996). Failure to treat depressed alcoholics with an appropriate medication is not simply benign neglect but also can contribute to a drinking relapse in patients trying to maintain abstinence. Research has consistently shown that serotonin (5-HT) plays an important role in alcohol consumption behavior and alcoholism.

The SSRIs produce modest decreases in alcohol consumption, even in the absence of depression. Fluoxetine (20 to 40 mg per day) has been found to reduce depressive symptoms and alcohol consumption in some studies of alcoholics. Buspirone, a 5-HT 1A agonist, also appears to be useful as an adjunct in the treatment of anxious alcoholics. It tends to enhance the patient's capacity to stay in treatment by decreasing anxiety and risk of relapse (Kosten and McCance-Katz, 1995; Meza and Kranzler, 1996).

4. Tricyclic antidepressants

Both imipramine and desipramine have been found useful in reducing depressive symptoms and relapse to heavy drinking. Some persons are able to maintain longer periods of abstinence and have enhanced psychosocial functioning with these drugs (Mason et al., 1996; Meza and Kranzler, 1996; Miller, 1997).

Some depressed alcoholics discontinue medication, despite improvement, because of the "medication-free" philosophy of some AA groups. Patients should be counseled about this potential bias and urged to stay on medication. As a preventive measure, the public must be educated about research findings that indicate beneficial effects from state-of-the-art pharmacotherapy as an important adjunct in comprehensive treatment planning for the alcoholic.

Other promising medications for alcoholics are being tested, including the opioid antagonist nalmefene and the European-developed acamprosate.

Employ Pharmacotherapy for Narcotic Addiction

1. Pharmacotherapeutic agents for narcotic addiction that may have advantages over methadone are naltrexone, *l*-alpha-acetylmethadol (LAAM, a longer-acting opioid than methadone), and buprenorphine (Buprenex). Clonidine, a nonopioid, alpha$_2$-adrenergic agonist, reduces the discomfort of withdrawal. It appears to increase tolerance for the unpleasant physiologic effects of the withdrawal syndrome (Kosten and McCance-Katz, 1995). Agents that affect dopaminergic transmission (e.g., amantadine, bromocriptine, L-dopa, bupropion) have been employed with limited success for acute treatment of cocaine withdrawal. Bupropion, an antidepressant that affects dopaminergic transmission, has been given with some success for treatment of cocaine addiction.
2. Primary care clinicians are referred to specific texts for the dosing schedules of these compounds (Miller, 1997). In all likelihood, new agents for the treatment of addictions will continue to evolve quickly as the biologic determinants of vulnerability to substance abuse become further elucidated. Combating drug abuse can be accomplished only when one understands the great variability that exists among individual patients. Specifically, further evaluation is required of the reasons that some women succumb to addiction after an initial exposure whereas others appear able to use highly addictive substances for recreation without developing dependence.

Understand the Limitations of Pharmacotherapy

1. Employ pharmacotherapy only within the context of a comprehensive treatment program. If using psychotropic medication, the clinician should refer patients to self-help groups and psychotherapists who support the use of appropriate pharmacotherapy. Because some 12-step fellowships advocate a medication-free philosophy, patients who would otherwise be helped may discontinue medication (Mason et al., 1996). Emphasize the recognized benefits of concomitant use of psychotherapy, pharmacotherapy, and 12-step fellowships.
2. Treatment programs that combine medication and psychosocial therapy have better results than medication therapy alone (see O'Malley, 1995; Woody et al., 1995b). In the absence of psychosocial support, medications are relatively ineffective (Blume, 1992; Gordis, 1996; Wallace, 1992). Although they do exert a powerful, positive effect, they are not a magic bullet. Most authorities believe they should not be given without a psychosocial treatment program in place to ensure or enhance compliance.
3. In the substance-abusing patient with comorbid anxiety or depression, psychopharmacology addresses a primary biologic diathesis that enables the patient to be more successful in addressing her problem and attaining sobriety. Such a woman may feel that she is fatally flawed because of her biologic vulnerability. Commending her for her courage in confronting her problems fulfills a crucial psychological need that builds self-esteem within the context of an affirming relationship. The primary care clinician is in an ideal position to be that essential supportive person.

Assess the Need for Residential Treatment, Particularly in Patients with Multiple Relapses

1. Even though resources for inpatient and residential treatment are becoming sparse in an era of managed care, some female alcoholics need to be hospitalized. Although detoxification is increasingly managed on an outpatient basis, acute withdrawal symptoms (anxiety, tachycardia, tremors, nausea, weakness, and sweating) are most conservatively treated on an inpatient basis, using benzodiazepines (e.g., chlordiazepoxide, lorazepam) as a substitute sedative agent (Crits-Cristoph and Sigueland, 1996; Wesson and Ling, 1996). Elderly or medically compromised patients, in particular, may require inpatient care (Goldstein et al., 1996; Liepman et al., 1993).
2. Female alcoholics may need to detach temporarily from household demands; it is difficult for them to put their own needs before the needs of others. Inpatient or residential treatment provides a haven for women in the early phases of recovery. They can then reevaluate priorities, set realistic goals, and begin to deal with life problems without turning to their drug (or drugs) of choice. The professional support provided by 24-hour care, although initially expensive in terms of time and health care dollars, often provides the essential groundwork to begin the painful work of rebuilding the self (Blume, 1986; Hall, 1994; Lex, 1995; McGovern, 1995; Moyar, 1987; Toneatto et al., 1992).

Remember Special Factors Related to Pregnancy

1. Stress the sequelae of alcoholism and drug abuse, but emphasize that the effects are greatest during the first trimester or in the weeks just before delivery. Research has yet to prove that drinking during pregnancy is safe, and not drinking is best for those patients wishing to conceive.
2. The postpartum period is an especially vulnerable time for relapse. Encourage psychosocial supports and emphasize that the patient's partner, who is also going through a time of change, must still reach out to support her. Both parents should participate in activities they find helpful and supportive.

SUMMARY

Primary care physicians are increasingly called upon to provide the first line of intervention for persons who misuse substances. This chapter focuses primarily on the distinct problems of alcohol and nicotine dependence, although many of the treatment principles described here can be applied to other addictions.

Considerable evidence demonstrates that women are prone to abuse of multiple substances, concurrently or in alternating fashion. There is also mounting evidence that a number of variables play a role in the origin and maintenance of drug abuse in women. Continued research must be done to identify those differences between men and women that have an impact on substance use and that can affect clinical care.

The ability to recognize the underdiagnosis of substance abuse in women and to be sensitive to their unique needs and problems is critical to treatment success. Although initial detoxification (increasingly done on an outpatient basis) plays an important role after diagnosis, the expanding pharmacopeia available for treatment of these disorders needs to be employed systematically. In particular, opioid antagonists and antidepressants will take on increasing importance in preventing relapse, particularly in alcoholism.

The treatment of women with substance use problems also involves education, family and couples therapy, individual psychotherapy, and psychosocial support. In order to comprehensively treat the female patient, primary clinicians should be aware of, and participate in, self-help groups such as AA, NA, and WFS. Other approaches include engaging the patient, making referrals to specialty care when appropriate, and employing general counseling and pharmacotherapeutic techniques.

It is also crucial to realize that special populations of chemically dependent women may require particular attention (e.g., minorities, elderly). Women who misuse substances are prone to be victims of domestic violence, have a higher incidence of homelessness, and have a greater difficulty parenting. Children born to women who abuse substances are at particular risk; they are subject to a number of developmental and social difficulties. Women who suffer chemical dependency have a range of emotional problems, especially depression, which can further complicate recognition and treatment. The treatment of addictions therefore presents the clinician with many formidable obstacles that can be overcome by increasing one's knowledge base.

Research demonstrates that women must have adequate, long-term support to stay substance free. In this respect, the primary care clinician who stays connected to the patient over a period of years plays a pivotal role in her recovery, especially should a relapse occur.

Finally, to accomplish the societal goal of preventing addiction, the primary clinician must work to combat reluctance (e.g., fear of stigma) on the patient's part about coming forward for treatment. Encouraging abstinence or moderate use in the childbearing population is especially important. Care must be taken to avoid iatrogenic drug dependence and thereby prevent a number of these disorders from taking hold in the first place. Principally, the clinician helps the patient take a more active role in assessing her alcohol and drug use and in recognizing and changing risky behavior. Even brief interventions can be enormously important, having a positive impact on the nation's epidemic public health problem of chemical dependency as well as on the lives of individual women.

Resources for Patients

Farquhar JW, Spiller GA: *The Last Puff: Ex-Smokers Share the Secrets of Their Success.* New York, WW Norton, 1991.
This popular paperback is a collection of more than 30 interviews with women and men who resolved to lick the smoking habit and did so. Unlike self-help manuals that offer guidelines for stopping smoking but are short on personal experience, these firsthand accounts are full of hard-won secrets and helpful suggestions. You cannot read this book without feeling hopeful about the human capacity to overcome serious addiction when the person is determined to do so. The most frequently asked questions of ex-smokers are addressed by the interviewees, including tips about avoiding weight gain (a particularly troublesome concern for women), establishing a realistic relapse prevention plan, and ways of diverting attention when compelled to smoke. These ex-smokers also discuss how life after smoking is indeed different from life before cessation. For example, some people must make a new circle of friends, adding to

reluctance to give up the habit and maintain abstinence. Readers will benefit from the sense of camaraderie conveyed by those who fought the battle with nicotine as they dig into these inspiring, funny, and life-affirming vignettes.

Kirkpatrick J: *Turnabout: New Help for the Woman Alcoholic.* New York, Bantam Books, 1990.

The author is the founder of the self-help fellowship Women for Sobriety. The powerful story of her recovery from alcoholism is a fast but gripping read. Kirkpatrick offers a thoughtful discussion of the special issues and conflicts of the woman alcoholic, making the book applicable to both the general and the professional audience. Helpful, practical advice on maintaining sobriety while developing a sense of personal competence is the cornerstone to overcoming addictive behavior. Kirkpatrick fleshes these steps out by describing her personal struggles, underscoring the wisdom of the "13 statements of acceptance" that are key to the success of the Women for Sobriety groups. Emphasis is placed on practicing new coping skills, overcoming destructive thought patterns and feelings of worthlessness, and striving for increased responsibility and competency in all avenues of a woman's life. Clinicians and support staff will glean additional insight into the particular burdens faced by women alcoholics, including specific patterns of abuse, interpersonal relationship struggles, and impaired self-esteem.

Knapp C: *Drinking: A Love Story.* New York, Dial Press, 1996.

Destined to become a classic autobiographic portrait of the obsession with alcohol, Knapp's book brilliantly illuminates the passion for drink as the ultimate search for external solutions to life's dilemmas. Viewing the disease as a multilayered, implacable physical and psychological foe, she relates her years of denial of addiction and her eventual engagement in the treatment process. She supplements her own insights with opinions from experts. Patients and clinicians alike will find her story a heart-wrenching tale of a family torn apart by multiple addictions. But embedded in the final chapters are guidelines and hope for recovery. Recognizing that alcoholism is a disease of relapse, Knapp views her sobriety as "less about 'getting better' in a clear linear sense than it is about subjecting yourself to change, to the inevitable ups and downs, fears and feelings, victories and failures, that accompany growth" (p. 235). For Knapp, putting down the bottle meant leaving the "passion, sensual pleasure, deep pools, lust, and fears" of her addiction to wrestle with personal growth and adult choices. Underscoring a point made by experts and buttressed by outcome studies, she credits AA and intensive residential treatment as pivotal points in her sobriety. She relishes her newfound joy in the hard work of living a substance-free life.

McGovern G: *Terry: My Daughter's Life-and-Death Struggle with Alcoholism.* New York, Plume, 1996.

Former Senator George McGovern's best-selling memoir of his daughter's valiant struggle with, and eventual death from, alcoholism is told with insight, compassion, courage, and great love. Particularly valuable for family members who have a loved one struggling with addiction, this book is also a resource for the patient herself. Although the senator's daughter struggled principally with alcohol, his message is applicable to those who deal with any addiction. The importance of the spiritual dimensions undergirding the disease, the need for long-term treatment follow-up, and the requirement of persistent involvement and support from family members are highlights of the book. Substance abuse is viewed as a disease that affects each member of the family, and the crucial needs for unconditional love, group and individual therapy, pharmacotherapy, and 12-step fellowships are viewed as playing key roles in recovery.

Peluso E, Peluso LS: *Women and Drugs: Getting Hooked, Getting Clean.* Minneapolis, Comp Care Publishers, 1988.

Although this book is now a bit dated, its personal accounts of women with drug addiction are easy to read and full of important information. The authors are counselors who themselves are recovering from addiction. Topics include addictions to alcohol, benzodiazepines, marijuana, cocaine, heroin, and diet pills. Important themes through-out the book are the alarming scope of drug problems among women (which has been minimized in our society), how addicted women tend to build their interpersonal relationships around the substances they misuse, and ways in which women have been able to break through the cycle of ravaging addictions. These chemically dependent women tell their stories in their own words, which makes this work particularly relevant and accessible for a wide variety of patients.

Resources for Clinicians

DuPont RL: *The Selfish Brain: Learning from Addiction.* Washington, DC, American Psychiatric Press, 1997.
This thoroughly engaging, comprehensive book about all facets of drug and alcohol addiction and the daunting road to recovery is one book that all professionals and recovering people should own and read. It includes topics such as the biology of addiction, codependency, intervention and treatment principles, public policy issues, and prevention measures. Sound, straightforward medical and psychotherapeutic ad-vice is offered throughout. The professional is given valuable tools to deal with the addicted patient as well as a balanced, authoritative perspective on contemporary, multidisciplinary treatment of addictions. DuPont covers alcohol, marijuana, cocaine, heroin, nicotine, inhalant, and hallucinogen abuse with an expert clinician's devoted heart and a scholar's expansive mind. Moreover, his down-to-earth writing style makes even the most technical aspects of the disorders accessible and interesting.
DuPont RL, McGovern JP: *A Bridge to Recovery: An Introduction to 12-Step Programs.* Washington, DC, American Psychiatric Press, 1994.
Because primary care physicians and care extenders are increasingly likely to provide the initial steps to treatment for patients with addictive disorders, this guide is an essential introduction to the wisdom, value, and rationale of 12-step fellowships. Emphasis is placed on becoming acquainted with and collaborating with local chapters of groups such as AA, NA, Al-Anon, and Alateen. The authors advise physicians to attend four or five open 12-step meetings to familiarize themselves with the basic purpose, format, and philosophy of the 12-step movement. Stressing that primary care clinicians play a unique role in offering support and perspective to patients and families seeking help for drinking or drug abuse, the authors make excellent recommen-dations about how to increase local access to 12-step programs and thereby intervene successfully with addiction problems. Additional essential information is provided about the family's role in addiction and recovery, hospital and transitional living programs, and legal and workplace issues. This practical reference is an excellent one to have on the bookshelf; much can be learned from it about addiction treatment in general.
Miller, NS (ed.): *The Principles and Practice of Addictions in Psychiatry.* Philadelphia, WB Saunders, 1997.
For clinicians who treat a number of substance-abusing patients and must stay abreast of the most up-to-date methods of detoxification, complications of withdrawal, and choice points in treatment planning, resources such as this can be an invaluable aid. This particular volume covers alcohol, sedative, opioid, cocaine, amphetamine, PCP, nicotine, and inhalant abuse. Therapeutics for the different phases of detoxification throughout long-range treatment are recommended. Approaches to specific populations at risk are included.

References

Anthony JC, Arria AM, Johnson EO: Epidemiological and public health issues for tobacco, alcohol, and other drugs. In: Oldham JM, Riba MB (eds.): *American Psychiatric Press Review of Psychiatry,* vol 14, pp. 15–50. Washington, DC, American Psychiatric Press, 1995.

Aponte H: Political bias, moral values, and spirituality in the training of psychotherapists. *Bull Menninger Clin* 1996;60:488–502.

Barnes HN, Bor DH: Substance use and abuse: Alcohol and other drugs. In: Woolf SH, Jonas S, Lawrence RS (eds.): *Health Promotion and Disease Prevention in Clinical Practice*, pp. 291–300. Baltimore, Williams & Wilkins, 1996.

Bepko C (ed.): Feminism and addiction. *Journal of Feminist Family Therapy* 1991;3:1–224.

Blum K, Cull, JG, Braverman ER: Reward deficiency syndrome. *American Scientist* 1996;84:132–145.

Blume SB: Women and alcohol: a review. *JAMA* 1986;256:1467–1470.

Blume SB: Alcohol and other drug problems in women. In: Lowinson JH, Ruiz P, Millman RB, et al. (eds.): *Substance Abuse: A Comprehensive Textbook*, pp. 794–807. Baltimore, Williams & Wilkins, 1992.

Blume SB, Counts SJ, Turnbull JM: Women and substance abuse. *Patient Care* 1992;26:141–156.

Borrelli B, Niaura R, Keuthen NJ, et al.: Development of major depressive disorder during smoking-cessation treatment. *J Clin Psychiatry* 1996;57:534–538.

Bradley KA, Boyd-Wickizer J, Powell SH, et al.: Alcohol screening questionnaires in women: A critical review. *JAMA* 1998;280:166–171.

Cirillo J: Prevention of family violence for the female alcoholic. In: Adler LL, Denmark FL (eds.): *Violence and the Prevention of Violence*, pp. 169–175. Westport, CT, Praeger Publishers/Greenwood Publishing Group, 1995.

Cirillo JM: Differential treatment: considerations for the female alcoholic. In: Sechzer JA, Pfafflin SM, Denmark FL, et al. (eds.): *Women and Mental Health*, pp. 83–99. New York, New York Academy of Sciences, 1996.

Crits-Cristoph P, Sigueland L: Psychosocial treatment for drug abuse: selected review and recommendations for national health care. *Arch Gen Psychiatry* 1996;58:749–756.

Dodes LM: The psychology of combined dynamic psychotherapy and Alcoholics Anonymous. *Bull Menninger Clin* 1988;52:283–293.

DuPont RL: Anxiety and addiction: a clinical perspective on comorbidity. *Bull Menninger Clin* 1995;59(suppl A):A53–A72.

DuPont RL: *The Selfish Brain: Learning from Addiction*. Washington, DC, American Psychiatric Press, 1997a.

DuPont RL: Psychotherapy in addictive disorders. In: Miller NS (ed.): *The Principles and Practice of Addictions in Psychiatry*, pp. 370–377. Philadelphia, WB Saunders, 1997b.

DuPont RL, McGovern JP: *A Bridge to Recovery: An Introduction to 12-Step Programs*. Washington, DC, American Psychiatric Press, 1994.

Ewing JA: Detecting alcoholism: the CAGE questionnaire. *JAMA* 1984;252:1905–1907.

Farquhar JW, Spiller GA: *The Last Puff: Ex-Smokers Share the Secrets of Their Success*. New York, WW Norton, 1990.

Ferguson DM, Lynskey MT, Horwood J: Comorbidity between depressive disorders and nicotine dependence in cohort of 16-year-olds. *Arch Gen Psychiatry* 1996;53:1043–1047.

Fleming MF, Barry KL, Manwell LB, et al.: Brief physician advice for problem alcohol drinkers: a randomized controlled trial in community-based primary care practices. *JAMA* 1997;277:1039–1045.

Frances RJ, Franklin JE: *Concise Guide to Treatment of Alcoholism and Addictions*. Washington, DC, American Psychiatric Press, 1989.

Frezza M, di Padova C, Pozzato G, et al.: The role of decreased gastric alcohol dehydrogenase activity and first-pass metabolism. *N Engl J Med* 1990;322:95–99.

Goldstein MZ, Pataki A, Webb MT: Alcoholism among elderly persons. *Psychiatr Serv* 1996;47:941–943.

Gordis E: Alcohol research: at the cutting edge [editorial]. *Arch Gen Psychiatry* 1996;53:199–201.

Greenfield SF: Women and substance use disorder: In: Jensvold MF, Halbreich U, Hamilton JA (eds.): *Psychopharmacology and Women: Sex, Gender, and Hormones*, pp. 297–322. Washington, DC, American Psychiatric Press, 1996.

Hajik P: Current issues in behavioral and pharmacological approaches to smoking cessation. *Addict Behav* 1996;21:699–707.

Hall SM: Women and drugs. In: Adesso VJ, Reddy DM, Fleming R (eds.): *Psychological Perspectives on Women's Health*, pp. 101–126. Philadelphia, Taylor & Francis, 1994.

Hall SM, Munoz RD, Reus VI: Cognitive-behavioral program increases abstinence rates for depressive-history smokers. *J Consult Clin Psychol* 1994;62:141–146.

Hill SY: Vulnerability to alcoholism in women: genetic and cultural factors. In: Galanter M (ed.): *Recent Developments in Alcoholism*, vol 12, pp. 9–28. New York, Plenum, 1995.

Harris-Offutt R: Cultural factors in the assessment and treatment of African-American addicts:

Africentric considerations. In: Wallace BC (ed.): *The Chemically Dependent: Phases of Treatment and Recovery*, pp. 289–297. New York, Brunner/Mazel, 1992.

Hesselbrock MN, Hesselbrock RM: Depression and antisocial personality disorder in alcoholism: gender comparison. In: Lisansky Gomberg ES, Nirenberg TD (eds.): *Women and Substance Abuse*, pp. 142–161. Norwood, NJ, Ablex, 1993.

Hurt RD, Offord KP, Croghan IT, et al.: Mortality following inpatient addictions treatment: role of tobacco use in a community-based cohort. *JAMA* 1996;275:1097–1103.

Khantzian EJ: Self-regulation vulnerabilities in substance abusers: Treatment implications. In: Dowling S (ed.): *The Psychology and Treatment of Addictive Behavior*, pp. 17–41. Madison, CT, International Universities Press, 1995.

Kirkpatrick J: *Turnabout: New Help for the Woman Alcoholic*. New York, Bantam, 1977/1990.

Knapp C: *Drinking: A Love Story*. New York, Dial Press, 1996.

Kosten TR, McCance-Katz E: New pharmacotherapies. In: Oldham JM, Riba MD (eds.): *American Psychiatric Press Review of Psychiatry*, vol 14, pp. 105–123. Washington, DC: American Psychiatric Press, 1995.

Lawford BR, Young RM, Rowell J, et al.: Bromocriptine in the treatment of alcoholics with the D2 dopamine receptor A1 allele. *Nat Med* 1995;1:337–341.

Levin JD: Psychodynamic treatment of alcohol abuse. In: Barber JP, Crits-Christoph P (eds.): *Dynamic Therapies for Psychiatric Disorders (Axis 1)*, pp. 193–229. New York, Basic Books, 1995.

Lex B: Some gender differences in alcohol and polysubstance users. *Health Psychol* 1991;10:121–132.

Lex BW: Alcohol and other psychoactive substance dependence in women and men. In: Seeman MV (ed.): *Gender and Psychopathology*, pp. 311–358. Washington, DC, American Psychiatric Press, 1995.

Liepman MR, Goldman RE, Monroe AD, et al.: Substance abuse by special populations of women. In: Lisansky Gomberg ES, Nirenberg TD (eds.): *Women and Substance Abuse*, pp. 214–257. Norwood, NJ, Ablex, 1993.

Lisansky Gomberg ES, Nirenberg TD (eds.): *Women and Substance Abuse*. Norwood, NJ, Ablex, 1993.

Little RE, Wendt JK: The effects of maternal drinking in the reproductive period: An epidemiologic review. In: Lisansky Gomberg ES, Nirenberg TD (eds.): *Women and Substance Abuse*, pp. 191–213. Norwood, NJ, Ablex, 1993.

Manley M. Tobacco use: Counseling and adjunctive treatment. In: Woolf SH, Jonas S, Lawrence RS (eds.): *Health Promotion and Disease Prevention in Clinical Practice*, pp. 163–173. Baltimore, Williams & Wilkins, 1996.

Mason BJ, Kocsis JH, Ritvo EC, et al.: A double-blind, placebo-controlled trial of desipramine for primary alcohol dependence stratified on the presence or absence of major depression. *JAMA* 1996;275:761–767.

McCrady BS, Langenbucher JW: Alcohol treatment and health care system reform. *Arch Gen Psychiatry* 1996;53:737–746.

McGovern G: *Terry: My Daughter's Life-and-Death Struggle with Alcoholism*. New York, Plume, 1995.

McLellan AT, Arndt IO, Metzger DS, et al.: The effects of psychosocial services in substance abuse treatment. *JAMA* 1993;269:1953–1959.

Mello NK: Some behavioral and biological aspects of alcohol problems in women. In: Kalant OJ (ed.): *Alcohol and Drug Problems in Women*, pp. 263–312. New York, Plenum, 1980.

Mello NK, Mendelson JH, Teoh SK: Neuroendocrine consequences of alcohol abuse in women, *Ann N Y Acad Sci* 1989;562:211–240.

Mermelstein RJ, Borrelli B: Women and smoking. In: Stanton AL, Gallant SJ (eds.): *The Psychology of Women's Health: Progress and Challenges in Research and Application*, pp. 309–348. Washington, DC, American Psychological Association, 1995.

Meza E, Kranzler HR: Closing the gap between alcoholism research and practice: the case for pharmacotherapy. *Psychiatr Serv* 1996;47:917–920.

Miller NS, Swift, RM: Primary care medicine and psychiatry: addictions treatment. *Psychiatr Ann* 1997;27:408–416.

Miller NS (ed.): *The Principles and Practice of Addictions in Psychiatry*. Philadelphia, WB Saunders, 1997.

Moyar M: Female alcoholism and affiliation needs. *Women and Therapy* 1987;6:313–321.

North CS: Alcoholism in women: more common—and serious—than you might think. *Postgrad Med* 1996;100:221–224, 230, 232–233.

Nouwen JHM: *The Wounded Healer: Ministry in Contemporary Society*. Garden City, NY, Doubleday, 1972.

Ockene J, Kristeller J: Tobacco withdrawal and tobacco dependence. In: Gabbard GO (ed.): *Treatments of Psychiatric Disorders*, vol 1, 2nd ed., pp. 733–742. Washington, DC, American Psychiatric Press, 1995.

O'Malley SS: Integration of opioid antagonists and psychosocial therapy in the treatment of narcotic and alcohol dependence. *J Clin Psychiatry* 1995;56(suppl 7):30–38.

O'Malley SS, Jaffe AJ, Chang G, et al.: Naltrexone and coping skills therapy for alcohol dependence. *Arch Gen Psychiatry* 1992;49:881–887.

O'Malley SS, Jaffe AJ, Chang G, et al.: Six-month follow-up of naltrexone and psychotherapy for alcohol dependence. *Arch Gen Psychiatry* 1996;53:217–224.

O'Malley SS, Jaffe AJ, Rode S, et al.: Experience of a "slip" among alcoholics treated with naltrexone or placebo. *Am J Psychiatry* 1996;153:281–283.

Parish DC: Another indication for screening and early intervention: problem drinking [editorial]. *JAMA* 1997;277:1079–1080.

Peluso E, Peluso LS: *Women and Drugs: Getting Hooked, Getting Clean*. Minneapolis, Comp Care Publishers, 1988.

Raskin VD: Treatment of addiction in childbearing populations. In: Miller NS (ed.): *The Principles and Practice of Addictions in Psychiatry*, pp. 297–301. Philadelphia, WB Saunders, 1997.

Rivara FP, Mueller BA, Somes G, et al.: Alcohol and illicit drug abuse and the risk of violent death in the home. *JAMA* 1997;278:569–575.

Stage KB, Glassman AH, Covey LS: Depression after smoking cessation: case reports. *J Clin Psychiatry* 1996;57:467–469.

Stammer ME: *Women and Alcohol: The Journey Back*. New York, Gardner Press, 1991.

Swift RM: Effect of naltrexone on human alcohol consumption. *J Clin Psychiatry* 1995;56(suppl 7):24–29.

Toneatto A, Sobell L, Sobell MD: Gender issues in the treatment of abuses of alcohol, nicotine, and other drugs. *J Subst Abuse* 1992;4:209–218.

Unumb TM: Under the influence: Early object representation and recovery in alcoholic women. In: Wallace BC (ed.): *The Chemically Dependent: Phases of Treatment and Recovery*, pp. 232–247. New York, Brunner/Mazel, 1992.

Vaillant GE: *The Natural History of Alcoholism*. Cambridge, MA, Harvard University Press, 1983.

Vaillant GE: A long-term follow-up of male alcohol abuse. *Arch Gen Psychiatry* 1996;53:243–249.

Volpicelli JR, Alterman AI, Hayashida M, et al.: Naltrexone in the treatment of alcohol dependence. *Arch Gen Psychiatry* 1992;49:876–880.

Volpicelli JR, Clay KL, Watson NT, et al.: Naltrexone in the treatment of alcoholism: predicting response to naltrexone. *J Clin Psychiatry* 1995a;56(suppl 7):39–44.

Volpicelli JR, Watson NT, King AC, et al.: Effect of naltrexone on alcohol "high" in alcoholics. *Am J Psychiatry* 1995b;152:613–615.

Wallace BC: Multidimensional relapse prevention from a biopsychosocial perspective across phases of recovery. In: Wallace BC (ed.): *The Chemically Dependent: Phases of Treatment and Recovery*, pp. 171–186. New York, Brunner/Mazel, 1992.

Wesson DR, Ling W: Addiction medicine. *JAMA* 1996;275:1792–1793.

Wilsnack SC: Alcohol use and alcohol problems in women. In: Stanton AL, Gallant SJ (eds.): *The Psychology of Women's Health: Progress and Challenges in Research and Application*, pp. 381–443. Washington, DC, American Psychological Association, 1995.

Wilsnack S, Beckman LS (eds.): *Alcohol Problems in Women*. New York, Plenum, 1980.

Windle M, Windle RC, Scheidt DM, et al.: Physical and sexual abuse and associated mental disorders among alcoholic inpatients. *Am J Psychiatry* 1995;152:1322–1328.

Winnicott DW: The capacity to be alone. In: *The Maturational Processes and the Facilitating Environment*, pp. 29–36. New York, International Universities Press, 1965 (original work published 1958).

Woody GE, McLellan AT, Bedrick J: Dual diagnosis. In: Oldham JM, Riba MD (eds.): *American Psychiatric Press Review of Psychiatry*, vol 14, pp. 83–104. Washington, DC, American Psychiatric Press, 1995a.

Woody GE, McLellan AT, Luborsky L, et al.: Psychotherapy in community methadone programs: a validation study. *Am J Psychiatry* 1995b;152:1302–1308.

Wurmser L: Psychology of compulsive drug use. In: Wallace BC (ed.): *The Chemically Dependent: Phases of Treatment and Recovery*, pp. 15–27. New York, Brunner/Mazel, 1992.

Chapter 5

Eating Disorders

Eating problems among women are ubiquitous but often go unrecognized. They are potentially very dangerous conditions (Bloom et al., 1994; Zerbe, 1993a, 1995). Because of the high rates of morbidity and mortality associated with these disorders, they must be detected early so that they can be treated rigorously. Although there is little evidence that these disorders have reached epidemic proportions, one need look no further than the latest fashion magazines and the multibillion-dollar diet industry to realize that the cultural ideal of attaining a slender, athletic body is implicated in the increasing prevalence of anorexia nervosa and bulimia nervosa.

Anorexia nervosa and bulimia nervosa affect both sexes, but they are nine times more common in women than in men (Hsu, 1996; Hsu et al., 1992). Although these disorders are assumed to be a syndrome of Caucasians in upper-middle- to upper-class social strata, they are increasingly observed in women of color and across all cultural and socioeconomic groups. Weight preoccupation and dieting behavior have been shown to be major risks for the pathogenesis of an eating disorder; in non-Western cultures, the prevalence of eating disorders has increased as dieting behavior has become more common (Hsu, 1996).

In Western cultures, anorexia nervosa affects about 0.5% of young women, and bulimia nervosa affects about 2%. These rates are based on case register and population studies for which full psychiatric criteria must be met (American Psychiatric Association, 1980, 1987, 1994). They do not take into account what clinicians believe to be the growing number of subsyndromal or subclinical cases that share many core features of the full-blown illness. Many of these subclinical cases, with time, may fulfill all criteria for anorexia nervosa or bulimia nervosa (Powers, 1996; Zerbe, 1992a, 1993a).

Women along this spectrum of eating disorders pay an enormous psychological price. They spend a substantial amount of time and money preoccupied with food, weight, body image, and body size, to the exclusion of other activities and fulfillments. Moreover, the medical complications (Table 5–1) affect all body systems and can quickly and without warning be implicated in the patient's sudden demise, even in the face of normal laboratory values (Carney and Andersen, 1996; Greenfeld et al., 1995; Herzog et al., 1997). Anorexia nervosa has a mortality rate of 8% to 18% when indexed cases are monitored for 10 to 20 years. Although the mortality rate of bulimia nervosa is not yet known (it has been thoroughly studied only during the past two decades), it is likely that long-term medical complications are just as severe and frequently underestimated (Halmi, 1994; Hsu, 1992; Zerbe, 1993a). Indeed, young women whose deaths are attributed to cardiac arrest, arrhythmia of unknown cause, gastric or esopha-geal tears, pancreatitis, or the numerous sequelae of osteoporosis may have a hidden, nonreported eating disorder as the root cause.

Table 5–1. **Medical Complications of Anorexia and Bulimia Nervosa**

Cardiovascular system
  Orthostatic hypotension
  Arrhythmias
  Peripheral cyanosis
  Sudden cardiac death
  Bradycardia (<60 beats/minute)
  Cardiomyopathy (e.g., purging from
    syrup of ipecac)
  Edema
  Congestive heart failure (e.g., after
    rapid nutritional refeeding)
Pulmonary system
  Pneumomediastinum
  Pulmonary edema (secondary to
    congestive heart failure)
Metabolic system
  Hypokalemia
  Hyponatremia (rare)
  Increased serum amylase
  Increased blood urea nitrogen
  Hypomagnesemia
  Hyperphosphatemia (bulimia)
  Hypophosphatemia (anorexia)
  Metabolic acidosis
Gastrointestinal system
  Dental caries
  Parotitis/hyperamylasemia
  Bloating/early satiety
  Constipation
  Diarrhea (e.g., laxative abuse)
  Esophageal or gastric dilation or
    rupture (rare)
  Pancreatitis
Endocrine system
  Increased growth hormone
  Increased cortisol
  Decreased triiodothyronine (T_3) and
    thyroxine (T_4)
  Osteopenia/osteoporosis
  Cold intolerance/hypothermia

Gynecologic system
  Amenorrhea/dysmenorrhea
  Infertility
Neurologic system
  Seizures
  Ventricular enlargement
  Brain atrophy
Musculoskeletal system
  Osteopenia/osteoporosis
  Generalized weakness
Hematologic system
  Acanthocytosis
  Mild anemia (e.g., normochromic/
    normocytic; microcytic/hypochromic)
  Folate deficiency
  Iron deficiency
  Low white blood cell count
  Low erythrocyte sedimentation rate
  Thrombocytopenia
Dermatologic system
  Dry or brittle skin
  Dry or brittle nails
  Callus formation on finger (Russell's
    sign)
  Lanugo hair
  Thinning scalp hair
  Loss of subcutaneous fat
  Pretibial edema without
    hypoproteinemia
  Irritation at corners of mouth
  Increased bruisability
  Carotene pigmentation

The primary care clinician must be alert to diagnose these underrecognized but devastating illnesses. Working in concert with mental health professionals, primary care clinicians can obtain the support and psychological help necessary to engage the patient and to begin to address the underlying cognitive distortions, psychodynamic bases, and medical sequelae. Once thought to be disorders of adolescence and young adulthood, eating disorders are now increasingly observed in midlife and late life. Vigilance about their surreptitious appearance must be maintained across the entire life cycle and, particularly, in those special populations at risk for an eating disorder (Table 5–2). These include the occupational risk groups, such as women athletes, models, and flight attendants. Also at high risk are women who have experienced other comorbid psychiatric difficulties (Halmi et al., 1991), sexual abuse (Kearney-Cooke and Striegel-Moore, 1994; Zerbe, 1992b, 1993a), or family discord (Bruch, 1974, 1978; Palazzoli, 1978) and those who have a relative with an eating disorder.

RECOGNIZING EATING DISORDERS IN PRIMARY CARE: SIGNS, SYMPTOMS, AND SECRETS

Fortunately, when *asked* by their primary care clinician, most patients are willing to talk about difficulties with food restriction, bingeing, overexercise, purging, diuretic or enema abuse, and related issues. To help the patient come forward while taking the history, let the patient know that you are aware that literally millions of women struggle with eating behaviors. In fact, weight preoccupation is almost a societal norm: 80% of women diet in any given year (Powers, 1996). Key screening questions that may help you determine whether a bona fide eating disorder is present include inquiries about (1) any change in weight; (2) meals eaten the day before the examination; (3) any binge episodes and compensatory actions to lose weight, such as self-induced vomiting or use of laxatives, diuretics, or enemas; (4) the amount of exercise in a typical week; and (5) regularity of menstrual periods (Blackburn et al., 1993; Kinoy, 1994; Powers, 1996; Zerbe, 1998).

Most importantly, the clinician must remember that eating disorders are best conceptualized as disturbances of personal identity and body image (Bloom et

---

Table 5–2. **Risk Factors for Development of an Eating Disorder**

Occupational risk groups
  Athletes, particularly gymnasts, runners, skaters, rowers
  Dancers
  Models
  Actresses
  Flight attendants
  Military personnel who must maintain a particular weight
Demographic risk factors
  Female sex
  Middle or upper class
Family emotional problems
  Overinvolvement
  Abandonment
  History of sexual abuse
  Complicated bereavement
History of weight problem/obesity in childhood or adolescence
History of eating disorder in family
Comorbid psychiatric problem (e.g., depression, anxiety disorder, chemical dependency, personality disorder)

al., 1994; Bruch, 1978; Fallon et al., 1994; Zerbe, 1993a, 1993c). These patients are preoccupied with their appearance and complain that they "feel fat" even when at a very low or normal body weight. They may ask you for advice about dieting or request some of the new medications for the treatment of obesity, even if they are not overweight.

However, detecting a body image disturbance can be frustrating and perplexing, because patients with anorexia use the defense mechanism of *denial*. You may pick up on the patient's fear of fatness only when you ask her to gain weight and she resists doing so (Powers, 1996; Rock and Curran-Celentano, 1996).

Secretiveness

Sometimes, despite the clinician's empathic approach, the patient keeps her symptoms hidden for a long time (Zerbe, 1992a, 1993a, 1998). It is not a clinical failure on your part if a patient that you suspect of having an eating disorder opens up only after months or years and tells you that she has engaged in periods of self-starvation and/or bingeing-purging behavior. She may finally have found the courage to trust in you that she needs to address the severe physical jeopardy she faces. In the Eating Disorders Program at The Menninger Clinic, we observed that a cohort of women came forward for the first time at midlife after 20 years of having a subsyndromal eating disorder! What prompted them to seek outpatient consultation was their recognition of an eating disorder in a younger family member (usually a daughter or a niece) and treatment of that person.

To increase your recognition of eating disorders, ask open-ended questions (e.g., "Are you doing anything special to lose weight, such as exercising or taking over-the-counter diet pills?"). Be sure to counsel the patient about the long-term medical consequences of anorexia and bulimia (see Table 5–1). Mentioning the inordinate pressure women face to attain personal, professional, and bodily perfection lets the patient know that you are sympathetic to the multiple demands and cultural ambiguities she may be experiencing. This tactful approach promotes an aura of acceptance and trust in the clinician-patient relationship and helps these women to be more open about their physical and emotional preoccupations.

History of Weight Fluctuations

For adolescents and young adults, a detailed weight history may be useful in detecting the onset of an eating disorder. Typically, children and adolescents with an eating disorder fail to gain weight when they should be having a growth spurt (Powers, 1996). On other occasions, you may note weight increasing, then decreasing, increasing again, and then dipping down. This saw-toothed pattern is typical of the patient with bulimia nervosa who attempts to diet, is unable to sustain rigid dietary restraint, then overeats to compensate, and subsequently purges. In young adult women, the most frequent cause of weight loss is anorexia, but other medical disorders should be ruled out (Table 5–3), particularly if the patient does not appear to be interested in, or denies concern about, her body image (Blackburn et al., 1993; Mickley, 1994; Powers, 1996).

Table 5–3. **Causes of Weight Loss in Young Adult Women**

Anorexia nervosa (most frequent cause)
Neoplasm
Cystic fibrosis
Pancreatic insufficiency
Hyperthyroidism
Diabetes mellitus
Inflammatory bowel disease
Occult infection (e.g., human immunodeficiency virus infection)
Drug abuse

Menstrual Problems and Infertility

Women with eating disorders report episodes of amenorrhea, dysmenorrhea, and a host of other gynecologic problems at a high rate. About 30% of bulimic patients experience some abnormality in their menstrual cycle, and they tend to have frequent premenstrual dysphoria (see Chapter 11). About 25% of anorectic patients actually have amenorrhea before losing weight; stress (e.g., leaving home for college) and neuroendocrine factors have been postulated to cause this aberrance (Frisch, 1988, 1996). After weight is restored, anorexia nervosa patients who regain their menses tend to have a better prognosis than those who do not (Hebebrand et al., 1997; Meyer et al., 1986).

Patients with subsyndromal, atypical, or full-blown eating disorders may initially present with infertility (Powers, 1996). One study (Stewart et al., 1990) found that 16.7% of 66 women who presented for an infertility consultation actually had an eating disorder.

Excessive Exercise

Anorectic patients are notorious for compulsive overexercise, even in the face of injury (Powers and Johnson, 1996). Indulging in extreme diets because they are never satisfied with their bodies, they also relentlessly stay active in order to "avoid getting fat." Sometimes only hospitalization and 24-hour-a-day skilled observation interrupts these compulsive behaviors (Yates, 1991; Zerbe, 1993a, 1993b, 1993c).

Animal research has implicated the combined influence of caloric restriction and strenuous exercise in behavioral and neurochemical alterations that mimic those found in eating disorders, obsessive-compulsive disorder, and various addictive behaviors. Clinical studies of patients with eating disorders have investigated the connections among obsessions, addictions, and exercise in the development, progression, and maintenance of eating disorders (Davis et al., 1995a, 1995b; Yates 1991). Results of these studies indicate that exercise, if taken to an extreme, may actually *initiate* or *perpetuate* an eating disorder. These findings should be used to educate women about how excessive physical exercise can make symptoms worse and more difficult to stop.

Bulimic patients exercise to compensate for a binge. Exercise actually becomes a method of purging. Although aerobic exercise (three to five times a week at a rate of 30 to 40 minutes per session) and strength training are recommended to promote health, patients with eating disorders literally exercise their lives away, often for hours a day, every day, even in the face of fever, fatigue, injury, or illness. One way to determine whether the exercise is excessive is to learn its purpose and frequency (Powers, 1996). As the primary care clinician, you need to maintain an attentiveness to these patients, because many of them are not aware or are unable to acknowledge that they are working out frenetically and compulsively. Understand this reaction as a symptom of illness, not as a lie intended to disrupt the treatment alliance or make you angry.

For these patients, exercising may be a result of a neurochemical alteration, or it may be a psychological coping strategy designed to provide an experience of the self as competent, strong, and effective (Zerbe, 1993b, 1993c). This pathologic identity can be corrected only with substantial psychological support over a period of time; from the patient's perspective, the eating and the "activity" (Yates 1991) provide a tenacious, albeit pathologic and ultimately life-threatening, hold on life itself (Crisp, 1980).

ADDITIONAL FACTORS TO ASSESS IN THE HISTORY

Primary care clinicians who screen and educate young women about eating disorders can play a significant role in the recognition and prevention of these illnesses (Graber and Brooks-Gunn, 1996; Paxton, 1996; Piran, 1996; Raphael, 1996; Steiner-Adair and Purcell, 1996). Particular attention should be paid to the following additional risk factors: family history (of an eating disorder or of significant problems or losses), depression and anxiety, substance abuse, and sexual abuse. These factors have been associated with poor prognosis and the need for additional collaboration with a mental health professional. (See Table 5-4 for criteria for referral to an eating disorders specialist.)

Family History

Eating disorders do run in families; there is a higher incidence of anorexia nervosa in monozygotic than in dizygotic twins (Halmi, 1992; Hsu, 1992; Kendler et al., 1991). Some researchers have emphasized the familial link between eating

---

Table 5–4. **Referral of Patients with Chronic Anorexia or Bulimia Nervosa**

1. Refusal to maintain weight at 85%–90% of ideal weight, despite physician counseling
2. Significant impairment in work, school, or family functioning
3. Comorbid psychiatric problems (e.g., depression, obsessive-compulsive disorder, dissociative disorder, personality disorder)
4. Comorbid substance abuse
5. History of physical or sexual abuse, including rape
6. Lack of comfort with using psychotropic medications (e.g., fluoxetine, 60–80 mg/day)
7. Frustration because the patient does not get well quickly and makes excessive demands on the physician's time and attention
8. Life-threatening medical complications and/or suicidal potential

disorders and affective disorders, citing in particular the response of both groups to antidepressants. Most authorities believe that anorexia nervosa and bulimia nervosa are distinct entities, but debate continues to rage as to whether either or both are related to depression (Edelstein and Yager, 1992; Halmi, 1992; Herzog et al., 1996; Mitchell et al., 1986, 1991).

Anorectic patients have been most thoroughly described as growing up in families where parental conflict is rife but covert. One of the parents, usually the mother, turns to her daughter for emotional support. The eating disorder patient-to-be is placed in a premature adult mode to serve as the confidant, pseudotherapist, or emotional buttress of a needful, demanding parent. Enmeshment results. The patient turns to self-starvation as the mode of asserting her autonomy and separating from her family of origin (Bruch, 1974, 1978, 1988; Crisp, 1980; Zerbe, 1993a, 1993b, 1996). In effect, through the eating disorder, the patient is unconsciously severing a bond with the stultifying parent. By focusing on weight and eating, the patient shields the family from working out more emotionally laden difficulties (Minuchin et al., 1978).

Bulimic patients, in contrast, describe a dearth of parental caretaking (Johnson and Connors, 1987). The patient turns to food as the ultimate caretaker. Eating offers a respite from the loneliness, feelings of abandonment and depression, and lack of soothing, supportive people in the patient's life. (See Table 5–5 for a list of the most commonly encountered psychological factors leading to an eating disorder.)

Unresolved loss and the inability to mourn may also underlie anorexia nervosa or bulimia nervosa. These dynamics are particularly important to recognize in primary care practice, because after a death family members frequently turn to their physicians or care extenders with psychosomatic complaints, requests for anxiolytic medications, and so forth (see Chapter 9). If the patient does not have the social support, family network, or coping skills to work through or even describe her loss, bereavement not only is perpetuated but also can be manifested in psychiatric or psychosomatic illness.

Table 5–5. **Psychological Factors Leading to Eating Disorders**

1. Separation-individuation issues in the family of origin
2. Covert family tension
3. Problems expressing feelings, particularly anger
4. Conflicts with sexual expression
5. Difficulty dealing with normal ambivalence in adult relationships
6. Difficulty achieving mature interdependency in relationships (e.g., has only one or no age-appropriate friendships)
7. Continued search for utopia (especially in the guise of achieving physical perfection)
8. Narcissistic pursuit of bodily perfection (e.g., cultural stereotype of attaining the "perfect body")
9. Inability to mourn losses
10. Tendency to be very self-critical and to engage in self-punishing behaviors
11. Tendency to avoid developing a sense of personal autonomy (e.g., finding "one's own voice")

For example, one patient with severe anorexia had never been able to talk about the meaning of her father's death from cancer 4 years before outpatient consultation. The family had been emotionally close, and the father's long illness had taken a huge toll on everyone. The patient's mother was exhausted but deeply grieved when her husband died; she felt she had nowhere to turn, and she had to work two jobs to take care of their four children. The patient identified with her father's cachexia, which became manifest concretely in her anorexia nervosa symptoms. In psychotherapy, she was able to talk about the experience of her father's death and work through it. Her anorexia then resolved, and she was able to return to college. She is functioning well today.

Depression and Anxiety Disorders

Depression is the most frequently and thoroughly described psychiatric co-morbidity accompanying the eating disorders (Edelstein and Yager, 1992; Herzog et al., 1996; Mitchell et al., 1991). Adequate nutrition frequently leads to remission of depressive symptomatology, even without the use of antidepressant medications such as tricyclic antidepressants (TCAs) or selective serotonin reuptake inhibitors (SSRIs). However, a subgroup of patients benefits from antidepressants, especially in higher doses than usual for the treatment of depression (e.g., fluoxetine, 60–80 mg/day). This clinical observation has led some investigators to wonder whether a different neurobiologic process is implicated in the eating disorders and in depression.

Studies have also linked eating disorders and the anxiety disorders, particularly obsessive-compulsive disorder (Halmi et al., 1991; Halmi, 1992). Observation reveals perfectionistic tendencies, obsessive preoccupation, ritualistic behaviors, and fastidiousness in some anorexia nervosa patients. Halmi and colleagues (1991) reported a greater prevalence of obsessive-compulsive disorder in mothers of anorectic patients and speculated about a possible connection with serotonin dysregulation. Panic disorder, agoraphobia, social phobia, and generalized anxiety disorder have also been reported at a higher frequency in bulimia and anorexia patients (Herzog et al., 1996).

Substance Abuse

Several studies have reported a higher incidence of substance abuse among patients with eating disorders. The primary care clinician must make it a priority to treat both the eating disorder and the drug and/or alcohol dependence when they coexist (see Chapter 4). Consultation with a clinician skilled in the treatment of chemical dependency is useful for these dually diagnosed patients. Prognosis is poor and the physical and emotional costs of illness are high unless both disorders are treated.

Bulimia nervosa and substance abuse share the common behaviors of addiction, such as craving, lack of control, impaired functioning, and denial (Mitchell et al., 1991; Wiederman and Pryor, 1996). The primary care clinician can help the patient to acknowledge the difficulty, even in the face of reluctance, by repeatedly asking her "just one more time" about any problems she has had with the use of illicit substances. Twelve-step fellowships such as Narcotics Anonymous and Alcoholics Anonymous often provide a crucial ingredient in a comprehensive treatment program to help curtail addiction and develop a relapse prevention plan (DuPont, 1997; DuPont and McGovern, 1994).

Sexual Abuse

In the past two decades, childhood trauma, especially physical and sexual abuse, has been implicated in the etiology of many psychiatric disturbances (see Chapter 6), including eating disorders. A history of trauma should always be taken, but the savvy clinician will not be surprised if this tragic aspect of a patient's life is acknowledged only after a sustained and comfortable relationship is established.

Do not neglect to inquire about a history of rape. Adult trauma of this kind may also lead to coping through an eating disorder, particularly bulimia nervosa. Individual psychotherapy is essential to help the patient address any feelings of self-reproach or other emotional sequelae of trauma.

A history of sexual or physical abuse complicates the treatment of an eating disorder. Patients may have difficulty expressing feelings and regulating tension, and they often tend to ruminate about the past and struggle with their interpersonal (particularly sexual) relationships. Because case reports of sexual and physical trauma are becoming almost daily fare in newspaper articles, television reports, and even scientific periodicals, the primary care clinician who does *not* see patients with this problem is rare. Providing support to and belief in the patient will help her to prevail despite the trauma. The clinician's empathy for the suffering of the patient may be facilitated by recalling these words by Rorty and Yager (1996), who eloquently summarize the impact of sexual abuse and eating disorders:

> The profound self-destructiveness and tenacity of eating disorders found among women abused and neglected in childhood become comprehensible when understood within a complex, posttraumatic conceptualization as desperate attempts to regulate overwhelming affective states and construct a coherent sense of self and system of meaning. . . . Abused patients' childhood experiences teach them that to *need* is to expose oneself to the pain of abandonment and betrayal at the hands of individuals responsible for their care. Consequently, needs— psychological, physical, and spiritual—come to be perceived as dangerous, and human relationships are simultaneously yearned for and feared. . . . Though reconnecting with humanity carries the risk of further pain, it opens up the opportunity for connection, healing, and growth (p. 785).

Probably the majority of eating disorder patients who have experienced such abuse will need psychotherapy to come to grips with the toll that sexual or physical abuse has taken on their lives. The primary care clinician should encourage the patient to participate in supportive group treatment or individual psychotherapy (Kearney-Cooke and Striegel-Moore, 1994). Family therapy is also useful in some cases, but blatant confrontations about abuse in family sessions have done more harm than good. An experienced family therapist can offer the nonjudgmental, commonsense advice that is essential to avoiding destructive family upheavals.

EATING DISORDERS IN SPECIAL POPULATIONS

Athletes

Eating disorders are increasingly common among competitive athletes, particularly in sports where appearance or performance rewards thinness (e.g., ballet, gymnastics, figure skating). Unique to the athletic community is an emphasis on "performance thinness" (Powers and Johnson, 1996). Coaches and trainers believe, despite scanty scientific evidence, that a low percentage of body fat enhances an athlete's competitive advantage. Athletes are therefore at high risk for loss of perspective about their bodies, believing they gain a competitive edge or will be amply rewarded both socially and athletically for achieving a low percentage of body fat.

Clinical experience now supports the view that competitive female athletes are a high-risk group for the development of subclinical or full syndromal eating disorders (Powers and Johnson, 1996). Primary care clinicians are in a unique position to prevent the emergence of eating disorders by speaking to athletes, family members, coaches, and trainers. Secondary prevention occurs when eating disorders among athletes are detected early, so it is essential to encourage the patient to develop a sense of self and meaning that is not attached solely to stellar athletic performance. When emphasis is placed on performing sports as a sign of strength and fitness (Powers and Johnson, 1996), as opposed to the pursuit of thinness or victory alone, athletes are less likely to feel driven to see their sport as the mainstay of their personal identity (Zerbe, 1993a, 1996).

When evaluating the athlete who may have an eating disorder, be sure to ask questions about any symptoms that might alert you, the coach, or the trainer to its presence (e.g., progressive weight loss, restriction of eating despite a high level of physical exertion, bingeing or purging before or after an event, undue emphasis on body image). In women athletes, disturbed eating behavior, amenorrhea, and osteoporosis have been identified as a common syndrome—the so-called female athlete triad. *By all means, discourage coaches from making comments about weight or assuming that a reduction in body fat or weight will enhance performance.* Provide accurate information about weight, weight loss, body composition, and nutrition. Emphasize the health risks of low weight, particularly for women with menstrual irregularities or amenorrhea. Educate athletes, team physicians, and coaches whenever possible; become involved in community outreach programs through the media, newspaper interviews, letters to the editor, or public speaking to provide another avenue toward greater public awareness of these syndromes.

Sometimes other athletes alert the clinician to the problem. They are often aware of a fellow athlete's restrictive eating or overexercising, or the smell of vomitus in the locker room. The primary care clinician can help the athlete herself, her coach, her parents, and significant others see the potential for disaster should the fixation on bodily perfection and an athletic identity lead to an eating disorder. Underscore how the triad of exercise, starvation, and purging is particularly perilous for women, occasionally even leading to sudden death (Yates, 1991).

Women at Midlife and Late Life

As noted previously, anorexia nervosa and bulimia nervosa usually are considered problems of late adolescence or early adulthood. They have, however, been increasingly observed from the fourth through the eighth decade. Some women have harbored a distorted body image since their youth and have engaged in various subclinical forms of an eating disorder. They seek out treatment at midlife and beyond, when they begin to experience the long-term physical side effects of the eating disorder (see Table 5–1) or when they desire relief from the isolation and interpersonal toll it has taken on their social, family, and work lives.

In the elderly, anorexia nervosa must be differentiated from major depression with melancholia. With melancholia, the patient has the delusional belief that eating food will poison her. Other somatic delusions about her body, such as the belief that she cannot eat because she does not possess a stomach, may indicate an unrecognized or undertreated major depression (Zerbe, 1998). In contrast, the older anorectic patient is preoccupied with a need to maintain a youthful appearance as long as possible, or else she may describe losses she has sustained over the life cycle. One patient, a 76-year-old anorectic woman who had had symptoms for 20 years, presented with a host of psychophysiologic complaints. She began to starve herself after the sudden death of her son. Her husband had also been unfaithful to her. She was unable to mourn and felt betrayed and anguished, but her dieting behavior gave her some sense of being in control of her life, which otherwise left her feeling as though she were fate's victim. In essence, the patient's eating disorder originated from two major losses—the death of her son and the loss of integrity in her marital relationship.

In the older patient with an eating disorder, it is important to first correct any nutritional deficiency and then refer the patient for psychotherapeutic intervention. In our culture, growing older is difficult for many women. The older woman must mourn the youthful body she has lost if she is to move through middle age and enter late life with grace and dignity. Encourage such patients to stay healthy and fit, which promotes psychological and physical well-being (Nelson and Wernick, 1997). Exploratory therapy can be useful in helping the patient look at and work through any losses, including the ideal of youth. Judicious psychotropic medication can be used adjunctively.

In contrast, treatments of choice for the older, delusional, depressed patient range from antidepressant and antipsychotic medications titrated to the appropriate levels to electroconvulsive therapy. The latter is again gaining favor among psychiatrists because it is safe, rapidly acting, and highly effective in reversing psychotic depression. It is particularly useful in the suicidal patient when there may not be time to wait for an antidepressant response.

CONCERNS ABOUT SEXUALITY AND PREGNANCY

Sexuality

Patients with eating disorders have a range of difficulties in the sexual arena. Some authorities believe that poor nutrition or the starvation state alone is the cause of this impaired sexual functioning (Keys et al., 1950). Although restoration of nutrition certainly helps patients to engage more fully in sexual relationships, interpersonal difficulties and conflicted feelings about intimacy inevitably impede these patients from engaging in affirming sexual relationships (Simpson and Ramberg, 1992; Zerbe, 1992b, 1995).

Patients with eating disorders tend to view their bodies as shameful and disgusting. Bulimic patients sometimes confide that they have engaged in sexually promiscuous activities without ever feeling emotionally satisfied in a relationship; this is part of a long-standing pattern of interpersonal impulsiveness. Anorectic patients tend to complain of feeling sexually inhibited or lacking desire or adventurousness. Anorectic and bulimic patients also complain of disengagement from the body, sometimes to the point of a frank dissociation of sexual experience (Zerbe, 1993a). When a history of childhood sexual abuse and/or rape is part of the clinical history, lack of sexual desire or responsiveness is common. Expert opinion converges to suggest that traditional sex therapy is not always helpful for patients with eating disorders (Simpson and Ramberg, 1992). First, the eating disorder must be tackled. Then psychotherapy that addresses problems with self-esteem, relationship conflicts, body image concerns, and guilty self-recrimination about sexual preference and response can help the patient regain a capacity to function sexually with a partner (Zerbe, 1992b, 1995).

Pregnancy

Despite their sexual conflicts and menstrual difficulties, patients with eating disorders do become pregnant. Many women who conceive are able to refrain from engaging in their eating disorder for the duration of the pregnancy, often because they do not wish to harm the fetus. A high-risk time occurs after the birth, when these new mothers must take on new roles and responsibilities. Feeding the baby and seeing it gain weight may be a struggle. One mother with a history of anorexia was worried that her 14-month-old son would not grow out of his "baby fat"; she told her primary care clinician that she chose a baby food with fewer fat grams than another brand so he would be slender!

Make sure the mother with a history of an eating disorder learns about appropriate nutrition for her child. Help her avoid obsessive concerns whenever possible. Shoring up any weaknesses in the marital bond is useful at this time of increasing workload and role transition; the father nurtures the mother, who nurtures the baby. This support helps the new mother cope without returning to her old pattern of maladaptive eating to get through stressful times. Support groups for mothers and group therapy with other eating disorder patients have been shown to be particularly effective adjuncts in treatment (Edelstein and King, 1992).

Pregnancy and birth inevitably reawaken issues from the past, including those with one's own mother. The new mother who is assured of her own competence and potential for success, and who is reminded of the human stressors of having a new baby, is less likely to return to her eating disorder as a form of emotional refuge and solace.

OBESITY AND BINGE EATING DISORDER

Despite the primacy that Western culture places on thinness as the quintessence of success and appeal, the prevalence of obesity in the United States increased by approximately 8% between 1976–1980 and 1988–1991 (Kucamarski et al., 1994). Women now weigh, on the average, 3.6 kg (about 8 pounds) more than they did 20 years ago. In addition, they are more prone to the major health risks of diabetes mellitus, hypertension, hyperlipidemia, and malignancy (Gortmaker et al., 1993). Moreover, obese women face enormous social and economic consequences. Psychosocial research has revealed that obese women marry less often, achieve lower academic success, and attain significantly lower incomes than women with other chronic medical conditions (Brownell and Wadden, 1992; Foreyt et al., 1996; Miller, 1996; Stunkard and Wadden, 1992).

This social discrimination and prejudice are real. Because primary care clinicians treat many obese persons in their practice, it is essential to recognize the substantially higher mortality rates and associated morbidities faced by obese women. Although obesity is not categorized as a bona fide eating disorder in the American Psychiatric Association's 1994 *Diagnostic and Statistical Manual of Mental Disorders* (*DSM-IV*), the medical and psychological consequences of obesity are such that it should be included in any pragmatic review of women's health concerns.

Binge eating disorder is a newly recognized condition characterized by uncontrolled binge eating in the absence of compensatory behaviors, such as vomiting, abuse of diuretics or laxatives, and overexercise (Devlin, 1996; Fairburn and Wilson, 1993; Marcus, 1993; Marcus et al., 1992). Not all binge eaters are overweight, but the majority are. Obese patients and those with binge eating disorder require a detailed clinical assessment that takes into account the behavioral, somatic, and psychological aspects of their disorder in the individual treatment plan.

Obesity is defined as being 20% to 30% above one's ideal weight. Although patients should be counseled about the genuine health risks and mortality that accompany obesity, physicians must discourage their patients from engaging in "yo-yo dieting," which some reports have shown exacerbates mortality in its own right. When working with obese women, it is important to empathize with the patient's feelings of bodily shame and humiliation. The primary care clinician can promote self-acceptance, a cornerstone for the alliance and treatment, by pointing out that other cultures value, and even laud, a full figure in a way that contemporary Western culture does not.

Education about how one's genetic heritage influences the nature of body problems is vital for all persons. In our society, both men and women tend to look at their body size as something they have achieved by dint of will or lack thereof. In reality, we must all reckon with our parental lineage as the principal harbinger of body size and type (Stunkard and Wadden, 1992). Looking at the size and shape of one's biologic relatives is the best guide for how much one will weigh in adulthood.

Nevertheless, environment plays a substantial role. One cannot gain weight without eating more calories than are used. Our society "provides access to and encourages consumption of a diet high in fat, high in calories, delicious, widely available and low in cost" (Battle and Brownell, 1996, p. 761). Treatment of obesity must aim at intervention in the patient's environment, increasing energy expenditure through exercise and reducing energy intake, or both (Battle and Brownell, 1996; Foreyt et al., 1996; National Task Force on Prevention and Treatment of Obesity, 1996).

Although our society may eventually move toward embracing a true diversity of body types and shapes that reflect the real variations in size in our population, obese patients should still be steered toward achieving modest (10%) reductions in body weight to promote health (St. Jeor, 1997). When engaging such patients in treatment, primary care clinicians must emphasize the benefits of achieving a healthy lifestyle rather than of merely improving one's appearance.

Considerations for Treatment of Obesity and Binge Eating Disorder

1. Emphasize that treatment must include a reduction in fat intake along with an increase in physical activity. The patient must participate in and become an active agent in permanent behavioral changes that support a healthier lifestyle (Brownell, 1988).
2. Because undertaking a gradual weight loss program can be discouraging, point out that research has shown that even small changes over a period of time make a difference in the long haul (St. Jeor, 1997).
3. Encourage the patient to take advantage of everyday routines to increase her daily activity, such as going up and down a few flights of stairs rather than using the elevator, standing rather than sitting, using free weights when speaking on the phone, walking rather than driving short distances, and doing housework. Over a period of a year, all these activities contribute to a small but significant weight loss and improved fitness. These adjustments in one's daily regimen also reflect a lifestyle change toward more activity that has overall healthful effects on the patient (Nelson and Wernick, 1997; St. Jeor, 1997).
4. Underscore the "10% solution" to the patient. By reducing body weight by as little as 10% over the course of 6 to 12 months, and maintaining that lowered weight, most of the critical health benefits can be achieved (e.g., lowered blood pressure, improved cardiovascular risk factors) (Blackburn et al., 1993; Brownell and Wadden, 1992). Here the clinician helps shift the patient's goal away from achieving an ideal body weight to the realistic, but healthier, adjunctive gradual weight loss and stepwise changes.
5. Identify any psychological issues such as depression that may contribute to the perpetuation of obesity. Treatment of any underlying comorbid or psychiatric conditions potentiates the possibility for success. Most authorities believe that up to 90% of properly screened obese patients can be helped (Brownell and Wadden, 1992).
6. Know the indications for the new obesity drugs (e.g., sibutramine), but use them only in conjunction with behavior modification programs. The decision to undertake ongoing medications for treatment of obesity is not to be made lightly because their long-term safety and efficacy has yet to be confirmed through controlled studies. The serotonergic agent dexfenfluramine (Redux) and the combined therapy of the serotonergic drug fenfluramine and the sympathomimetic drug phentermine (fen-phen) brought new hope to many patients (National Task Force on Prevention and Treatment of Obesity, 1996; Weintraub, 1992). In one study, twice as many patients taking the combination fen-phen as those taking the placebo achieved a given weight loss, although more patients taking the medication had transient side effects,

such as tiredness, diarrhea, dry mouth, polyuria, and drowsiness (Guy-Grand, et al., 1989). The combination drug fen-phen and Redux were taken off the market because of the potential lethal effects of pulmonary hypertension. Sibutramine or phentermine alone continued to be used in selected cases for severe obesity.

7. Have as a goal the prevention of weight gain after 6 months. If this goal is met, patients are more likely to stick with other aspects of the weight reduction program (e.g., increased exercise). Sibutramine, a drug structurally related to amphetamine, has been approved by the FDA for obesity (10 mg per day starting dose; increase to 15 mg per day in 4 weeks). Naltrexone (ReVia) has also been provided as an adjunct in the treatment of binge eating disorder (50 mg per day). Naltrexone apparently works by reducing food craving by action on the endogenous opioid system (Marrazzi, et al., 1995; Mercer and Holder, 1997).

8. Anticipate that patients tend to be disheartened because they have not attained ideal weight. To help them overcome discouragement, educate patients about medical goals and improvement in comorbid conditions. Suggest that they consider the medication as a "jump start" in a three-part regimen of weight loss that includes diet modification and increased exercise. Phentermine or sibutramine is recommended for patients who are 30% (20% in the presence of other health problems) above their ideal weight. The drug should never be used in combination with monoamine oxidase inhibitors (MAOIs) and should be used with caution with the SSRIs or TCAs, lest untoward medical complications and psychosis be provoked.

9. Keep in mind that fluoxetine (Prozac) and sertraline (Zoloft) have not been approved for the treatment of obesity. Nevertheless, physicians have empirically noted weight loss when prescribing the SSRIs for depression, and these drugs have been employed in practice for treating obese patients with some modestly good results (Greeno and Wing, 1996). Usually, weight is regained after a few months. Clinical experience with substantial weight maintenance using the fenfluramine-related drugs is more extensive.

10. Be aware that most experts believe that obesity and weight control require lifetime management. Success also requires a high level of commitment to eating wisely, regular aerobic exercise, and avoidance of binging on high calorie/high fat foods (National Task Force for the Prevention and Treatment of Obesity, 1996). For most women, weight loss levels off after 6 months and weight is regained once a drug regimen is discontinued. Some patients regain lost pounds even while taking the medication. New drug therapies may offer long-term hope for these patients, supporting the concept that obesity is a lifelong disorder to be monitored, not necessarily cured (Walsh and Devlin, 1995; Weintraub, 1992). Studies that assess the use of anorexiant medications for longer than 1 year are few. Information about long-term safety and efficacy, including the potential for addiction, is limited.

11. Give less consideration to surgical procedures as a way to reduce weight. Although a stomach or an intestinal bypass was once considered an effective treatment for the severely obese (patients more than 100% above normal body weight), these methods are currently less favored (Kral, 1992). Although such procedures produce large weight loss in some cases, they can also produce significant side effects of vitamin and mineral deficiencies, anemia, vomiting, and diarrhea. These patients must also undergo behavioral

and lifestyle changes in order for the operation to be truly successful (Kral, 1992).

12. Maintain the basic principle of individualized treatment planning for the patient. Other important points for the patient to consider as part of comprehensive care are the following: (1) eat small but frequent meals to avoid hunger, (2) avoid fatty foods while partaking generously of carbohydrates, (3) learn new behavioral strategies to augment self-monitoring, and (4) increase exercise and general activity levels (Foreyt et al., 1996; Levine et al., 1996; Miller, 1996). These steps help to reshape the patient's mindset (such as during times of high risk for overeating). In addition, the development of a relapse prevention plan is essential, because these patients often feel demoralized when they backslide (Brownell et al., 1986; Carter and Fairburn, 1995; Devlin, 1996; Guy-Grand et al., 1989; Weintraub et al., 1992).

PATIENT GUIDELINES FOR COPING WITH AN EATING DISORDER

Learn about the physical costs of the eating disorder and how they can be corrected.

1. Be aware that eating disorders have the highest mortality rate of any psychiatric illness. Although this striking fact can lead to discouragement, remember that most people benefit by returning to normal eating patterns. The newer medications and psychological techniques can also help you cope with your eating disorder.
2. Become knowledgeable about good nutritional practices and implement them. Many patients with an eating disorder also experience anxiety or depression. Often a return to good nutritional practices reverses these symptoms without the use of medication. This commonsense approach has actually been scientifically studied; volunteers who were starved exhibited the same behaviors and mood disturbances as patients with eating disorders (Keys et al., 1950).
3. As a first step to feeling better, learn how to eat wisely and well. Healthy eating patterns are met when you follow at least four of these six requirements every day (Rock and Curran-Celentano, 1996; Zerbe, 1993a):
   a. Two or more servings of fruits per day.
   b. Three or more servings of vegetables per day.
   c. Two or three servings of milk, yogurt, or cheese per day.
   d. Two to three servings of meat, poultry, fish, dry beans, eggs, or nuts per day.
   e. Six to ten servings of bread, cereal, rice, and pasta per day.
   f. Less than two servings of fats, oils, and sweets per day.
4. Even if it means gaining some weight, increase your caloric intake under skilled medical supervision to achieve a healthy weight range (at least 90% of low-average body weight).
5. Avoid using over-the-counter and prescribed diuretics, laxatives, syrup of ipecac, or other purgatives. Although purging may help you feel better temporarily after a binge or as a strategy for coping with stressful feelings,

these activities can actually be life-threatening. At the very least, they lead over the long term to ineffectual coping patterns and numerous medical complications.
6. Follow your clinician's advice to learn as much as you can about the physical effects of having a long-term eating disorder, and remind yourself of these when you are tempted to relapse.

Challenge widely held social and cultural norms.

1. Do not diet. Most women begin their eating disorder behaviors by going on a stringent diet. Positive health practices, such as maintaining a normal weight range, performing moderate exercise, and eating a low-fat, varied diet, are to be encouraged. Too much dietary restraint leads to bingeing later. Eating too few carbohydrates also leads to craving and binge eating.
2. If you must lose weight, seek out consultation from a dietitian or your doctor. Go slowly. Develop patience so you can follow an individualized plan that works for you. Avoid becoming immersed in the destructive binge-purge cycle or the highly restrictive eating pattern of anorexia nervosa. Realize that the same approach does not work for everyone. Your best friend's perfect diet and exercise plan probably will not meet your own unique needs.
3. Recognize that contradictory cultural messages place you in a dilemma about weight and eating. Research shows that our society's emphasis on beauty and physical perfection is a leading contributor to eating disorders. As a woman, you are pulled in conflicting directions—to be sexual and voluptuous while paradoxically being fit and thin. Counteract these mixed signals by putting more emphasis on values and meaning in your life rather than on attaining the stereotypical ideal. Embrace a sense of developing strength and power, not of being perfect.
4. Place less emphasis on external appearance and outward success. The quest to have a "perfect body" may be addressed in other ways. Although the tremendous changes in Western society have given women greater freedom and new roles, women, like men, can get caught up in the "Nobel Prize conflict." That is, the pursuit of success, professional goals, and worldly acclaim can take on a life of its own. Sometimes eating is a way to deal with confusion about what constitutes a life well lived.

Find ways to feel more assertive and empowered in life, even if you are the only person who "sees" them. Develop a relapse prevention program.

1. Figure out those times when you are most likely to engage in your eating disorder. Your physician or mental health professional can help you define those high-risk times when you are likely to starve yourself, binge, or purge. Identifying those situations will enable you to feel more powerful and less hopeless and to develop new skills to maintain reasonable expectations.
2. Identify, admit, and express your feelings. It is essential for recovery to recognize the feelings that trigger your tendency to binge, purge, and so forth and to find new ways of handling them. Many times it is particularly difficult for women to recognize and express anger. This potent emotion may be intimately tied to disordered eating.

3. Find healthy ways, such as using a support group or talking with a therapist, to begin to express your feelings. Then translate the lessons you learn into your interpersonal relationships, working toward more honest expression of feelings with family members and friends.

Learn new coping skills.

1. Maintain a sense of humor. Poke fun at your own foibles. Take life less seriously. Try to see the comic element; it will lighten your spirit.
2. Develop a support system of people you can call when under stress. Sometimes the 12-step fellowships (Overeaters Anonymous or even Alcoholics Anonymous or Narcotics Anonymous) or other support groups can help you with your eating disorder, and usually they are free. However, if members talk *only* about food or cling to one dietary plan, the group will not be as useful as when individual differences are encouraged and championed.
3. Challenge and think through your tendency to "catastrophize" situations. At times we all tend to overestimate the likelihood of negative situations or terrible consequences (e.g., "I will get fat if I eat that brownie"; "My husband will leave me if I gain more weight"). Reason with yourself to avoid these broad, usually unfounded, generalizations.
4. Look carefully at each situation that you fear and discuss it with your clinician. Develop a dialogue with yourself about how to cope more effectively with your problems. In essence, you will learn to rehearse how to handle a problem and cope with it without being overwhelmed. Feelings of competency and mastery grow when you repeat these activities, so you are less likely to return to the old, maladaptive solutions of eating that make you feel so bad about yourself.
5. Try to be less rigid. Confront your tendency to think in absolutes. People with eating problems tend to see things in a "black-and-white, either/or" mode. You may find yourself magnifying your faults, minimizing your strengths, and viewing the world negatively. Become aware of the times that you use the words *must*, *should*, and *ought* and thereby put great pressure on yourself to attain perfection.
6. Don't expect perfection in dealing with high-risk occasions. Eating disorders are an ongoing vulnerability for many women, particularly at times of stress. Recognize this reality and incorporate a plan to deal with setbacks.
7. Read some of the many good self-help books, articles, and testimonials by other women who have had an eating disorder. They are available at your local library or bookstore. Take the suggestions that work for you. Remember that the same approach does not work for every person. An individualized treatment plan and relapse prevention program is essential because each person's issues with eating are unique.

Look at the psychological issues that lie behind your eating disorder.

1. Disavow the commonly held notion of attaining perfection. Hilde Bruch, a pioneer in the study and treatment of eating disorders, once remarked that a goal for recovery from an eating disorder toward healthy living occurs only when patients "discover that they have substance and worth and do not

need the strain and stress of artificial perfection" (1988, p. 8). Recovery means that you mourn the loss of your symptom because it has been an important source of personal identity. As Bruch further asserts, a patient with an eating disorder can "make important progress in finding a less painful way of living when a warm, human relationship develops between her and the therapist and when their verbal exchange has the openness and directness of ordinary conversation" (p. 12).

2. Develop the courage to allow yourself to become a person who is at peace with yourself, even if you are not at your ideal weight. Recognize your strength in adversity.

3. Develop patience to confront the particular emotional issues that underlie your eating disorder. Remain committed in your recovery, even during setbacks, which are unavoidable aspects of every woman's life.

4. Develop trust in yourself as the one who will find the personal path to recovery. Some people find their personal path by writing in a journal because it provides a useful outlet for their feelings. It also helps them note progress over a period of time. Others find that medication plays a very helpful role in their treatment. The important point to emphasize is to find what works for you.

5. Try not to "go it alone." Instead, seek out an experienced, trusted psychotherapist who, most importantly and fundamentally, will listen to you and help you listen to yourself, your body, and your feelings.

Don't be afraid to look at family issues.

1. Because anorexia tends to run in families, be sure to tell your doctor about any emotional disturbance, such as depression or an eating disorder, that has occurred in other family members.

2. Consider how family emotional patterns may play a role in your eating disorder. Some anorectic patients describe their families as rigid, overprotective, and riddled with conflicts. Bulimic patients, in contrast, often report the experience of abandonment, lack of warmth, and loneliness. Sexual and physical assault have also been linked to bulimia nervosa. Other patients with eating disorders find that the disorder is their only way of expressing dissatisfaction with life itself. Take a risk to learn more about yourself and the roots of your eating disorder by seeking out psychotherapy.

Be aware of how your eating disorder affects your children.

1. Avoid placing your baby or child "on a diet" without medical consultation. Although obesity in children is certainly to be discouraged, women with an eating disorder or body image problem may be excessively focused on their infant's or child's weight. Encourage your child to be more physically active if excess weight is a concern.

2. Recognize that young children are receiving the same messages from the media as you are about the physical standards of perfection. Try to address some of these at home by opening up good communication between you and your child about societal norms. Younger and younger children are dieting, potentially leading to an increase in eating disorders. This alarms parents, teachers, and medical professionals alike.

3. Reinvent family mealtime. It is hard with today's family structure to eat together, but this is a time when children not only learn to eat wisely but also develop social skills (Gilbert 1986). Eating with your children will help you observe any early tendency toward restriction of food intake or overeating.

4. Recognize that certain occupations or activities increase the risk for eating disorders. Athletes, gymnasts, dancers, models, actresses, and girls who attend boarding schools have a higher incidence of eating disorders. Children who participate in these activities must be considered at risk for an eating disorder. More education is needed to resist stereotypes, and the pressures placed on these girls must be acknowledged and confronted.

5. Avoid telling your child that he or she "looks fat," needs to lose (or maintain) weight, or needs to "take off a few inches" for a sport or activity. Such comments can lead to an eating disorder. Parents must also be aware of such untoward messages delivered by others and counter them by discussing them at home with their children and by making sure that educators are aware of how eating disorders start.

SPECIAL GUIDELINES FOR PREGNANT PATIENTS AND NEW MOTHERS

1. View pregnancy and the postpartum period as high-risk times. You will tend to do well during pregnancy, as you "care for the baby" by eating healthfully. But your symptoms may reappear after the birth (Edelstein and King, 1992). Be aware that you may be struggling with changes in body image, stressors or conflicts with your role as a mother, or interpersonal issues with your spouse or partner.

2. Realize that you may be sensitive to having a baby who is "too fat." You may indicate your preoccupation with food by talking about differences in fat grams of particular baby foods, excessively worrying about the child's weight, demanding that your doctor put the baby "on a diet," and so forth. Because eating disorders are on the rise in children, be alert to the potential of inadvertently promoting an unhealthy focus on weight and potentially causing an eating disturbance in your child.

3. Rather than placing your child on a diet, encourage more exercise. If possible, participate with your child in some form of exercise (e.g., walking, bicycling, aerobic exercise, dance classes).

4. Eat family meals together at least several times per week. Try to resist current societal norms, which would seem to dictate that families not eat together in the structured, routine ways of years ago. Encourage eating breakfast regularly; skipping breakfast promotes later bingeing on high-calorie foods (Carter and Fairburn, 1995; Paxton, 1996; Raphael, 1996; Steiner-Adair and Purcell, 1996). At mealtimes, stay away from emotionally charged topics. Discourage discussions about food or family conflicts; instead, encourage socialization and dialogue about family activities, especially children's interests and successes (Gilbert, 1986).

5. Remember that obese children sometimes eat to counter their feelings of insecurity or to cope with boredom. Again, make a concerted effort to eat

together as a family several times a week. Some authorities believe that the decline in family mealtimes has increased the incidence of eating problems, particularly obesity, because children turn to high-fat snack foods that are readily available to them.

6. In general, spend time interacting with your children about non-food-related topics and activities. This encourages them to socialize with other children and adults and helps them to develop a range of interests for which food is not the central focus.

ADDITIONAL GUIDELINES FOR PRIMARY CARE CLINICIANS

Restore Weight and Normal Eating Patterns

1. Focus first on weight restoration. There is general agreement that this should come early in the treatment of the anorectic patient, with the aim of restoring menstrual periods. Sometimes as much as 3,500 calories per day is necessary to initiate weight restoration; daily calories can be decreased as weight moves toward the normal range.
2. Suggest nutritional counseling and supervised mealtimes. Research demonstrates that anorectic patients with a body mass index less than 13 kg/m² have a poor prognosis and are at risk for substantial medical problems, even death, from emaciation (Hebebrand et al., 1997). They know how to sabotage refeeding programs by behaviors such as cutting food into little bits, smearing condiments or pats of butter under the table, or restricting their food choices to a very narrow range (e.g., refusing anything but vegetables and avoiding fat) (Densmore-John, 1988; Zerbe, 1993a). Nutritional counseling and supervised meals promote the goal of weight gain by increasing energy intake, expanding the diet, encouraging social skills at meals, confronting self-destructive eating patterns, and introducing formerly forbidden foods with reassurance and sensitivity.
3. Urge the patient to participate in individual or group therapy. Although most patients benefit from treatment in which the primary care clinican plays a focal role, the majority need ongoing support in the form of individual or group therapy. A 12-step fellowship may provide an adjunctive, cost-effective treatment; participation in such groups is gaining favor among some experts who view it as a component of a truly multifocal treatment plan (Johnson and Taylor, 1996).
4. If the patient is having severe difficulties, recommend hospital treatment or a structured outpatient program. In practice, many of these patients have difficulty eating 3,500 calories per day. A program that includes supervised, structured mealtimes is important in reestablishing normal eating patterns.

Become Familiar with and Utilize Psychopharmacologic Agents

1. Consider a trial of fluoxetine. Although no single psychopharmacologic agent has been demonstrated to be satisfactory as a sole or even primary treatment

for eating disorders, fluoxetine appears to have some success in (1) preventing relapse in weight-restored anorectic patients (Kaye et al., 1997); (2) decreasing the frequency of binge episodes and self-induced vomiting in patients with bulimia nervosa; and (3) helping those who fail to respond to psychotherapy or who present with concurrent major depression or anxiety (Agras et al., 1992; Jimerson et al., 1996; Walsh and Devlin, 1995; Walsh et al., 1997).

2. Be aware that the long-term use of fluoxetine for relapse prevention in bulimia nervosa is still undergoing clinical trial. Some physicians do use it long-term because of its safety and low side-effect profile. To curtail bulimic symptoms, many patients need up to 80 mg of fluoxetine per day (in contrast to the usual 20 mg for major depression).

3. Some patients respond to TCAs or MAOIs but not to the SSRIs. You may need to try several agents sequentially. Cyproheptadine has been used with some success to stimulate the appetites of anorexics. Zinc and naloxone (Narcan) are two miscellaneous drugs used with some success in the treatment of bulimia. Refer to specific pharmacologic texts or the latest summary of practice guidelines when deciding to employ these or other less commonly prescribed agents for eating disorders (Agras et al., 1992; Halmi, 1992; Kinoy, 1994; Zerbe, 1993a).

Consider Other Psychiatric Comorbidities and Refer to Appropriate Specialties

1. Identify any comorbid conditions. About 30% to 40% of patients with an eating disorder have a comorbid condition of depression, obsessive-compulsive disorder, alcoholism and/or substance abuse, personality disorder, or a history of physical and/or sexual abuse. Identification of any comorbidity is essential for recovery, because these patients will not respond unless both the eating disorder and the comorbid problem are addressed.

2. Reestablish adequate nutrition. Semistarvation impairs cognition, perhaps irreversibly (Golden et al., 1996; Katzman, et al., 1996; Krieg et al., 1988; Swayze et al., 1996). The patient cannot focus on psychological, family, or other issues until nutrition is attended to. When patients receive adequate nutrition, many symptoms remit, and the patient can then engage in therapy.

3. Be aware of factors found to be predictive of good and poor outcomes. Good outcome is associated with early age of onset, early intervention, friendships, and motivation for and response to treatment. Poor outcome is related to severe eating pathology, high frequency of vomiting, extreme weight fluctuations, impulsivity, suicidal behaviors, and poor self-esteem (Bemporad et al., 1992a; Herzog et al., 1996; Keel and Mitchell, 1997).

SUMMARY

Eating problems are increasing in frequency in all socioeconomic groups, yet they frequently go unrecognized and, consequently, are undertreated. Anorexia nervosa and bulimia nervosa are pathologic extremes of a continuum of weight-related attitudes and behaviors that are so common among young women in the United States and in cultures influenced by Western weight and dieting standards as to be considered normal (Friday, 1996; Hsu, 1996; Zerbe, 1993a). If primary care clinicians express stereotypical attitudes about nutrition and ideal weight, they can reinforce body preoccupation and dieting behavior in susceptible patients, thus contributing to the development of eating disorders. Primary prevention and the treatment process require that clinicians sensitively confront messages that promote an unhealthy focus on weight and diet composition. At the same time, clinicians must support guidelines for a healthy weight range, development of an exercise and muscle strengthening plan, and understanding of why patients struggle with body image and eating and how they get better.

Because these disorders occur across the life cycle, the primary care clinician is often the first person the patient seeks out for diagnosis and treatment. However, many patients are reluctant to reveal their symptoms because they feel shame, guilt, and embarrassment. Consequently, the primary care clinician must have a high index of suspicion about eating problems in women and must repeatedly ask questions about dietary restriction, modes of purging (including the life-threatening use of syrup of ipecac), laxative and diuretic abuse, and excessive exercise to control weight. Although anorexia nervosa and bulimia nervosa have been described most frequently in the early adolescent and late adolescent populations, these disorders are also seen with increasing frequency at midlife and late life, as well as in specific groups (e.g., models, athletes).

Frequently, a parent, spouse, sibling, or concerned friend turns to the primary care clinician with observations on the patient's disruptive eating patterns and preoccupation with body image. This involvement can be quite supportive in the overall treatment, particularly if education is given regarding the long-term physical and psychological effects of the eating disorder.

The first line of treatment is a thorough medical evaluation and nutritional stabilization. Laboratory values may be normal despite a severe eating disorder (Greenfeld et al., 1995; Mickley, 1994; Powers et al., 1995). Although new pharmacologic interventions (e.g., fluoxetine) are useful for many patients with anorexia nervosa or bulimia nervosa, nutritional stabilization and psychotherapy are the mainstays of contemporary intervention. These disorders are likely to be the final result of a host of intertwined biologic, societal, and psychological factors, and their treatment requires sensitivity to cultural and family issues and skilled psychotherapeutic support.

The long-term morbidity and mortality of eating disorders are among the highest of those for any psychiatric illness. Quality of life is dramatically diminished by the physical sequelae of the eating disorder and the psychological toll taken by the patient's preoccupation with her physical appearance. Long-term follow-up studies demonstrate that employment, relationships, sexual functioning, and parenting are compromised and not easily remediated (Bemporad 1992a, 1992b; Clinton, 1996; Keel and Mitchell, 1997).

As with other psychological and medical disorders, early intervention appears to be the key to a more favorable prognosis. The primary care clinician plays a significant role in both primary and secondary prevention of these illnesses by educating family members, teachers, and coaches. Early intervention by the primary care clinician also helps the patient avoid progressing to a more entrenched position, which is harder to tackle and carries a greater risk of physical, social, and psychological complications. The physician should maintain a high index of suspicion when patients request prescriptions for diuretics and appetite suppressants. The clinician should share information about self-help organizations and make appropriate referrals to mental health professionals when the problem does not abate quickly.

Studies now show that in 40% to 60% of cases eating symptoms are long-term. In these situations, the primary care clinician oversees medical management and handles treatment integration with mental health professionals. Even a patient who has been very ill for an extended period can improve when she addresses how she has used the eating disorder to cope with a variety of psychological stressors. Encouraging family members to address areas of overt or covert conflict is an important strategy. Patients still place great stock in the advice and perspective of their physician, and the primary care clinician who stresses development of a sense of control and effectiveness in life can help patients to overcome their sense of personal inadequacy, denial, and secrecy. Ultimately, this approach leads to a reduction in the frequency and tenacity of these pernicious symptoms, enlarges patients' capacity to enter and maintain affirming relationships, and thereby enhances recovery and resiliency.

Resources for Patients

Hall L (ed.): *Full Lives: Women Who Have Freed Themselves from Food and Weight Obsession.* Carlsbad, CA, Gürze Books, 1993.
This series of autobiographical accounts of women who have had, and recovered from, a serious eating disorder is a straightforward, fast, and inspiring read. The authors, themselves entrepreneurs, teachers, artists, clinicians, and speakers, address why they developed problems with food. These issues include sexual abuse, struggles with love and intimacy, society's obsession with thinness and beauty, the need for companionship, conflicts about becoming a parent, and the search for personal meaning and self-understanding. Struggles with anorexia, bulimia, binge eating, and obesity are covered. Practical suggestions and coping strategies are offered to help the patient come to terms with the role of eating in her own life and find her personal, individual path to recovery.
Nelson ME, Wernick F: *Strong Women Stay Young.* New York, Bantam Books, 1997.
Drawing on research from the Tufts University Nutrition Center, this program of twice-weekly strengthening exercises shows women how they can attain more energy, improve balance and physique, have greater body tone and flexibility, and live longer. For eating disorder patients, tips on how to "bone up the skeleton" are particularly important for reversing osteopenia. Exercises for aerobic and strength training help women of all ages develop a step-by-step program that is realistic but moderate. Tips for regular workouts will help obese patients tone and lose weight. Persons with anorexia and bulimia will be guided by the sensible dietary advice and scientifically tested exercise recommendations.
Zerbe KJ: *The Body Betrayed: Women, Eating Disorders, and Treatment.* Washington, DC, American Psychiatric Press, 1993 (softcover edition: Carlsbad, CA, Gürze Books, 1995).
Considered a comprehensive book that addresses all aspects of diagnosis, medical management, and psychiatric treatment of eating disorders, this book was written for patients, parents, significant others, and professionals who desire understanding and strategies that aid in recovery. Eating disorders are looked at across the life span, from childhood to old age. Special concerns for "at risk" groups such as athletes are reviewed. Containing numerous case examples of women who have struggled valiantly, although at first reluctantly, with eating disorders, the book offers a hopeful perspective on contemporary treatments and many practical suggestions for patients and treaters.

It also specifically tackles the impact of sexual and physical abuse, the relationship with chemical dependency and other psychiatric disorders, medical complications, the biology of nutrition, and special problems of sexuality and pregnancy. Conflicts in mother-daughter and father-daughter relationships that can lead to eating problems are discussed from a cultural, family, and individual perspective.

Resources for Clinicians

Kinoy BP (ed.): *Eating Disorders: New Directions in Treatment and Recovery*. New York, Columbia University Press, 1994.
> *For the primary care clinician who wishes to have a concise reference available on the bookshelf, this book is ideal. It includes an insightful discussion of the medical aspects of eating disorders and wise advice for successful psychotherapy and outpatient management. Topics include nutritional counseling, the benefit of psychiatric consultation, family intervention, therapeutic use of humor, and recovery tools. Written for physicians, nutritionists, nurses, and psychotherapists, this series of essays demonstrates many useful techniques that aid patients in recovery.*

Yager J (ed.): Eating disorders. *Psychiatr Clin North Am* 1996;19(4):639–882.
> *The chapters in this special journal issue cover assessment and evaluation, epidemiology, comorbidity and outcome, and the roles of cognitive-behavioral, 12-step, and feminist psychodynamic psychotherapy. Although written with the specialist in mind, this volume is a helpful reference for the primary care clinician who has a number of patients with eating disorders. Particularly applicable in the primary care setting are the chapters that address early treatment options for anorexia nervosa and bulimia nervosa, including special assessment techniques for athletes. Physical manifestations of eating disorders and medical complications are reviewed in excellent chapters on patient evaluation and the initial medical workup.*

Zerbe KJ: *The Body Betrayed: Women, Eating Disorders, and Treatment*. Washington, DC, American Psychiatric Press, 1993 (softcover edition: Carlsbad, CA, Gürze Books, 1995).
> *A comprehensive review of the current knowledge regarding eating disorders, this book is also a resource for additional information about obesity, the medical complications of eating disorders, pharmacotherapy of eating disorders, the biology of nutrition, and the psychiatric comorbidities that so often accompany eating disorders (e.g., chemical dependency, sexual and physical abuse, depression). Special sections on how eating disorders affect the pregnant patient and can occur over the entire life cycle (in infants, children, athletes, and older women) aid in the recognition and understanding of these disorders, which are frequently underrecognized in the primary care practice.*

References

Agras WS, Rossiter EM, Arnow B, et al.: Pharmacologic and cognitive-behavioral treatment for bulimia nervosa: A controlled comparison. *Am J Psychiatry* 1992;149:82–87.

American Psychiatric Association: *Diagnostic and Statistical Manual of Mental Disorders (DSM-III)*, 3rd ed. Washington, DC, American Psychiatric Association, 1980.

American Psychiatric Association: *Diagnostic and Statistical Manual of Mental Disorders (DSM-III-R)*, 3rd ed., revised. Washington, DC, Author, 1987.

American Psychiatric Association: *Diagnostic and Statistical Manual of Mental Disorders (DSM-IV)*, 4th ed. Washington, DC, Author, 1994.

Battle EK, Brownell KD: Confronting a rising tide of eating disorders and obesity: Treatment vs prevention and policy. *Addict Behav* 1996;21:755–765.

Bemporad JR, Beresen E, Ratey JJ, et al.: A psychoanalytic study of eating disorders: I. A developmental profile of 67 index cases. *J Am Acad Psychoanal* 1992a;20:509–532.

Bemporad JR, O'Driscoll G, Beresin E, et al.: A psychoanalytic study of eating disorders: II. Intergroup and intragroup comparisons. *J Am Acad Psychoanal* 1992b;20:533–542.

Blackburn GL, Brotman AW, Rosofsky WG: Why and how to stop weight cycling in overweight adults. *Eating Disorders Review* 1993;4:1–3.

Bloom C, Gitter A, Gutwill, S, et al.: *Eating Problems: A Feminist Psychoanalytic Treatment Model.* New York, Basic Books, 1994.

Brownell KD: *Lifestyle, Exercise, Attitudes, Relationships: The Learn Program for Weight Control.* Philadelphia, PA, University of Pennsylvania, 1988.

Brownell KD, Marlatt GA, Lichtenstein E, et al.: Understanding and preventing relapse. *Am Psychol* 1986;41:765–782.

Brownell KD, Wadden TA: Etiology and treatment of obesity: Understanding a serious, prevalent, and refractory disorder. *J Consult Clin Psychol* 1992;60:505–517.

Bruch H: *Eating Disorders.* London: Routledge & Kegan Paul, 1974.

Bruch H: *The Golden Cage: The Enigma of Anorexia Nervosa.* Cambridge, MA, Harvard Universities Press, 1978.

Bruch H: *Conversations with Anorexics.* Czyzewski D, Suhr MA (eds.). New York, Basic Books, 1988.

Carney CP, Andersen AE: Eating disorders: Guide to medical evaluation and complications. *Psychiatr Clin North Am* 1996;19:657–679.

Carter JC, Fairburn CG: Treating binge eating problems in primary care. *Addict Behav* 1995;20:765–772.

Clinton DN: Why do eating disorder patients drop out? *Psychother Psychosom* 1996;65:29–35.

Crisp AH: *Anorexia Nervosa: Let Me Be.* London, Academic Press, 1980.

Davis C, Durnin JVGA, Elliott S: Social, psychological, and behavioral factors related to body size in adult men and women: a comparison of methods. *Ann Behav Med* 1995a;17:25–31.

Davis C, Kennedy SH, Ralevski E, et al.: Obsessive compulsiveness and physical activity in anorexia nervosa and high-level exercising. *J Psychosom Res* 1995b;39:967–976.

Densmore-John J: Nutritional characteristics and consequences of anorexia nervosa and bulimia. In: Blinder BJ, Chaitin BF, Goldstein RS (eds.): *The Eating Disorders: Medical and Psychological Bases of Diagnosis and Treatment,* pp. 305–313. New York, PMA Publishing, 1988.

Devlin MJ: Assessment and treatment of binge-eating disorder. *Psychiatr Clin North Am* 1996;19:761–772.

DuPont RL: *The Selfish Brain: Learning from Addiction.* Washington, DC, American Psychiatric Press, 1997.

DuPont RL, McGovern JP: *A Bridge to Recovery: An Introduction to 12-Step Programs.* Washington, DC, American Psychiatric Press, 1994.

Edelstein CK, King BH: Pregnancy and eating disorders. In: Yager J, Gwirtsman HE, Edelstein CK (eds.): *Special Problems in Managing Eating Disorders,* pp. 163–184. Washington, DC, American Psychiatric Press, 1992.

Edelstein CK, Yager J: Eating disorders and affective disorders. In: Yager J, Gwirtsman HE, Edelstein CK (eds.). *Special Problems in Managing Eating Disorders,* pp. 15–50. Washington, DC, American Psychiatric Press, 1992.

Fairburn CG, Wilson GT (eds.): *Binge Eating: Nature, Assessment, and Treatment.* New York, Guilford, 1993.

Fallon P, Katzman MA, Wooley SC (eds.): *Feminist Perspectives on Eating Disorders.* New York, Guilford, 1994.

Foreyt JP, Poston WS 2nd, Goodrick GK: Future directions in obesity and eating disorders. *Addict Behav* 1996;21:767–778.

Friday N: *The Power of Beauty.* New York, Harper Collins, 1996.

Frisch RE: Fatness and fertility. *Sci Am* 1988;258:88–95.

Frisch RE: The right weight: body fat, menarche, and fertility [editorial]. *Nutrition* 1996;12:452–53

Gilbert S: *The Pathology of Eating: Psychology and Treatment.* London, Routledge & Kegan Paul, 1986.

Golden NH, Ashtari M, Kohn MR, et al.: Reversibility of cerebral ventricular enlargement in anorexia nervosa, demonstrated by quantitative magnetic resonance imaging. *J Pediatr* 1996;128:296–301.

Gortmaker SA, Must A, Perrin JM, et al.: Social and economic consequences of overweight in adolescence and young adulthood. *N Engl J Med* 1993;329:1003–1012.

Graber JA, Brooks-Gunn J: Prevention of eating problems and disorders: including patients. *Eating Disorders: Journal of Treatment and Prevention* 1996;4:348–363.

Greenfeld D, Mickley D, Quinlan DM, et al.: Hypokalemia in outpatients with eating disorders. *Am J Psychiatry* 1995;152:60–63.

Greeno CG, Wing RR: A double-blind placebo-controlled trial of the effect of fluoxetine on dietary intake in overweight women with and without binge-eating disorder. *Am J Clin Nutr* 1996;64:267–273.

Guy-Grand B, Appelbaum M, Crepaldi G, et al.: International trial of long-term dexfenfluramine in obesity. *Lancet* 1989;2(8672):1142–1145.

Hall L (ed): *Full Lives: Women Who Have Freed Themselves from Food and Weight Obsession.* Carlsbad, CA, Gürze Books, 1993.

Halmi KA: *Psychobiology and Treatment of Anorexia Nervosa and Bulimia Nervosa.* Washington, DC, American Psychiatric Press, 1992.

Halmi KA: Eating disorders: anorexia nervosa, bulimia nervosa, and obesity. In: Hales RE, Yudofsky SC, Talbott JA (eds.): *American Psychiatric Press Textbook of Psychiatry*, 2nd ed., pp. 857–875. Washington, DC, American Psychiatric Press, 1994.

Halmi KA, Eckert E, Marchi P, et al.: Comorbidity of psychiatric diagnoses in anorexia nervosa. *Arch Gen Psychiatry* 1991;48:712–718.

Hebebrand J, Himmelmann GW, Herzog W, et al.: Prediction of low body weight at long-term follow-up in acute anorexia nervosa by low body weight at referral. *Am J Psychiatry* 1997;154:566–569.

Herzog W, Deter HC, Fiehn W, Petzold E: Medical findings and predictors of long-term physical outcome in anorexia nervosa: A prospective, 12-year follow-up study. *Psychol Med* 1997;27:269–279.

Herzog DB, Nussbaum KM, Marmor AK: Comorbidity and outcome in eating disorders. *Psychiatr Clin North Am* 1996;19:843–859.

Hsu LK: Critique of follow-up studies. In: Halmi KA (ed.): *Psychobiology and Treatment of Anorexia Nervosa and Bulimia Nervosa*, pp. 125–147. Washington, DC, American Psychiatric Press, 1992.

Hsu LK: Epidemiology of eating disorders. *Psychiatr Clin North Am* 1996;19:681–700.

Hsu LK, Crisp AH, Callender JS: Psychiatric diagnoses in recovered and unrecovered anorectics 22 years after onset of illness: a pilot study. *Compr Psychiatry* 1992;33:123–127.

Jimerson DC, Wolfe BE, Brotman AE, et al.: Medications in the treatment of eating disorders. *Psychiatr Clin North Am* 1996;19:739–754.

Johnson C, Connors ME: *The Etiology and Treatment of Bulimia Nervosa: A Biopsychosocial Perspective.* New York, Basic Books, 1987.

Johnson C, Taylor C: Working with difficult-to-treat eating disorders using an integration of twelve-step and traditional psychotherapies. *Psychiatr Clin North Am* 1996;19:829–842.

Katzman DK, Lambe EK, Mikulis DJ, et al.: Cerebral gray matter and white matter volume deficits in adolescent girls with anorexia nervosa. *J Pediatr* 1996;129:794.

Kaye WH, Weltzin TE, Hsu G, et al.: Relapse prevention with fluoxetine in anorexia nervosa: a double-blind placebo-controlled study. Paper presented at the 150th Annual Meeting of the American Psychiatric Association, San Diego, California, May 21, 1997.

Kearney-Cooke A, Striegel-Moore RH: Treatment of childhood sexual abuse in anorexia nervosa and bulimia nervosa: A feminist psychodynamic approach. *Int J Eat Disord* 1994;15:305–319.

Keel PK, Mitchell JE: Outcome in bulimia nervosa. *Am J Psychiatry* 1997;154:313–321.

Kendler KS, MacLean C, Neale M, et al.: The genetic epidemiology of bulimia nervosa. *Am J Psychiatry* 1991;148:1627–1637.

Keys A, Brozek J, Herschel A, et al.: *The Biology of Human Starvation.* Minneapolis, MN, University of Minnesota Press, 1950.

Kinoy BP (ed.): *Eating Disorders: New Directions in Treatment and Recovery.* New York, Columbia University Press, 1994.

Kral JG: Surgical treatment of obesity. In: Wadden TA, Van Itallie TB (eds.): *Treatment of the Seriously Obese Patient*, pp. 496–506. New York, Guilford, 1992.

Krieg J-C, Pirke K-M, Lauer C: Endocrine, metabolic, and cranial computed tomographic findings in anorexia nervosa. *Biol Psychiatry* 1988;23:377.

Kucazmarski RJ, Flegal KM, Campbell SM, et al.: Increasing prevalence of overweight among U.S. adults: The National Health and Nutrition Examination Surveys, 1960 to 1991. *JAMA* 1994;272:205–211.

Levine MD, Marcus MD, Moulton P: Exercise in the treatment of binge eating disorder. *Int J Eat Disord* 1996;19:171–177.

Marcus MD: Binge eating in obesity. In: Fairburn CG, Wilson GT (eds.): *Binge Eating: Nature, Assessment, and Treatment*, pp. 77–96. New York, Guilford, 1993.

Marcus MD, Smith D, Santelli R, et al.: Characterization of eating disordered behavior in obese binge eaters. *Int J Eat Disord* 1992;12:249–255.

Marrazzi MA, Markham KM, Kinzie J, et al.: Binge eating disorder: Response to naltrexone. *Int J Obes Relat Metab Disord* 1995;19:143–145.

Mercer E, Holder MD: Food cravings, endogeneous opioid peptides, and food intake: A review. Appetite 1997;29:325–352.

Meyer AE, von Holtzapfel B, Deffner G, et al.: Psychoendocrinology of remenorrhea in the late outcome of anorexia nervosa. *Psychother Psychosom* 1986;45:174–185.

Mickley DW: Medical aspects of anorexia and bulimia. In: Kinoy B (ed.): *Eating Disorders: New Directions in Treatment and Recovery*, pp. 7–14. New York, Columbia University Press, 1994.

Miller PM: Redefining success in eating disorders. *Addict Behav* 1996;21;745–754.

Minuchin S, Rosman BL, Baker L: *Psychosomatic Families: Anorexia Nervosa in Context*. Cambridge, Harvard University Press, 1978.

Mitchell JE, Hatsukami DK, Pyle RL, et al.: Bulimia with and without a family history of depressive illness. *Compr Psychiatry* 1986;27:215–219.

Mitchell JE, Specker SM, de Zwaan M: Comorbidity and medical complications of bulimia nervosa. *J Clin Psychiatry* 1991;52(Suppl):13–20.

National Task Force on the Prevention and Treatment of Obesity: Long-term pharmacotherapy in the management of obesity. *JAMA* 1996;276:1907–1915.

Nelson ME, Wernick F: *Strong Women Stay Young*. New York, Bantam Books, 1997.

Palazzoli MD: *Self-Starvation: From the Intrapsychic to Transpersonal Approach*. New York, Jason Aronson, 1978.

Paxton SJ: Prevention implications of peer influences on body image dissatisfaction and disturbed eating in adolescent girls. *Eating Disorders: Journal of Treatment and Prevention* 1996;4:334–347.

Piran N: The reduction of preoccupation with body weight and shape in school: a feminist approach. *Eating Disorders: Journal of Treatment and Prevention* 1996;4:323–333.

Powers PS: Initial assessment and early treatment options for anorexia nervosa and bulimia nervosa. *Psychiatr Clin North Am* 1996;19:639–655.

Powers PS, Johnson C: Small victories: prevention of eating disorders among athletes. *Eating Disorders: Journal of Treatment and Prevention* 1996;4:364–377.

Powers PS, Tyson IB, Stevens BA, et al.: Total body potassium and serum potassium among eating disorder patients. *Int J Eat Disorders* 1995;18:269–276.

Raphael F: The prevention of eating disorders. In: Kendrick T, Tylee A, Freeling PA (eds.): *The Prevention of Mental Illness in Primary Care*, pp. 207–222. Cambridge, Cambridge University Press, 1996.

Rock DL, Curran-Celentano J: Nutritional management of eating disorders. *Psychiatr Clin North Am* 1996;19:701–713.

Rorty M, Yager J: Histories of childhood trauma and complex post-traumatic sequelae in women with eating disorders: *Psychiatr Clin North Am* 1996;19:773–791.

Simpson WS, Ramberg JA: Sexual dysfunction in married female patients with anorexia and bulimia nervosa. *J Sex Marital Ther* 1992;18:44–54.

St. Jeor ST (ed): *Obesity Assessment: Tools, Methods, Interpretations. A Reference Case: The RENO Diet-Heart Study*. New York, Chapman & Hall, 1997.

Steiner-Adair C, Purcell A: Approaches to mainstreaming eating disorders prevention. *Eating Disorders: Journal of Treatment and Prevention* 1996;4:294–309.

Stewart DE, Robinson GE, Goldbloom DS, et al.: Infertility and eating disorders. *Am J Obstet Gynecol* 1990;163:1996.

Stunkard AJ, Wadden TA (eds.): *Obesity: Theory and Therapy*, 2nd ed. New York, Raven Press, 1992.

Swayze VW II, Andersen A, Arndt S, et al.: Reversibility of brain tissue loss in anorexia nervosa assessed with a computerized Talairach 3-D proportional grid. *Psychol Med* 1996;26:381.

Walsh BT, Devlin MJ: Pharmacotherapy of bulimia nervosa and binge eating disorder. *Addict Behav* 1995;29:757–764.

Walsh BT, Wilson GT, Loeb KL, et al.: Medication and psychotherapy in the treatment of bulimia nervosa. *Am J Psychiatry* 1997;154:523–531.

Weintraub M: Long-term weight control study. *Clin Pharmacol Ther* 1992;51(5):642–646.

Weintraub M, et al.: Long-term weight control study. I-VII. *Clin Pharmacol Ther* 1992;51(5):586–641.

Wiederman MW, Pryor T: Substance use among women with eating disorders. *Int J Eat Disorders* 1996;20:163–168.

Yager J (ed.): Eating disorders. *Psychiatr Clin North Am* 1996;19(4):639–882.

Yates A: *Compulsive Exercise and the Eating Disorders: Toward an Integrated Theory of Activity*. New York, Brunner/Mazel, 1991.

Zerbe KJ: Eating disorders in the 1990s: clinical challenges and treatment implications. *Bull Menninger Clin* 1992a;56:167–187.

Zerbe KJ: Why eating-disordered patients resist sex therapy: a response to Simpson and Ramberg. *J Sex Marital Ther* 1992b;18:55–64.

Zerbe KJ: *The Body Betrayed: Women, Eating Disorders, and Treatment.* Washington, American Psychiatric Press, 1993a. (Softcover edition: *The Body Betrayed: A Deeper Understanding of Women, Eating Disorders, and Treatment.* Carlsbad, CA, Gürze Books, 1995.)

Zerbe KJ: Selves that starve and suffocate: the continuum of eating disorders and dissociative phenomena. *Bull Menninger Clin* 1993b;57:319–327.

Zerbe KJ: Whose body is it anyway? Understanding and treating psychosomatic aspects of eating disorders. *Bull Menninger Clin* 1993c;57:161–177.

Zerbe KJ: The emerging sexual self of the patient with an eating disorder: implications for treatment. *Eating Disorders: Journal of Treatment and Prevention* 1995;3:197–215.

Zerbe KJ: Feminist psychodynamic psychotherapy of eating disorders: theoretic integration informing clinical practice. *Psychiatr Clin North Am* 1996;19:811–827.

Zerbe, KJ: Eating disorders. In: Wallis L (ed.): *Women's Health*, pp. 839–848. New York, Lippincott-Raven, 1998.

Chapter 6

Trauma and Violence

At the outbreak of World War II, the poet W. H. Auden captured in one short stanza a horrifying but indisputable hallmark of the residual effects of trauma and violence:

I and the public know what all school children learn.
Those to whom evil is done do evil in return.

(From *September 1, 1939*, p. 57)

Psychological trauma is a formidable clinical and societal problem. It tends to repeat itself from generation to generation because its victims defensively reenact the evil that has been done to them by vicariously or overtly repeating it with those they hold most dear, especially significant others and children (Davidson, 1993; Plakun, 1998). The distress of the traumatized patient is palpable, manifesting itself in a range of feelings, from anger to depression, and in a range of psychological defenses, such as aggressive outbursts, verbal provocation, disavowal (e.g., "This never really happened to me"), and guilt feelings. Posttraumatic stress disorder (PTSD) is one of the most commonly discussed psychiatric syndromes in the popular press. Women and men are increasingly open about the damaging effects of inappropriately sexualized and abusive relationships, and the mass media take us into the lives of people who have survived natural and manmade disasters. Rarely does a day go by without some reference to the painful effects of trauma on people's lives and how they attempt to navigate away from it or adapt to its consequences. Moreover, increasingly in our society, violence is moving out of the home and into the schoolyard, workplace, and neighborhood. No one is immune to the impact of trauma and its potentially devastating effects, and no physician can avoid seeing its ravages in practice.

Trauma's victims are often debilitated because their capacity to cope is overwhelmed. What is particularly beguiling to clinicians is the fact that no two persons handle overwhelming stress in the same way (Tables 6–1 and 6–2). Whether a woman develops psychiatric symptoms within days, months, or even years—or not at all—after a traumatic event depends on her characteristics, her psychological health before the trauma, her age, the unique personal meaning she attaches to the event, and her support system during recovery.

In the course of a lifetime few escape traumatic events, but often victims are left to deal with the psychological consequences alone. Overwhelming rage and a sense of helplessness are the most common responses, but they erupt particularly when a catastrophe comes out of the blue, is experienced as malevolent and random, or takes the life of a loved one. For example, Susan Cohen is the mother of 20-year-old Theo Cohen, who was murdered when terrorists blew up Pan Am Flight 103 over Lockerbie, Scotland, on December 21, 1988. Mrs.

Table 6–1. **Hallmark Signs of Posttraumatic Reaction**

Reaction	Manifestation
Hyperalertness/hyperarousal	Anger
	Inability to sleep; hyperirritability
	Exaggerated startle response
Intrusive thoughts	Flashbacks, nightmares, memories
	Provoked by anything that symbolizes or reminds the patient of the trauma
Emotional constriction	Numbing, avoiding situations
	Feeling "cut off" from friends or loved ones
	Withdrawal from social events

Cohen poignantly captures for many the "nightmare world" of personal catastrophe when she writes:

> Of all the emotions I have held since Theo's murder, anger is the best. Rage gives me energy. Rage makes me strong. . . . I live my diminished life. But grief is always there. I am in pain all the time. . . . Call it living defensively, this always being prepared for the unexpected reminder, always being on guard against the shock that creates panic, this eternal vigilance against the innocent remark that will bring on depression. . . . Like a child going through nightly rituals to ward off fear of the dark, I too must be especially careful at bedtime. . . . If I fall asleep, I dream: Catastrophic dreams, sad dreams, dreams of searching for Theo.
>
> (Cohen, 1996, p. 50)

This chapter describes the diagnosis and treatment of the effects of trauma and violence from a biologic, cultural, and psychological perspective, suggesting practical ways in which the primary care clinician can intervene. The unbroken cycle of abuse and violence that eventuates in battery, domestic violence, emotional/physical and sexual violation of children, and rape can be severed only when each person takes responsibility for ending it. The primary care clinician plays a pivotal role in making the diagnosis and in urging victims (and sometimes perpetrators) to invest themselves in comprehensive treatment approaches (Leeder, 1994).

The residual effects of domestic violence, sexual abuse, and rape are emphasized here because they are the principal causes of PTSD in women. However, the diagnostic and treatment principles apply to any traumatic event that leaves

Table 6–2. **Psychiatric Problems Associated with Trauma**

Depression
Anxiety and phobias
Alcoholism and/or chemical dependency
Eating disorders
Increased lifetime rate of attempted suicide
Dissociative disorders/complex posttraumatic stress disorder
Self-harm and risk-taking
Sexual dysfunction (e.g., lack of sexual desire)

a patient with residual symptoms. In studies of community samples, many stressors were found to precipitate the syndrome of PTSD, including motor vehicle accidents, catastrophic medical illnesses (e.g., burns, myocardial infarction), and various types of employment. PTSD may develop in any occupation where the individual is exposed to "life-threatening situations and violent or grotesque scenes" (Davis and Breslau, 1994, p. 293).

ROLE OF THE PRIMARY CARE CLINICIAN

Once again, the primary care clinician is on the front line in recognizing and intervening with an epidemic public health problem. The personal and societal sequelae of child maltreatment and adult abuse are enormous. Between 3 and 4 million women are victims of domestic abuse annually. Murder by an intimate is a major cause of death among women and the leading cause of death for African-American women age 15 to 34 years (Campbell, 1992; Farley, 1986; Vasquez, 1996). Depression, anxiety disorders, and eating disorders are frequent comorbid symptoms of trauma and tend to be refractory to psychiatric intervention unless the trauma is addressed (Allen, 1995; Breslau et al., 1997; Campbell et al., 1996; Davidson, 1993; Zerbe, 1993/1995).

It is estimated that violence occurs at least once in 66% of all marriages. Ninety-five percent of domestic abuse victims are women, who are also three times as likely as men to be victims of a violent crime by a family member. Indeed, wife beating results in more injuries requiring medical treatment than do sexual assaults, automobile accidents, and robberies. Twenty-one percent of pregnant women are abused, and these women are twice as likely to miscarry compared with nonabused women. Both men and women who have been physically or sexually abused in childhood are likely to become perpetrators in adulthood (Campbell et al., 1996; Eby et al., 1995; Freund, 1995; Radford and Russell, 1992).

Rigorous epidemiologic research indicates that 1 woman in 4 in the United States will be raped at some time during her life, and that 1 in 3 has been sexually abused in childhood (Campbell, 1992; Radford and Russell, 1992; Russell, 1986). But even these stark findings do not take into account the high rate of verbal abuse and physical violence missed by even the most thorough studies. Experts in the field of domestic violence estimate that 1 in 4 women presenting at an urban emergency room has actually experienced domestic or sexual battery within the past year (Campbell, 1995; Feldhaus et al., 1997). The risk of "femicide" (Radford and Russell, 1992) increases when there is a history of beating and the woman decides to leave. As Campbell elucidates regarding issues of power and control in the relationship between battered women and their spouses, the woman's partner is essentially saying, "If I can't have you, no one can" (Campbell, 1992, p. 111).

EFFECTS ON CHILDREN

This women's health problem naturally carries over to affect the lives of our nation's children. In at least 50% of families where the mother is abused, the child is also abused (Freund, 1995; Leeder, 1994; Olds et al., 1997). Children who witness incidents of violence are inevitably traumatized, but they rarely receive counseling or emotional support. In addition, abused children may have severe behavioral and emotional problems but are often inaccessible to intervention. They make psychological adaptations "to abusive situations and to enduring relationship patterns that present both impediments and opportunities for treatment" (Barber et al., 1994, p. 64). Physicians fail to identify the problem because of time constraints, because of lack of training and experience, and especially because they know that they will be required to report such situations to legal authorities (Flitcraft, 1998). This failure to identify child abuse produces long-term effects on children's development and behavior, including learning problems, depression and anxiety, tendency to express pent-up feelings in somatic problems, and imitative violent behavior (see Table 6–2).

Children naturally want to be like adults. Those who repeatedly witness or experience violence by adults do not learn how to contain their own aggressive behavior because they have poor role models. Children in such situations often have poor peer relationships, bully other children, and in extreme cases engage in animal torture and killing. In one controlled study of 68 sexually abused children and 75 control subjects, Swanston and colleagues (1997) found significant behavioral problems, including depression, anxiety, and eating disorders in the victimized group; these children also suffered from poorer self-esteem, fewer social networks, and more attempted suicides, and they had a higher incidence of smoking and other self-injuries than did control subjects. The impaired children were more likely to have parents with drug and alcohol problems (see Chapter 4). None of these research findings will surprise any clinician who has worked for even a short time in an emergency room setting or office-based practice and has seen the immediate and long-term psychological, physical, and social difficulties associated with child abuse.

WHY THE PATIENT DOES NOT TELL: THE ROLE OF SHAME AND STIGMA

Both abused women and abused children have a tendency to believe that they "caused" the abuse, leading to a vicious cycle of self-blame and shame. Consequently, it is difficult for them to tell the clinician about what has happened, particularly if they are not asked openly and repeatedly. Often a diagnosis of abuse is missed, not because the clinician does not ask, but because the patients cannot bring themselves to tell. For example, the abused woman may worry about recrimination from her partner and her clinician. As Alice Brand Bartlett (1996), a psychoanalyst at The Menninger Clinic, aptly observed, "Due to shame and her wish to avoid painful memories and feelings, she may not mention the experience again unless the clinician can create a safe and supportive treatment environment" (p. 148). In such an environment, details of the history can be elicited and heard. The most important steps for primary care clinicians to take are to (1) recognize the pervasiveness of childhood and adult abuse; (2) learn to suspect its occurrence, particularly when other physical or emotional problems are present; and (3) ask about abuse—and ask again if you suspect that the patient is denying that it happened or is unable to tell you.

Clinicians wonder why so many patients fail to reveal a problem and, when they do, why they refuse to accept the offer of support or assistance. This dilemma leads clinicians to feel frustrated, and they often become convinced that the problem is unsolvable. Understanding the patient's reluctance helps clinicians bear the long periods of reticence during which a woman may not be verbally forthcoming even while she nonverbally or psychosomatically indicates a history of violence, abuse, assault, or catastrophe (e.g., accident). For example, one primary care clinician suspected abuse for a long time and frequently questioned his patient about it despite her repeated denials. The clinician did not know how he knew—"I just knew." After several years of developing an alliance with the patient, the clinician enabled her to share her plight.

Even when clinicians provide a safe, nonjudgmental environment, patients may repeatedly deny ongoing or past domestic violence or a history of childhood abuse or adult rape. Such denial is pervasive because women tend to blame themselves for incurring the abuse. Furthermore, the abused woman suspects that you will react "like everybody else and not believe me." This impression inadvertently exacerbates her already low self-worth. She suspects that you are asking, under your breath, "What did you do to bring this on yourself, and why didn't you stop it?"

TRAUMATIC BONDS

Clinicians have long been perplexed about why traumatized persons stay in abusive relationships. Attachment theory (Allen, 1995, 1996a, 1996b; Bowlby 1973, 1979; Goldberg et al., 1995) has helped therapists to understand the tenacious role of the familiar in our lives and the pervasive need humans have for contact with others. An abusive relationship is difficult for the patient to disengage from because without it she feels even more anxious, disconnected, and alone. Many patients clearly state that they fear what their partner will do if they leave, but they also fear being without them because this is what they know. They have grown comfortable with the familiar—and with the intermittent periods of security and kindness when the partner vows "never to do it again" (Walker, 1979). In essence, in abusive relationships women become attached to a traumatic bond instead of a healthy one (Vasquez, 1996). Women persist in their attachment to abusive relationships, despite even malignant consequences, because they provide the security of the known and familiar.

Obviously, to dislodge such a vicious and long-established relationship requires first the formation and nurturing of a "secure base" (i.e., the psychotherapeutic relationship). Treatment of trauma and abuse can take a long time, depending on the internal resources of motivation, intelligence, and hopefulness of the patient. Contemporary psychodynamic psychotherapy has integrated attachment theory research and has demonstrated how remembering and openly discussing unhappy, stifling, and frankly abusive attachment experiences does lead to change in many victims of abuse. In essence, the patient forms a secure, nonabusive attachment with the psychotherapist, who not only provides "the feeling of well being and security" but facilitates "exploration of the world and of oneself" (Eagle, 1995, p. 128). But primary care clinicians must strongly and consistently express the idea that change is possible and offer initial guidance in helping the patient form new, healthier connections in which her needs are recognized. The personal reminiscence of one former victim speaks to the crucial role her primary care clinician played in moving her toward recovery, healing, and ultimately more satisfying relationships:

"Nobody has the right to hurt you," said the doctor. Terrorized by my husband, I had believed that I, indeed, deserved the punishment. I must be a very bad person. My self-esteem was at bottom low. The phrase reassured me that nobody, myself included, deserves to be beaten. It started to build up my self-confidence. On the other hand, I was lucky that morning in the emergency room, not to hear two questions that frequently plague victims of domestic violence. Nobody asked "What did you do to provoke it?" and "Why have you not left him?"

(Seaman, 1998, p. 259)

CREATING A "SAFE PLACE"

Although it is important for the primary care clinician to be able to (1) inquire privately about the source of injury, (2) document it carefully, (3) make referrals to shelters and other agencies that can provide support, and (4) help protect the survivor from the perpetrator by drawing on the resources of local social service agencies, it is also essential to provide a calm and stable relationship over time in order to reduce anxiety and feelings of disconnection. Patients who have been traumatized have grown comfortable with the familiar. They are so locked into the trauma that all relationships are experienced based on the past, but it is inaccurate to describe such persons as masochistic. They do not find pleasure in suffering. With respect to victims of sexual trauma and domestic abuse, senior psychologist Jon Allen of The Menninger Clinic, explains: "Patients are far more likely to feel helped and supported by the assumption that they are trying to suffer less, although they may not be going about it in the best way. . . . They are more comfortable with the familiar" (1996b, p. 7). Thus abused women gravitate to relationships that are emotionally intense (violent) or isolated and disconnected. Over time, they must learn that benign relationships can be formed, and that within these relationships they can be cared for with compassion and respect. For these reasons, long-term psychotherapy is indicated, even though it is difficult for such persons to engage in it.

Having no role model for a calm, stable, and durable relationship, the patients may actually miss the intense personal contact that an abusive interaction provides. They tend to feel lonely, bored, or anxious when extricating themselves from the damaging bond. Hence, even when you have done your best to encourage them to get into and continue an individual or group psychotherapy process, it is not uncommon to witness a patient sabotaging herself. Learning how to form a secure attachment to "interrupt the continual repetition of abusive relationships and their perpetuation into further generations" (Allen, 1996b, p. 13) occurs only after frequent reassurances that you respect and appreciate the patient's attempts to form a better life for herself. This task is neither dramatic nor curative, but it is enormously helpful in indicating to the patient that you care and understand the complexity of her experience.

SCREENING FOR VIOLENCE AND ABUSE IN PRIMARY CARE: WHAT A BUSY PRACTITIONER CAN DO QUICKLY

Several clinical assessment tools are now available to help clinicians assess for domestic abuse and/or posttraumatic stress after rape, natural disaster, or sexual or physical abuse (Bartlett, 1996; Campbell, 1986, 1995; Feldhaus et al., 1997). Because a thorough assessment usually takes 1 to 3 hours, primary care clinicians should have ready access to specialty consultation and community support services (e.g., hotlines, support groups, battered women's shelters). However, a few questions that take only several minutes to ask usually uncover what needs to be known to begin office management. Nonabused patients will not become irritated when you ask these questions; they will understand that you are paying attention to a pervasive social malady. For the woman who has been or is being abused, your acknowledgment of the problem as a real event underscores your concern and advocacy position.

Begin by asking questions directly but in a safe place where privacy and confidentiality can be maintained. Let the patient know that you are inquiring because violence against women is a rampant societal ill. In this way, you are essentially saying that she is not alone and should not judge herself as harshly as she otherwise might.

You might begin by asking the following: (1) Have you been hit, kicked, or otherwise hurt by someone in the past year and, if so, by whom? (2) Do you feel safe in your current relationship? (3) Is there a partner from a previous relationship who is making you feel unsafe now? These queries, from the Partner Violence Screen (PVS), have a predictive value of almost 90% for domestic abuse (Feldhaus et al., 1997). In the review of systems, look for clusters of physical health symptoms frequently reported by victims of trauma; these are outlined in Table 6–3 (Abbott et al., 1995; Campbell, 1995; Feldhaus et al., 1997; McAfee, 1995).

If you have time, you could inquire further about the quality of relationships in the family. Particularly relevant are how close to each other family members feel, whether they eat dinner together, and how disputes are resolved. In the history taking, be particularly alert for the associated comorbid psychiatric problems of depression, substance abuse, and eating disorders (e.g., bulimia), which are often linked with past or ongoing trauma (see Table 6–2).

WHAT DO I DO BEFORE THE PATIENT LEAVES MY OFFICE?

Most patients with a history of trauma or ongoing domestic abuse will need the help of additional resources. Be aware of shelter programs in your commu-

---

Table 6–3. **Physical Health Symptoms Reported by Battered Women**

Weight changes
Chronic pain (old injuries that have not healed)
Symptoms suggesting neurologic damage (especially headache, blurred vision, ringing in ear, dizziness)
Gynecologic symptoms (pelvic pain, missed periods, painful intercourse, vaginal bleeding or discharge)
Gastrointestinal complaints (irritable bowel syndrome)
Anxiety/posttraumatic stress disorder symptoms (nightmares, difficulty sleeping, trembling, dyspnea, heart pounding and/or palpitations)
Burns
Fractures
Damaged viscera

---

nity. If possible, acquaint yourself with community agencies and have materials from them available (Keller, 1996). If there is no local resource, refer the patient to the National Domestic Violence Hotline (1-800-799-SAFE/1-800-799-7233). In some jurisdictions, you may be required to report the abuse. Marjory Braude, MD, an expert in the diagnosis and treatment of domestic violence, reminded clinicians that despite the burden this kind of medical and social activism places on their shoulders, such interventions are potentially as lifesaving as in any other disease. She stated, "Yes, it is more work to investigate and assess the situation properly. It is also work to investigate and treat a cancer or rare disease as we are trained to do. To assist a woman to develop the resources to help herself can equally save her life and health" (1998, p. 142).

IS THERE ANYTHING I SHOULD *NOT* ASK OR DO?

There are some real pitfalls in working with victims of acute or chronic trauma, be it childhood abuse, domestic violence, or natural disaster. Every clinician knows of or has read about a dedicated physician who became overly involved with a patient in order to "rescue" him or her from a horrific past or unsatisfactory relationship. The primary care clinician must be aware of these occurrences and remain mindful of unhelpful overinvolvement in office practice (Figley, 1995; Plakun, 1998).

First, because patients tend to reenact rather than remember their abuse, sexually traumatized patients can be beguiling and seductive during the clinical encounter. Through no fault of their own, they are attempting to master anxiety and/or the actual traumatic experience. Think of it this way: Poor modeling of how to deal with sexual feelings, intense anger, and the like has led these patients to act on their feelings rather than put them into words. Your ability to model professional boundaries (e.g., not to become sexually involved; not to believe that you can "rescue" the patient by doing all the treatment by yourself) actually helps the patient find an appropriate place (e.g., psychotherapy) where she can develop a capacity to reflect rather than act on her feelings.

Also pervasive is the tendency for some women who have experienced trauma to "just want to get all the feelings out of my system." People handle overwhelming stress in very different ways, but most can benefit from a systematic processing of the events (see Bartlett, 1996; Peebles, 1989; Peebles-Kleiger, 1989).

The patient must learn to trust her world and her emotional reactions again (Foa and Riggs, 1993; Menninger and Wilkinson, 1988). This takes time and patience, which "help reverse the paralytic passivity caused by acute trauma" (Peebles-Kleiger and Zerbe, 1998, p. 188). Social and family supports are also crucial in helping the patient face any tendency for guilt or self-blame. Those who have a social network fare better than those who do not, particularly in situations such as physical catastrophe or rape.

When a victim survives and a close friend or relative does not, the patient is left to deal with the aftermath of "survivor guilt" (Foa and Riggs, 1993; Menninger and Wilkinson, 1988). Those who can validate the victim's symptoms and encourage her to talk and to go on with her life despite the catastrophe enable her to overcome a tendency for self-blame while she processes the trauma.

Social supports assist the woman by counteracting a self-accusation that "the symptoms represent inadequate coping" (Foa and Riggs, 1993, p. 292).

The clinician must avoid what psychologists and psychiatrists call "overwhelming and retraumatizing abreaction" (Bartlett, 1996, p. 151). In the early part of the 20th century, therapists routinely recommended emotional catharsis (Peebles, 1989); now it is generally conceded that abreaction can be damaging. Most people cannot simply purge intense feelings and move on with life. If this were the case, posttraumatic problems could be solved by reading a book, seeing a movie, or attending a couple of therapeutic sessions. Consequently, skilled psychotherapists have shifted the focus of trauma treatment from abreaction or catharsis to learning to handle "a small package of intense feelings" one step at a time. Bartlett (1996) likens this approach to taking a "biopsy of the patient's representational world" (p. 154), which helps construct a narrative of what has actually happened to her. This approach of slowly reconstructing the patient's personal story avoids the untoward consequences of becoming unwittingly and traumatically overwhelmed. It also respects the victim's autonomy and provides her with a psychological holding environment while she regains her perspective and strength.

HELPING THE PATIENT FIND COURAGE

Do not minimize the strength it takes for a woman to leave an abusive situation or to decide to work with her past traumas in therapy. Many patients have been retraumatized by clinicians who have inadvertently wondered out loud, "Why do you stay in this abusive relationship?" Instead, this question should be reframed as, "What does my patient need in order to leave?" (Silverman-Yam, 1996, p. 5).

Underscore the patient's desire to protect herself and her children, and convey to her your own appreciation of the enormity of her decision. She has lost the belief that others can understand or tolerate her experience. Help her regain control and put into place healthier defenses. This approach includes listing concrete resources she will need, such as finances, housing, health care, and child care (Braude, 1998; Marmar et al., 1993; Reubens, 1996; Stewart and Robinson, 1996). The ongoing involvement of a skilled social worker and/or social services staff member is usually essential. The expertise of these professionals in knowing how to navigate the judicial and community support system so that the patient can obtain needed financial and housing resources astounds medical personnel, whose adroitness lies in other arenas.

For example, a batterer frequently denies his partner access to bank accounts, credit cards, or cash. A mother agonizes that leaving her spouse may introduce her to the complex web of child protective agencies. She worries that she will lose her parental rights, because she knows these are sometimes contested (Bassuk et al., 1996; Freund, 1995). Your role is to help her take one step—and one day—at a time. Empower her by pointing her in the right direction, toward the social networks that are available to help. This degree of support, encouragement, and concrete direction gives the patient a path toward affirming her own sense of competency and conveys your trust that she can eventually resolve her problem at an acceptable pace.

BURDENS FACING THE CLINICIAN

Even though the primary care clinician's role is mainly one of medical assessment and triage to mental health professionals, working with victims of abuse and violence can take a heavy emotional toll. One group of mental health clinicians systematically addressed the residual effects of helping trauma victims to cope (see Figley, 1995). Their recommendations can be adapted to a primary care clinician's practice and are summarized later in this chapter to help you care for yourself and your practice extenders. In particular, if you treat several of these patients in your practice, or if your community experiences a natural or a manmade catastrophe (e.g., a bombing), you are likely to be "vicariously traumatized" and may fall victim to "compassion fatigue" (see Figley, 1995).

In medical school and residency, physicians often are not taught to give credence to their own personal feelings of anger, beleaguerment, sexual arousal, and even outrage. These human reactions cannot be disavowed, however, because they tend to emerge in one's working relationships with patients. Because they occur frequently, the clinician needs to know that they are not only legitimate but also are a potential key to understanding patients' feelings. Awareness of your feelings can help you work more effectively and efficiently with your patients. While maintaining objectivity—and professional boundaries—the clinician can empathize more fully with the travails of patients.

When working with a traumatized patient, be aware of your tendency to vicariously experience that person's anger or anxiety. Although medications can be enormously helpful to these patients, some clinicians rush to prescribe because they themselves become overly anxious about the patient's experience of helplessness. A better tack is to help the victim understand her experiences one step at a time and to avoid overidentification with her as the victim. Clinicians who treat such patients need support themselves (Peebles-Kleiger, 1994; Powers et al., 1994; Robb, 1995). To manage feelings of anguish and stress and avoid secondary PTSD, you should talk through your feelings with a colleague whenever possible (Figley, 1995; Keller, 1996; Powers et al., 1994).

Mental health professionals are urged to seek out supervisors or their own personal psychotherapy resources to cope with issues their work with patients brings up, but in primary care these opportunities may not be as readily available. You may have to ask for care from others in your practice or even from your support staff. Bartlett (1996) describes a female clinician who began to distrust men because of her intense work with one woman who had been severely abused. In psychotherapy she became aware that her feelings were in part an overreaction to what she had heard, an insight that enabled her to step back and remind herself of the positive attributes of most men. A particularly vexatious reaction for a clinician is the tendency to seek to "rescue" the victim of abuse. A patient's troubles may be especially compelling to one clinician but not to another; this may lead a particular clinician to "champion" the patient, to the neglect of other patients or even the treater's own family. Although the tendency to want to rescue the patient is a professional hazard, especially early in one's career, patients who have been abused incite this fantasy routinely. In essence, the victim wants to be cared for and projects this need onto the clinician (Plakun, 1998). Finding a safe space to acknowledge and talk through these powerful feelings enables the clinician to effectively care for the patient and "protects the clinician and the patient from unhelpful or damaging enactments" (Bartlett, 1996, p. 157).

NEUROBIOLOGY OF TRAUMA: PRACTICAL IMPLICATIONS FOR TREATMENT

A number of landmark studies describe the complex neurobiologic sequelae of childhood and adult trauma (Perry, 1994; Perry et al., 1995; Perry and Pate, 1994; van der Kolk, 1996). It is now generally assumed that the endogenous stress hormones (e.g., catecholamines, corticosteroids, serotonin, endogenous opioids) affect how memories are stored in the brain. Traumatized individuals tend to remember only bits and pieces of an experience because of the massive secretion of these neurohormones, particularly norepinephrine.

Trauma disrupts the functional integration of widespread cortical and subcortical regions, as suggested by electroencephalography, positron emission tomography, and cortical event-related potentials (Perry, 1994; Perry et al., 1995; Perry and Pate, 1994; van der Kolk, 1996). These neuroanatomic effects include decreased hippocampal volume, activation of the amygdala and its connected structures, and lateralization to the right hemisphere when traumatic events are remembered. Decreased activation of Broca's area during flashbacks supports the clinical observation that traumatized persons cannot use words to describe their experience. Apparently, Broca's area actually "switches off" when traumatic memories are activated (see van der Kolk et al., 1996).

Stimulation of the amygdala interferes with hippocampal functioning, but the actual effects on brain structure are complex and difficult to unravel. Permanent changes in the limbic system also impair cortical control and tend to be indelible. Hence, the trauma victim is unable to consolidate, process, and work through traumatic memories. Disruptions in the limbic structure cause an array of problems, including amnesia, exaggerated startle response, hyperarousal, and dissociation (see Tables 6–1 and 6–3).

Patients with PTSD have decreased hippocampal volumes, leading to a loss of verbal memories. Furthermore, traumatic memories are activated in the right hemisphere of the brain, which processes emotion; hence, the clinically observable phenomenon of traumatized patients who "suffer from speechless terror" (van der Kolk, 1996, p. 234). Apparently, in the left hemisphere, Broca's area (which is responsible for language and communication) has diminished oxygen utilization; the right hemisphere independently recalls and facilitates emotional responses and sensory impressions based only on fragments and unintegrated bits of information. The patient who is reminded of traumatic events has compounded neurophysiologic vulnerability that affects her capacity to name feelings, describe what has happened, and work through trauma.

CLINICAL OFFICE MANAGEMENT

These brain-based mechanisms also can account for some of the commonly observed experiences in primary care. You may inadvertently retraumatize a patient during history taking or a clinical examination, even though you are trying to be gentle and kind. How does this happen? One clinician knew that her patient had been brutally raped several times. The patient would dissociate during her annual gynecologic examination. This psychological defense can terrify even the most experienced clinician who is unsuspecting or unaware of adult or childhood trauma. In essence, the patient dissociates, or at the very least cannot access her words to tell you about her experience. You are unable to be helpful because she cannot yet let you into her inner world.

Peebles-Kleiger described the case of a woman who developed PTSD after she became conscious while supposedly under anesthesia. Peebles-Kleiger found that querying the patient on her experience retraumatized her but that hypnotherapy helped her work through the shock. Peebles-Kleiger recommends that primary care clinicians who observe a traumatized patient dissociate, cry uncontrollably, or appear oblivious during an examination should reorient the patient as quickly as possible to the present. Speak in a firm, calm voice and remind the patient of who you are, where she is, and that she is "remembering" but not repeating the experience (Peebles and Fisher, 1987; Peebles-Kleiger and Zerbe, 1998).

In these patients, higher cortical processing is impaired. Unresolved, traumatic memories remain "in limbo," prone to flashback recurrence. Any situation that causes physiologic arousal or that brings back the context of the trauma creates the intrusive quality of that memory. It is useful for the clinician to remember that neurocircuits established via the amygdala are tenacious. Behavioral changes tend to be remembered "for a lifetime." Change occurs when various forms of therapy (e.g., psychodynamic psychotherapy, eye movement desensitization and reprocessing, hypnotherapy) are undertaken to enable the patient to override the "emotional memories" of the subcortical structures.

PHARMACOLOGIC CONSIDERATIONS

Psychopharmacologic agents are increasingly used in comprehensive treatment of PTSD (Davidson et al., 1996) to reduce hyperarousal and reexperiencing of symptoms (e.g., numbing, flashbacks, insomnia) and to relieve anxiety and depression (Table 6–4). Most will recommend that pharmacotherapy be tailored to the stage of the illness. For example, a benzodiazepine may initially be needed to deal acutely with hyperarousal; in patients who are depressed, a selective serotonin reuptake inhibitor (SSRI) or tricyclic antidepressant may be continued for 1 year or longer. PTSD patients may not be responsive to traditional doses of medication; in each case, medication should be seen as an adjunct to treatment. In most cases, psychotherapy is necessary "to help the victim reintegrate the traumatic experience into the self and world view in a more fruitful manner" (Marmar et al., 1993, p. 258).

SPECIAL CONSIDERATIONS FOR PREGNANCY AND THE POSTPARTUM PERIOD

Violence occurs frequently among pregnant women and may be even more prevalent in the postpartum period than during pregnancy. In primary care, evidence for this situation should be routinely sought and evaluated (Gazmararian et al., 1996), particularly because pregnancy and the postnatal period are times when women frequently come in contact with the health care system. Questions about violence or abuse in the home at this time may help ameliorate a tendency for the problem to become chronic. However, health care providers may neglect to ask the questions because of their own unresolved personal

Table 6–4. **Psychopharmacologic Considerations in the Treatment of PTSD**

Drug Class	Target Symptoms
Antidepressants Tricyclic antidepressants (e.g., amitriptyline, imipramine) Monoamine oxidase inhibitors (e.g., phenelzine) SSRI (e.g., fluoxetine)°	Overall PTSD symptoms, especially numbing, flashbacks, nightmares, insomnia
Benzodiazepines Clonazepam°	Insomnia, nightmares, anxiety, panic attacks Hyperarousal and startle response in some cases
Anticonvulsants Carbamazepine Valproic acid	Arousal and reexperiencing Avoidance and numbing
Antihistamines Diphenhydramine Cyproheptadine	Nightmares Insomnia
Beta-blockers Propranolol	Hyperarousal, startle response, intrusive thoughts
Alpha$_2$-agonists Clonidine	Hyperarousal (may improve sleep, decrease nightmares)

°Most commonly used, first-line agents.

histories of abuse. A study by de Lahunta and Tulsky (1996) showed that at least 14% of medical students and their faculty had experienced physical or sexual abuse in their lifetime. This may negatively influence the capacity of clinicians to be aware of the problem.

Family violence crosses all socioeconomic and educational boundaries, but homeless and low-income mothers are particularly vulnerable to traumatic and disruptive life events. In one study, 86.7% of homeless and low-income mothers experienced multiple episodes of physical and sexual assaults over their lifespan, and the resulting posttraumatic effects greatly affected "the already challenging tasks of being alone and needing to support a family, find a job, and be a parent" (Bassuk et al., 1996, p. 644). Because of the high prevalence of PTSD among these mothers and the increased rates of comorbid depression, substance abuse, and cumulative effects of past trauma, Bassuk and her research team recommended medical programs that link women with community services and "strong partnerships among health and mental health professionals" (p. 645).

Clinicians may ask about family violence and psychological trauma less than they should, not only because they are likely to unveil a sensitive and difficult issue but also because of their own personal experiences with family violence. Identification of abuse and intervention on behalf of patients is thus undermined. In contrast, minimal intervention by home nurses may ultimately reduce child abuse and neglect and help the mothers themselves avoid victimization (Olds et al., 1997). Primary care clinicians who inquire about a history of trauma and suggest supportive, adjunctive maneuvers such as nurse visits or support groups can make a difference in preventing domestic violence (McAfee, 1995). Psychological consultants can instill hope at a crucial developmental phase and "ameliorate these self-destructive interactions with authority figures, which can all too often be reflected in the patient's relationship with the physicians and health care providers who are treating her for her obstetrical or gynecological condition" (Josephs, 1996, p. 25). In essence, the primary care clinician addresses the trauma issue because it has wreaked havoc on the woman's sense of self as whole and competent. When self-esteem, sexual and maternal functioning, and intimacy are sensitively approached, the patient will be much more capable of nurturing her child, seeing herself as capable, and avoiding a propensity to be revictimized (Josephs, 1996).

PATIENT GUIDELINES FOR COPING WITH TRAUMA AND VIOLENCE

1. Acknowledge the trauma. You have been a victim of a catastrophic experience you could not control. In most situations help is available, but you must take the first steps to ensure your own safety by your willingness to get help. Ask your doctor about community resources (e.g., shelters for domestic violence, psychotherapists with experience in dealing with trauma).
2. Find a safe place to talk about what has happened to you. Many victims keep abuse secret even after the death of the perpetrator because of threats or knowledge that someone they love could be hurt. Although our society is still less responsive than it should be to women who have been victims of abuse or violence, more avenues for help are available than ever before. Most communities now have a number of local resources available that will protect your privacy.
3. Begin to talk with people who are most likely to be supportive but avoid blurting out details of abuse to family members or friends who may be reluctant to hear your story. Disrupted relationships have been known to occur and can be devastating. You do not want to feel minimized, vulnerable, and disbelieved because your story places others in uncomfortable loyalty binds. Go slowly. Try to develop a positive sense of yourself by finally coming forward. It will benefit you to talk openly as much as you can about your situation and to face down the sense of shame, humiliation, and powerlessness that accompany victimization.
4. Avoid social isolation. Friends and family may have been neglected because you have felt ashamed of your problem. You may also be frightened to see them because you have been forbidden to by a spouse or partner. Satisfying social relationships are emotionally supportive and essential; they will help you develop a sense of security. By all means, if you have been battered and feel at risk, try as much as possible *to not be alone*. This is not only a protective maneuver but also one that can be emotionally sustaining.
5. Take advantage of treatment opportunities, including medications. Many symptoms of anxiety and depression disappear when victims find a safe place to deal with their problems. Your doctor may also recommend some of the

new medications to help you deal with the depression and/or anxiety disorders that are frequently related to trauma. Your difficulty sleeping, fretfulness about minor events, and tendency to always be on the alert or feeling that you are in a dangerous situation can be significantly alleviated with medication. Remember that most experts believe these medications are not an end in themselves. Therapy is also essential to help you master your trauma.

6. If you are the victim of childhood or adult trauma (e.g., rape, physical disaster, catastrophic event), your clinician will encourage you to seek psychotherapy. Depending on your needs and preferences, individual and group therapies have been found to be enormously helpful.

7. Consider reading some of the excellent texts, self-help workbooks, and patient guides (see end of chapter) that are now available. They can be supportive by helping you feel less alone and by providing excellent advice you may not have considered. In essence, reading is an excellent adjunct in your care.

8. If you are a victim of domestic violence, always have a plan for safety and/ or exit from your home. This safety plan should include: (1) a change of clothes for you and your children; (2) cash, checkbook, and savings account; (3) identification papers, such as birth certificate, social security card, and driver's license; (4) any financial papers, such as a mortgage and an automobile title; (5) something familiar or special to each child, such as a book or a toy (Braude, 1998), and (6) going to a safe destination such as a shelter.

9. Women who have been battered tend to *underestimate* that the abuse will happen again. The batterer is often quickly forgiven when he or she apologizes. Often the batterer gets you to feel that you have done something wrong to bring the violence on yourself. Although it is difficult to do, try to remember that no one has the right to hit you. Avoid finding fault with yourself and try to remember that the future can be much brighter. There are many examples of battered women who made their way out of traumatic partnerships and survived. Try to read about their stories and learn from them to support your own plan.

10. To get better, the victim of domestic abuse must learn to empower herself. This means learning as much as you can about yourself through treatment. A comprehensive treatment program will help you address financial issues, worries about your children, your need for companionship and social outlets, and your fears about what the abuser is likely to do.

11. Learn as much as you can about the effects of trauma, violence, or any catastrophic natural event. You will see that you are not alone. Most women and men experience trauma at some point in life. People have different ways of handling it, but treatment can teach you about your own resilience. Although therapy is difficult, it will also help you learn about yourself and your rights as a human being. Knowledge is power. The more information you have about your situation, the less likely it is that you will feel vulnerable and fragile, and the more effective you will be in changing your life.

12. Work to identify safe, helpful individuals to create a healthy support system. If you have never felt such support, use your therapist to help you learn who can be trusted.

ADDITIONAL GUIDELINES
FOR PRIMARY CARE CLINICIANS

1. Be aware of the signs and symptoms that bring abuse victims into the medical system (see Tables 6–1, 6–2, and 6–3). Ask about abuse and document any injuries. Be sure to list the patient's personal strengths, not just her pain, because this helps her be a partner with you in the recovery process (Campbell, 1995; Campbell et al., 1996).

2. Take time to listen and be sure to ask questions. But if you ask, be prepared to hear the answers. Be sure to have available a list of community resources, such as hotlines, shelters, or any free support groups. Write down the National Domestic Violence Hotline number (1-800-799-SAFE/1-800-799-7233). The patient will then have this number available if a crisis arises, even if she has not had an opportunity to take advantage of your other suggestions.

3. Know the requirements of your state about reporting suspected abuse. Physicians who document injuries also increase awareness and help prevent future violence. In some jurisdictions, training is becoming mandatory in order to comply with state laws requiring medical documentation and reporting of domestic violence injuries. The new Partner Violence Screen-Polaroid instant camera is an invaluable tool in primary care (Stapleton, 1997). Having a photograph enhances your records, boosts victims' confidence to press charges against perpetrators, and minimizes the need for you to testify in court.

4. Question the patient about the symptoms of anxiety, depression, substance abuse, and suicidality that often accompany PTSD. Whenever possible, make a referral to a mental health professional and judiciously use psychotropic medications. Remember that 30% to 50% of attempted suicides by women occur after an incident of domestic abuse (Campbell, 1995; Fontanarosa, 1995; McCauley et al., 1997).

5. Be sure to ask the woman how she is faring with her children. In homes where the mother is abused, children also tend to be abused. Children who witness domestic abuse are inevitably traumatized themselves and learn to imitate the violent behavior they see. Preventing violence in society begins by intervening early in the lives of children who may later become perpetrators of violence because they have been abused and/or traumatized in childhood (Swanston et al., 1997).

6. Do *not* expect the patient to find you trustworthy. Remember that her subjective experience may have been darkened by those in power or authority who have not been helpful. She must develop new memories, capacities, and esteem in order to eventually trust. Consider the development of a good therapeutic alliance with you an achievement, not an entitlement.

7. Be aware of the highly personal, suggestive nature of human memory. Much has been written in the lay and professional literature about "true" and "false" memories. Although there is still much to be learned about the neurophysiologic base and psychological underpinnings of memory, clinicians must realize that it is normal for humans to try to fill in the gaps of memory. They elaborate a story so that it makes sense. The brain-based disruptions that occur with trauma make it entirely possible that victims do distort or

elaborate some memories. However, although specific details of the trauma may not be historically accurate, it is nonetheless crucial for you to believe the patient and the overall intent of the history she tells you.

8. Remember that your interest, compassion, and open-mindedness will help the patient, but that she will inevitably need additional psychotherapeutic support to work through traumatic memories and learn new adaptation skills. Psychotherapy with victims of trauma requires additional skills on the part of even experienced therapists. For this reason, it is recommended that clinicians know those psychotherapists in their communities who have interest and experience in working with the condition. Iatrogenic damage has occurred from well-meaning but unskilled psychotherapists who put pressure on the patient to retrieve old memories, reconstruct "actual" events, and abreact horrific experiences in the office. This experience can retraumatize the patient who has already felt helpless and emotionally overwhelmed. Be suspicious of a therapist who thinks every patient can be healed by one particular modality. For some patients, cognitive-behavioral therapy, hypnosis or eye movement desensitization and reprocessing is key; others benefit from psychodynamic (exploratory) therapy. EMDR or eye movement desensitization and reprocessing is a technique that is gaining in popularity for the treatment of trauma. It ". . . combines exposure, cognitive therapy, and stress management in a highly systematic and efficient fashion" (Allen and Lewis, 1996; Shapiro, 1995).

9. Help the patient to master trauma by seeing herself as being in control of her life. As Smith (1993, 1996) has opined regarding the use of hypnotherapy as one tool to help victims overcome terrifying experiences, the goal is to help the patient be more in control, not less. An experienced therapist paces the treatment so that memories become more emotionally tolerable and "the experience can now be linguistically encoded and made sensible, rather than having the memory be dominated by emotion and jumbled images" (Smith, 1995, p. 367).

10. Recognize that for the patient to improve she must grieve. What psychotherapists term the "working-through process" means the remodeling of an often-idealized sense of the self or of a significant other. The greater the threat to the self, the more powerful will be the patient's resistance to change. People tend to preserve their attachments to others, even if they are not beneficial or supportive (Vasquez, 1996); after all, these are the relationships that are familiar. Resolving trauma (i.e., finding relief from the intrusive images, nightmares, and flashbacks) takes time and is painful. It means reworking attachments to others and developing a new sense of self. Psychotherapy for the trauma victim is rarely a short-term process, because the individual must develop a sense of self-agency, coherence, and continuity and must also grieve for old, but inherently pathologic, relationships to others.

11. Recognize that working with victims of trauma, natural catastrophe, and domestic abuse can cause vicarious victimization in caregivers. Even in a primary care setting, where clinicians play a less central role in helping patients rework and master horrific experiences, you may find yourself identifying with the victim, feeling angry at the perpetrator, becoming intensely curious about details, and feeling moved to "rescue" the patient.

Although working with these patients ultimately can be rewarding and lifesaving, be aware of any tendency to blur professional boundaries or to spend excessive time with these patients. Overinvolvement can disrupt your practice or even your personal life. For these reasons, it is wise to steer the patient to an experienced psychotherapist who can "differentiate feelings originating in the patient from feelings originating in himself or herself" (Peebles-Kleiger, 1989, p. 523).

12. Encourage the patient to take advantage of new psychopharmacologic treatments. Tricyclic antidepressants (e.g., imipramine, amitriptyline), monoamine oxidase inhibitors (e.g., phenelzine), and particularly SSRIs (e.g., fluoxetine) have been shown to reduce symptoms of PTSD in a number of clinic populations. Benzodiazepines (e.g., clonazepam) are particularly useful in damping the patient's startle response and hyperarousal symptoms. Amelioration of these symptoms can often help the patient both participate in treatment and work more effectively, ultimately promoting greater ego integrity (see Davidson and van der Kolk, 1996).

13. Be alert to the possibility of addiction or misuse of psychotropic drugs. Chronic administration must be watched carefully because of the addictive potential of some agents (i.e., benzodiazepines) and the tendency to create very disturbing withdrawal symptoms when quickly discontinued.

14. If you treat a number of trauma-related problems in your practice, be alert to new trends in pharmacotherapy. Clonidine (Catapres) has been helpful in decreasing autonomic arousal, thereby helping the patient avoid nightmares and other intrusive thoughts; beta-adrenergic blockers have also been observed to relieve hypervigilance, hyperarousal, explosiveness, nightmares, and startle symptoms.

15. Help the patient understand the rationale of pharmacotherapy. Explain that, theoretically, medication interrupts kindling phenomena that can perpetuate trauma via long-term psychophysiologic effects. In general, medications can improve the quality of life of many women with PTSD symptoms by reducing intrusive thoughts, improving depressed or anxious mood, reducing impulsive aggression against self or others, and ameliorating hyperarousal. The latter symptom is particularly important because it leads many women to self-medicate with drugs or alcohol; to be prone to sleep problems, including traumatic nightmares; and to be unable to participate in psychotherapy. When panic and anxiety symptoms are treated, the patient is better able to describe her emotional experience in words and to develop a narrative continuity of self in therapy.

16. Stay involved in the total care of the patient, even if you refer her for specialty consultation. Trauma victims are exquisitely sensitive to feelings of abandonment and the fantasy that they have hurt another person. Although referral to a mental health professional can be enormously helpful, you must let the patient know that you also are interested in knowing how treatment is going and that you are available for medical needs.

SUMMARY

The impact of domestic violence, rape, physical and sexual trauma, and natural disaster on the lives of women is astounding. Few individuals are immune to the impact of traumatic events, because life is a high-risk proposition. By recognizing and treating victims of abuse and posttraumatic stress, physicians can make enormous inroads toward improving the mental and physical health of women.

Despite this massive public health problem, physicians need guidelines for patients who suffer the consequences of natural disaster, childhood abuse, adult trauma (e.g., rape, robbery, kidnapping, bombing), or domestic violence. Many problems remain unrecognized because symptoms can be triggered months and even years after the event. When a problem is identified, the clinician must be prepared to work with the patient as part of a team. Ultimately, this care is enormously cost-effective. Screening and early intervention are becoming incorporated into the preventive health services of some insurance and managed care plans, because the persistent health and emotional problems that abused women experience lead to so many other physical and psychological problems. These difficulties can be minimized if effective help is offered early.

Intervention begins by creating a safe environment where the clinician can ask the patient in privacy if abuse has occurred. Once the traumatic stress is identified, the clinician can work to stabilize the symptoms. Sometimes the patient denies the abuse, only to confide it months or years later because of the shame and guilt it causes. When the woman is able to express her pain or to acknowledge a traumatic experience, crying may be her first release. Soon afterward she may begin to vent her anger and sense of hopelessness about what to do next. The primary care clinician must provide the patient with a sense of safety and help her formulate a plan of what steps to take, including finding extra emotional support.

Usually the patient benefits from individual and/or group psychotherapy, which helps her to process the traumatic events and to integrate the trauma into her world view. During this process, the primary care clinician plays a pivotal role by offering support and encouragement while providing medical care. You promote mastery by reminding the patient that trauma and violence are about control and power. Calmly use phrases such as, "You have survived and are working hard to recover in your therapy. As terrible as it was, you are simply remembering now. You are now in control." In cases of domestic violence, remind the patient of the feminist slogan: "Whatever he says you did, he had no right to hit you."

Primary care clinicians must be vigilant about the occurrence of PTSD when highly functioning patients are exposed to natural disasters, motor vehicle accidents, and even catastrophic medical illnesses such as burns or myocardial infarctions. These patients also are likely to benefit from treatment interventions that include individual and group psychotherapy and pharmacotherapy. For those patients who survive or recover from a disaster or catastrophic stressor, available community resources are extremely important. Support from family, relatives, and friends helps them cope better than those who do not have such support. Although mental health personnel are often available immediately after an event, patients may experience delayed effects, and they should be urged to seek out professional support. Family members can be helpful when they listen empathically but then redirect attention to the present and the future.

For those patients who lose a loved one in an unanticipated, cataclysmic personal event (e.g., automobile accident), survivor guilt about being alive when someone beloved has died can take a heavy toll. Often these survivors develop a plethora of somatic complaints, depression, anxiety, or lack of zest for living because they have not been able to effectively work through their loss. These patients need help in channeling their aggression constructively, as in social activism (e.g., Mothers Against Drunk Driving), and in fighting the tendency to blame themselves. They must learn that the trauma was beyond their control. A treatment principle essential for all forms of trauma is the working through and mastery of the residual effects in psychotherapy. In the process, psychopharmacologic modalities (e.g., SSRIs, clonazepam, clonidine) can be very useful to reduce arousal, insomnia, and anxiety. Most believe that psychotherapy is key to processing traumatic events and memories and to adaptively integrating what has happened into the trauma survivor's world view.

The diagnosis and treatment of trauma can be a challenge to even the most experienced clinician. Treaters who care for victims also pay a heavy price by confronting directly what human beings can do to each other. Treaters also are faced with the fact that, in the midst of particularly devastating and personal catastrophes, there often is relatively little they can do to help. But actively listening to patients as they face events they could not control does help them make gains in their everyday lives. In essence, you are reminding them that they have survived and are better now. This perspective on one's personal history, replete with scars from the trauma-induced experience, gives a patient new will to carry on, by working through anger, mourning, and finding power to add to life achievements. W. H. Auden (1926) presciently captured the position of those who know or work with traumatized persons, urging us to stand shoulder to shoulder with those who may otherwise lose hope, because: "Evil is always personal and spectacular, but goodness needs the evidence of all of our lives" (p. 686).

Resources for Patients and Family Members

Allen JG: *Coping with Trauma: A Guide to Self-Understanding.* Washington, DC, American Psychiatric Press, 1995.
  Written to teach patients about all aspects of trauma and the psychiatric aftermath that arises from it, this lucid and thoroughly researched volume also addresses the essentials of treatment. From his years of clinical experience in the Trauma Recovery Program at The Menninger Clinic, Dr. Allen bases his book on a series of lectures he gives to patients to help them understand the neurologic, family, and personal effects of trauma. Readers will benefit from the thorough description of the effects of trauma on their emotions, memory, self-concept, and relationships; there are also excellent discussions of the process of dissociation and a rationale for why patients experience it as both a blessing and a curse (pp. 81–84). Because trauma is a complex problem, it usually requires long-term, multifaceted treatment involving individual, group, family, or hospital modalities in addition to psychotropic medication.
  Drawing on clinical cases and research-based studies, Allen explains the importance of having "a secure base" from which children and adolescents receive emotional and physical nourishment that enables them to grow. It is this secure base that is disrupted by natural disasters such as earthquakes or tornadoes, manmade catastrophes such as bombings or fires, and sexual, physical, or emotional abuse. To get better, the patient must reestablish a secure base in treatment, because "secure attachment is the antidote for trauma" (p. 39).
  In addition to providing practical pointers about how the patient can overcome

trauma (e.g., "understand your brain and be gentle on your mind; develop supportive relationships to help you tolerate distressing emotions"), Allen gives a balanced understanding of the recovery process, "false" memories, the causes of PTSD and dissociation, and the biology of trauma. Ultimately, patients are helped to "cope with trauma" by learning as much as they can about it, which helps them to take better care of themselves. But for the trauma victim, pleasure must come in small doses. Allen explains why such positive emotions as joy and pride are achievable goals but difficult tasks for persons who have been maltreated or who have endured atrocities.

Herman JL: *Trauma and Recovery: The Aftermath of Violence—From Domestic Abuse to Political Terror.* New York, Basic Books, 1992.

This widely available, influential resource reviews the most important aspects of childhood and adult trauma. Dr. Herman includes case examples from her own practice and some actual segments of dialogue from treatment sessions to demonstrate how forming human relationships is essential to helping "the damaged self" (p. 52) overcome trauma. She helps her reader appreciate the ravaging of the soul when human connections are violated. Although the author believes that full recovery from trauma is never complete, resolution of trauma can occur when the damaged self begins to view itself as repaired and begins to reestablish important relationships. Patients will be reassured and sustained as they learn from the stories of others who have survived horrific abuse.

For Herman, the therapeutic process rarely follows "a simple progression but often detours and doubles back" (p. 213). She believes that a trauma victim must get to know herself again in order to reconnect with others and lead a healthier life. She suggests that survivors can benefit from engaging in positive social actions and heartfelt causes. The victim is in a unique position to help others because "she has a clear sense of what is important and what is not. Having encountered evil, she knows how to cling to what is good. Having encountered the fear of death, she knows how to celebrate life" (p. 213). Assisting others abets the patient's recovery.

Terr L: *Too Scared to Cry: Psychic Trauma in Childhood.* New York, Harper & Row, 1990.

In 1976, 26 California children were kidnapped from their school bus and buried alive. Although all the children survived, they sustained long-term, multifaceted traumas, which are described at length in the author's seminal Chowchilla Research Studies. This book is primarily about the author's experience as a clinician and researcher dealing with the virulent effects of trauma on children, but any adult who wants to learn about the emotions, behaviors, and treatment of psychic trauma will find Terr a sympathetic and adept guide.

To demonstrate the sequelae of terror, rage, denial and numbing, unresolved grief, and shame, Terr includes reports from adults who have survived various forms of traumatic stress. Her case histories elucidate the side effects of natural or manmade disaster. Because most of the examples are about children, the woman who has been traumatized may be able to read this book and gain new understanding of herself while taking ample distance from her unique situation and painful recollections. In this way, the tendency toward posttraumatic reenactment or retraumatization may be avoided. The author explains how children and adults respond differently to traumatic incidents (e.g., children often have problems with learning). She points out how each of us carries the residual effects of some degree of trauma that contribute to our mental development. Because patients who have been victimized so often feel alone and believe their experiences make them "different" and deviant, recognizing the ubiquity of the problem facilitates a broader perspective. In essence, victims learn that trauma is a matter of degree and hence they are less likely to feel alone and defiled.

Terr L: *Unchained Memories: True Stories of Traumatic Memories, Lost and Found.* New York, Basic Books, 1994.

Because of the debate about "true" and "false" memories, many patients with a history of abuse or trauma search for an authoritative book to explain the nature and vicissitudes of memory. Relying on her experience as a psychiatrist, researcher, and expert witness, Dr. Terr explains why we remember some details about traumatic events and forget others. In the context of fascinating case histories and stories of survivors, she describes state-of-the-art research on the neurobiology of memory and the circumstances under which memories are retained or forgotten. Her humanistic tone is also balm for the patient who desires a deeper understanding of what happens to memory during trauma. She includes biographic vignettes about authors and artists (e.g., Stephen King) who have withstood enormous trauma and learned to creatively adapt by reworking them in their artistic productions.

Resources for Clinicians

Allen JG: *Coping with Trauma: A Guide to Self-Understanding.* Washington, DC, American Psychiatric Press, 1995.

Herman JL: *Trauma and Recovery: The Aftermath of Violence—From Domestic Abuse to Political Terror.* New York, Basic Books, 1992.

Terr L: *Too Scared to Cry: Psychic Trauma in Childhood.* New York, Harper & Row, 1990.

Terr L: *Unchained Memories: True Stories of Traumatic Memories, Lost and Found.* New York, Basic Books, 1994.

Each of the books listed above for patients also serves as an ideal primer for the primary care clinician who wants to gain a greater appreciation of the ravages of trauma and what contemporary psychiatry and psychotherapy offer patients.

The books by Dr. Allen and Dr. Herman provide the best overview of treatment modalities, combined with practical suggestions that can be employed in primary care practice. Either of Dr. Terr's books gives an ample description of what it is like to sustain and live creatively despite trauma. To diagnose phenomena such as dissociation, fugue states, intrusive memories, and dissociation, the clinician can get a compelling and memorable glimpse through Terr's case examples (she includes the early life stories of Virginia Woolf, Alfred Hitchcock, Edgar Allen Poe, and Stephen King, to name a few).

van der Kolk BA, McFarlane AC, Weisaeth L (eds): *Traumatic Stress: The Effects of Overwhelming Stress on Mind, Body, and Society.* New York, Guilford Press, 1996.

For the clinician who desires a clinical handbook about the workup, neurobiologic and psychodynamic mechanisms, and treatment of PTSD, this book is ideal. Particularly interesting for the primary care clinician are the chapters reviewing brain-based changes that PTSD patients undergo (e.g., decreased hippocampal volume, impaired functioning of Broca's area). The arousal and activation of the amygdala that disrupts hippocampal functioning leads to the clinically observable phenomena of speechless terror and the inability to put feelings into words.

Also included are state-of-the-art reviews on psychopharmacology, preventive interventions for acute trauma (e.g., after an accident), and the rationale for cognitive-behavioral and psychoanalytic psychotherapies. The importance of a strong therapeutic alliance to help the patient feel safe is underscored.

Because treatment of the traumatized patient is often punctuated by relapses and remissions, the primary care clinician will benefit from this comprehensive review of the importance of patience in the treatment to help counter "intense feelings of helplessness, rage, rescue, and sadness" (p. 555). Because trauma and psychosomatic problems also go hand in hand, the primary care clinician will be aided by the mental and psychobiologic hypotheses about the co-occurrence of the two conditions (see especially Chapter 10: "The Body Keeps the Score: Approaches to the Psychobiology of Posttraumatic Stress Disorder," pp. 214–241).

References

Abbott J, Johnson R, Koziol-McLain J, et al.: Domestic violence against women: incidence and prevalence in an emergency department population. *JAMA* 1995;273:1763–1767.

Allen JG: *Coping with Trauma: A Guide to Self-Understanding.* Washington, DC, American Psychiatric Press, 1995.

Allen JG: Review of Goldberg S, Muir R, Kerr J (eds.): *Attachment Theory: Social, Developmental and Clinical Perspectives. Bull Menninger Clin* 1996a;60:554–559.

Allen JG: Loosening traumatic bonds. *Renfrew Perspective* 1996b;2:7, 8, 13.

Allen JG, Lewis L: A conceptual framework for treating traumatic memories with EMPRO. *Bull Menninger Clin* 1996;60:238–263.

Auden WH: *The Collected Poems of W. H. Auden.* New York, Random House, 1945.

Auden WH: Journey to war. In: Mendelson E (ed.): *The Complete Works of W. H. Auden: Prose and Travel Books, vol 1 (1926–1936),* pp. 667–689. Princeton, NJ, Princeton University Press, 1926.

Barber CC, Colson DB, McPartland MQ, et al.: Child abuse and treatment difficulty in inpatient treatment of children and adolescents. *Child Psychiatry Hum Dev* 1994;25:63–64.

Bartlett AB: Clinical assessment of sexual trauma: interviewing adult survivors of childhood sexual abuse. *Bull Menninger Clin* 1996;60:147–159.

Bassuk EL, Weinreb LF, Buckner JC: The characteristics and needs of sheltered homeless and low-income housed mothers. *JAMA* 1996;276:640–646.

Bowlby J: *Attachment and Loss,* vol 2. London, Hogarth Press, 1973.

Bowlby J: *The Making and Breaking of Affectional Bonds.* London, Routledge, 1979.

Braude M: Domestic Violence Workshop. Presented at the First International Conference on Women's Health, Miami, Florida, March 21, 1998. Unpublished lecture notes and outline, pp. 138–146.

Breslau N, Davis GC, Peterson EL, et al.: Psychiatric sequelae of posttraumatic stress disorder in women. *Arch Gen Psychiatry* 1997;54:81–87.

Campbell JC: A nursing assessment for risk of homicide with battered women. *Advances in Nursing Science* 1986;8:36–51.

Campbell JC: "If I can't have you, no one can": power and control in homicide of female partners. In: Radford J, Russell DEH (eds.): *Femicide: The Politics of Woman Killing,* pp. 99–113. New York, Twayne Publishers, 1992.

Campbell JC (ed.): *Assessing Dangerousness: Violence by Sexual Offenders, Batterers, and Child Abusers.* Thousand Oaks, CA, Sage Publications, 1995.

Campbell J, Kub JE, Rose L: Depression in battered women. *J Am Med Womens Assoc* 1996;51:106–110.

Cohen S: Rage makes me strong. *Time,* July 29, 1996, p. 50.

Davidson J: Issues in the diagnosis of posttraumatic stress disorder. In: Oldham JM, Riba MB, Tasman A (eds.): *Review of Psychiatry,* vol 21, pp. 141–156. Washington, DC, American Psychiatric Press, 1993.

Davidson JR, Hughes DC, George LK, et al.: The association of sexual assault and attempted suicide within the community. *Arch Gen Psychiatry* 1996;53:550–555.

Davidson JRT, van der Kolk BA: The psychopharmacological treatment of posttraumatic stress disorder. In: van der Kolk BA, McFarlane AC, Weisaeth L (eds.): *Traumatic Stress: The Effects of Overwhelming Experience on Mind, Body, and Society,* pp. 510–524. New York, Guilford, 1996.

Davis GC, Breslau N: Post-traumatic disorder in victims of civilian trauma and criminal violence. *Psychiatr Clin North Am* 1994;17:289–299.

de Lahunta EA, Tulsky AA: Personal exposure of faculty and medical students to family violence. *JAMA* 1996;275:1903–1906.

Eagle M: The developmental perspectives of attachment and psychoanalytic theory. In: Goldberg S, Muir R, Kerr J (eds.): *Attachment Theory: Social, Developmental, and Clinical Perspectives,* pp. 123–152. Hillsdale, NJ, The Analytic Press, 1995.

Eby KA, Campbell JC, Sullivan CM, et al.: Health effects of experiences of sexual violence for women with abusive partners. *Health Care for Women International* 1995;16:563–576.

Farley R: Homicide trends in the United States. In: Hawkins DF (ed.): *Homicide Among Black Americans,* pp. 13–27. New York, University Press of America, 1986.

Feldhaus KL, Koziol-McLain J, Amsbury HL, et al.: Accuracy of three brief screening questions for detecting partner violence in the emergency department. *JAMA* 1997;277:1357–1361.

Figley CR: Compassion fatigue as secondary traumatic stress disorder: an overview. In: Figley CR (ed.): *Compassion Fatigue: Coping with Secondary Traumatic Stress Disorder in Those Who Treat the Traumatized,* pp. 1–20. New York, Brunner/Mazel, 1995.

Flitcraft A: Violence, abuse and assault over the life phases. In: Wallis LA (ed): *Textbook of Women's Health,* pp. 249–258. Philadelphia, Lippincott-Raven, 1998.

Foa EB, Riggs DS: Posttraumatic stress disorder and rape. In: Oldham JM, Riba MB, Tasman A (eds.): *Review of Psychiatry,* vol 12, pp. 273–303. Washington, DC, American Psychiatric Press, 1993.

Fontanarosa PB: The unrelenting epidemic of violence in America: truths and consequences. *JAMA* 1995;273:1992–1993.

Freund KM: Domestic violence. In: Carr PL, Freund KM, Somani S (eds.): *The Medical Care of Women,* pp. 722–728. Philadelphia, WB Saunders, 1995.

Gazmararian J, Lazorick S, Spitz AM, et al.: Prevalence of violence against pregnant women. *JAMA* 1996;175:1915–1920.

Goldberg S, Muir, R, Kerr J (eds.): *Attachment Theory: Social, Developmental, and Clinical Perspectives.* Hillsdale, NJ, Analytic Press, 1995.

Herman JL: *Trauma and Recovery: The Aftermath of Violence—From Domestic Abuse to Political Terror.* New York, Basic Books, 1992.

Josephs L: Women and trauma: a contemporary psychodynamic approach to traumatization for patients in the OB/GYN psychological consultation clinic. *Bull Menninger Clin* 1996;60:22–38.

Keller LE: Invisible victims: battered women in psychiatric and medical emergency rooms. *Bull Menninger Clin* 1996;60:1–21.

Leeder EJ: *Treating Abuse in Families: A Feminist and Community Approach.* New York, Springer, 1994.

Marmar CR, Foy D, Kagan B, et al.: An integrated approach for treating posttraumatic stress. In: Oldham JM, Riba MD, Tasman A (eds.): *Review of Psychiatry,* vol 12, pp. 239–272. Washington, DC, American Psychiatric Press, 1993.

McAfee RE: Physicians and domestic violence: Can we make a difference? *JAMA* 1995;273:1790–1791.

McCauley J, Kern D, Kolodner K, et al.: Clinical characteristics of women with a history of childhood abuse: Unhealed wounds. *JAMA* 1997;277:1362–1368.

Menninger WW, Wilkinson CB: The aftermath of catastrophe: The Hyatt Regency disaster. *Bull Menninger Clin* 1988;52:65–74.

Olds DL, Eckenrode J, Henderson CR, et al.: Long-term effects of home visitation on maternal life course and child abuse and neglect: fifteen-year follow-up of a randomized trial. *JAMA* 1997;278:637–643.

Peebles MJ: Posttraumatic stress disorder: a historical perspective on diagnosis and treatment. *Bull Menninger Clin* 1989;53:274–286.

Peebles MJ [writer], Fisher V [producer]. *Diagnosis of Posttraumatic Stress Disorder: A Case of Awareness Under Surgical Anesthesia* [videotape]. Topeka, KS, Menninger Video Productions, 1987.

Peebles-Kleiger MJ: Using countertransference in the hypnosis of trauma victims: a model of turning hazard into healing. *Am J Psychother* 1989;43:518–530.

Peebles-Kleiger MJ: Traumatic stress principles applied to the medical-surgical setting: helping PICU/NICU staff help families at risk. Presented at the Joshua Stouck Memorial Symposium, Children's National Medical Center, Washington, DC, May 20, 1994.

Peebles-Kleiger MJ, Zerbe KJ: Office management of posttraumatic stress disorder: A clinician's guide to a pervasive problem. *Postgrad Med* 1998;103:181–196.

Perry BD: Neurobiological sequelae of childhood trauma: PTSD in children. In: Murburg MM (ed.): *Catecholamine Function in Posttraumatic Stress Disorder: Emerging Concepts,* pp. 233–255. Washington, DC, American Psychiatric Press, 1994.

Perry BD, Pate J: Neurodevelopment and the psychobiological roots of post-traumatic stress disorder. In: Koziol LF, Stout CE (eds.): *The Neuropsychology of Mental Disorders: A Practical Guide,* pp. 129–146. Springfield, IL, Charles C Thomas, 1994.

Perry BD, Pollard RA, Blakeley TL, et al.: Childhood trauma, the neurobiology of adaptation, and "use-dependent" development of the brain: how "states" become "traits." *Infant Mental Health Journal* 1995;16:271–289.

Plakun EM: Enactment and the treatment of abuse survivors. *Harv Rev Psychiatry* 1998;5:318–325.

Powers PS, Cruse CW, Daniels S, et al.: Posttraumatic stress disorder in patients with burns. *J Burn Care Rehabil* 1994;15:147–153.

Radford J, Russell DEH (eds.): *Femicide: The Politics of Woman Killing.* New York, Twayne Publishers, 1992.

Reubens M: Issues in the treatment of domestic violence. *Renfrew Perspective* 1996;2:1–4.

Robb E: Post-incident care and support for assaulted staff. In: Kidd B, Stark C (eds.): *Management of Violence and Aggression in Health Care,* pp. 140–162. London, Gaskell, 1995.

Russell DE: *The Secret Trauma*. New York, Basic Books, 1986.

Seaman B: A survivor's view. In: Wallis LA (ed.): *Textbook of Women's Health*, p. 259. Philadelphia, Lippincott-Raven, 1998.

Shapiro F: *Eye Movement Desensitization and Reprocessing: Basic Principles, Protocols, and Procedures*. New York, Guilford, 1998.

Silverman-Yam B: An agency-based perspective on domestic violence. *Renfrew Perspective* 1996;2:5–9.

Smith WH: Hypnotherapy with rape victims. In: Rhue JH, Lynn SJ, Kirsch I (eds.): *Handbook of Clinical Hypnosis*, pp. 479–491. Washington, DC, American Psychological Association, 1993.

Smith WH: Hypnosis in the treatment of sexual trauma: a master class commentary. *Int J Clin Exp Hypn* 1995;43:366–368.

Smith WH: The use of hypnosis in diagnosis and treatment. In: Spira JL, Yalom ID (eds.): *Treating Dissociative Identity Disorder*, pp. 219–238. San Francisco, Jossey-Bass, 1996.

Stapleton S: Domestic violence intervention still elusive. *AMA News*, December 1, 1997, pp. 3, 21.

Stewart DE, Robinson GE: Violence and women's mental health. *Harv Rev Psychiatry* 1996;4:54–57.

Swanston HY, Tebbutt JS, O'Toole BI, et al.: Sexually abused children five years after presentation: a case-control study. *Pediatrics* 1997;100:600–608.

Terr L: *Too Scared to Cry: Psychic Trauma in Childhood*. New York, Harper & Row, 1990.

Terr L: *Unchained Memories: True Stories of Traumatic Memories, Lost and Found*. New York, Basic Books, 1994.

van der Kolk B: The body keeps the score: approaches to the psychobiology of posttraumatic stress disorder. In: van der Kolk BA, McFarlane AC, Weisaeth L (eds.): *Traumatic Stress: The Effects of Overwhelming Experience on Mind, Body, and Society*, pp. 214–241. New York, Guilford, 1996.

van der Kolk BA, McFarlane AC, and Weisaeth L (eds.): *Traumatic Stress: The Effects of Overwhelming Experience on Mind, Body, and Society*. New York, Guilford, 1996.

Vasquez CI: Spousal abuse and violence against women: the significance of understanding attachment. In: Sechzer JA, Pfafflin SM, Denmark FL, et al. (eds.): *Women and Mental Health*, pp. 119–128. New York, New York Academy of Sciences, 1996.

Walker LE: *The Battered Woman*. New York, Harper & Row, 1979.

Zerbe KJ: *The Body Betrayed: Women, Eating Disorders, and Treatment*. Washington, DC: American Psychiatric Press, 1993. Washington, American Psychiatric Press, 1993. (Softcover edition: *The Body Betrayed: A Deeper Understanding of Women, Eating Disorders, and Treatment*. Carlsbad, CA, Gürze Books, 1995.)

Chapter 7

Insomnia

Each year insomnia affects more than 60 million adults in the United States (30% to 50% of the general population). It is one of the most common presenting complaints in primary care.

It is generally believed that insomnia is more prevalent among women, but real gender differences remain unclear. In both men and women, a good night's sleep is essential to overall physical and mental health. Sleep needs among individuals vary a great deal, but a basic step anyone can take to feel healthy, increase energy, and even fight physical disease is to get as much sleep as needed (Hobson, 1994).

Insomnia is defined as a disturbance or perceived disturbance in one's usual sleep pattern. It may have a number of troublesome consequences, most frequently daytime fatigue, drowsiness, irritability, anxiety, depression, and somatic complaints. Motor vehicle accidents are among the most serious possible consequences. Despite the widespread prevalence and numerous consequences of insomnia, its physiologic causes are not well understood.

As is true of most other emotional disorders, women with insomnia are more likely than men to seek help for their sleep problems. Psychiatric comorbidity, particularly affective disorders, substance abuse disorders, anxiety disorders, and the effects of domestic violence, frequently manifest in patients encountered in general medical practice as "trouble falling asleep and staying asleep" (Table 7–1). Indeed, the clinician should be particularly alert to the possibility that battering and domestic discord may underlie sleep problems in women. Patients may not easily volunteer this information unless asked—and asked repeatedly—because they are ashamed of and frightened about this aspect of their personal history (Krakow et al., 1995). Sleep disturbances also are correlated with the postpartum period (Cox et al., 1982; Salzarulo and Rigoard, 1987) and with menopause (Ballinger, 1976; Gonen et al., 1986).

Treatment should focus on the primary complaint or disorder; specific pharmacologic or psychotherapeutic interventions often culminate in improvement (see "Patient Guidelines for Improved Sleep"). However, a significant percentage of sleep problems among women that are *not* caused by major life crises or emotional difficulties can be improved with some simple strategies.

Changing one's environment, taking a vacation, leaving an acute environmental stress, or making minor adjustments in sleep hygiene may improve the quality of sleep—and life—without further pharmacologic or behavioral intervention. Education about the importance of sleep hygiene addresses the maladaptive behaviors that interfere with sleep.

A basic step all women can take to improve their physical health and mental well-being is to determine how much sleep they need and then make sure they get it. This is often easier said than done in our contemporary society. Although

165

Table 7–1. **Sleep Disorders Related to Mental Disturbances**

Major depression	Generalized anxiety disorder
Fitful sleep	Trouble falling asleep and staying
Insomnia	asleep
Early-morning awakening	Insomnia
Lack of feeling refreshed after sleep	Nightmares
Waking up in middle of night sobbing	Panic disorder
(rare, but classic sign)	Trouble falling asleep and staying
Hypersomnia	asleep
Nightmares	Insomnia; abrupt awakenings with panic
Dysthymia	attacks
Insomnia	Posttraumatic stress disorder
Daytime sleepiness	Insomnia
Hypersomnia	Nightmares
Nightmares	Eating disorders
Lack of feeling refreshed after sleep	Insomnia
Mania	Frequent awakenings
Short periods of sleep	Early-morning awakening
Sleep loss may induce mania	Substance abuse disorders
Schizophrenia/psychosis	Alcoholism
Insomnia	
Disorganized sleep-wake schedule	

women have always had to juggle multiple roles of spouse, homemaker, mother, and worker, the modern world places new burdens on men and women and gives less sanction for the need all of us have for rest. Most persons get 1 to 2 hours less sleep each night than they actually need; this sleep deficit leads to increased daytime sleepiness, irritability, fatigue, and interference with the normal sleep-wake cycle. An affliction of contemporary society is getting less sleep than actually needed (a chronic state of sleep deprivation) because our culture so highly prizes continual activity, work, and accomplishments at the price of carving out space for the self to rest, reflect, and renew.

The primary care clinician should suspect sleep deprivation as the underlying cause in any patient who complains of irritability, lack of energy, anxiety, daytime sleepiness, or depression. Yet sleep habits are rarely an aspect of a routine health evaluation (Schramm et al., 1995). Physicians often fail to suspect sleep difficulties as an underlying cause of discord, perhaps, in part, because their own training and professional life has required them also to forgo sleep. The sleep deprivation that normally accompanies medical training and residency therefore may be one complicating factor in the generally poor recognition physicians have of their patients' chronic sleep complaints. As part of all routine health evaluations, physicians must become more vigilant in asking about sleep patterns and problems—realizing that many poor sleepers have been "closeted" about their difficulties, only to respond when asked concretely about their nighttime habits.

To correct many sleep difficulties, clinicians can employ simple counseling techniques in the office setting (see "Additional Guidelines for Clinicians"). Often even minor adjustments can help avoid elaborate psychiatric evaluation, polysomnographic studies, or referral to a specialty sleep disorder clinic. Most important, the primary care clinician who takes seriously the role of good sleep hygiene counters the societal notion that overwork and lack of sleep can be endured endlessly without a significant toll on the body or mind.

PATIENT GUIDELINES FOR IMPROVED SLEEP

1. *Keep a regular sleep schedule:* Go to bed and get up at the same time every day, including weekends. This helps develop a regular sleep-wake rhythm.
2. *Reduce unwanted noise and light in the bedroom:* As much as possible, minimize unwanted sound. Although airplane and traffic noise, loud music, and lights can be eliminated in some instances, those caring for young children will not be able to fully eliminate background noise; their vigilance inclines them to get less sleep. A partner who snores may also disrupt sleep. Make sure to check with your primary care clinician about some simple steps to take to reduce snoring (e.g, plastic nasal strips).
3. *Minimize use of caffeinated beverages:* Avoiding caffeine is particularly important after the evening meal or for several hours before going to bed. This includes coffee, tea, cola beverages, and chocolate.
4. *Do not work at falling asleep:* Trying too hard to get to sleep creates the vicious circle of increasing anxiety, which only perpetuates wakefulness. Get out of bed for 15 to 30 minutes, then return to bed only when sleepy.
5. *Do not go to bed hungry:* Although overeating before bedtime should be avoided, women who are dieting or watching their weight for health reasons will be prone to hunger pangs then. They should have a light snack of low-calorie food such as carrots, pretzels, or skim milk; one cannot rest well on an empty stomach.
6. *Avoid having a "nightcap":* Alcohol disrupts the normal sleep-wake cycle. Although it may help some people fall asleep because of its depressive action, alcohol disrupts normal sleep architecture and can lead to early awakenings.
7. *Use the bed and bedroom only for sleep and sex:* Avoid reading, watching TV, eating, or working there. This practice develops the mental association between restful time and the bedroom.
8. *Exercise regularly in the late afternoon or early evening:* Avoid exercising too close to bedtime. Leading an active life generally produces better and deeper sleep.
9. *Keep the bedroom at a comfortable temperature:* A room that is too warm or too cold interrupts good sleep. If your partner has a different preference for what the temperature should be, try to accommodate each other. Even simple unresolved relationship conflicts like this may interfere with sleep.
10. *Avoid smoking in the evening:* Nicotine is a central nervous system stimulant best discontinued 4 to 6 hours before bedtime.
11. *Avoid worrying:* When you are trying to go to sleep, make a conscious effort to relax. Imagine yourself resting in a peaceful place.
12. *Let go of emotional pain:* Many women try to swallow their emotional pain and relationship conflicts by keeping everything to themselves, only to find that they can never "let go." To promote your overall well-being, talk

about these issues with a trusted friend, in individual counseling, or in group therapy.

ADDITIONAL GUIDELINES FOR PRIMARY CARE CLINICIANS

1. Urge the patient to practice relaxation techniques or cognitive-behavioral strategies (see description in text).
2. Empathize with the unique burdens women have in getting adequate rest. Help the patient problem solve. Can her partner compromise about nighttime child care so that she can sleep at least a couple of nights a week? Can she carve out at least a few hours of time every week for her own personal relaxation and growth? If family supports are unavailable, could she consider treating herself to professional respite care a few times a month (e.g., having a babysitter at home while she sleeps; using daycare for children or elderly persons for whom she has primary responsibility)?
3. Ask the sleep partner (if one is available) whether the patient has any of these symptoms: loud snoring or episodes of interrupted breathing, leg movements, kicking inadvertently but often. Consideration must be given to sleep apnea, restless legs syndrome, or periodic limb movement disorder, respectively. Diagnosis is made by polysomnography after referral to a sleep disorder center.
4. Ask the patient about her partner's sleep habits. A woman's sleep may be disrupted if she herself or her partner has any of the above conditions. Overweight, middle-aged men, in particular, are predisposed to sleep apnea, which goes unrecognized and underdiagnosed until their spouses complain of concomitant sleep disturbances. For both women and men, the sleeping partner, when available, may provide the most accurate historical confirmation regarding poor sleep habits, substance abuse, sleep apnea, caffeine use, restless legs, and nocturia.

When a female patient acknowledges having sleep difficulties, the clinician must pay attention to the special role conflicts and competing demands women face. Even the best recommendations will go unheeded if the patient cannot realistically put them into practice. For example, women with babies or young children and those who do shift work or carry two jobs are often sleep deprived (Lee, 1992; Lee and DeJoseph, 1992). Because she cannot quickly change her lifestyle, such a woman must instead find creative approaches and elicit support from her environment to get the rest she needs. It can be very difficult for her to have to acknowledge that she is not "superwoman" and turn to other family members, friends, or caregivers for respite. One patient, a single mother in her late 30s, found she had to "treat" herself to a babysitter for her two youngsters while she slept; twice monthly, the sitter came to the patient's home so that she could rest without the intrusions of her work and her children's needs.

Women are particularly prone to having sleep difficulties as a result of an underlying substance abuse disorder. This includes dependence on or abuse of alcohol or other psychoactive drugs used to promote sleep.

Be mindful of all the physical disorders and life cycle changes that may erode a woman's capacity to sleep through the night (Table 7–2). A frequent complaint signaling the menopause is fitful, wakeful sleep, which may be accompanied by

Table 7–2. **Medical Conditions Causing Sleep Difficulties**

Cardiovascular disease	Neurologic disorders
Congestive heart failure	Epilepsy (sleep deprivation may trigger
Angina	seizures)
Endocrine disorders	Parkinson's disease
Hyperthyroidism	Headaches, cluster (avoid sleep
Diabetes	deprivation to prevent headaches)
Hypothyroidism	Migraine
Musculoskeletal disorders	Gastrointestinal disorders
Arthritis	Esophagitis/heartburn
Fibromyalgia	Obstetric/gynecologic changes
Respiratory disorders	Menopause
Emphysema	Postpartum depression/psychosis
Bronchitis	

hot flashes. There is no substitute for a thorough physical evaluation and clinical judgment to rule out the most common medical causes of sleep difficulties before undertaking more specific polysomnographic study. A significant number of patients have an underlying physical illness (e.g., migraine, hyperthyroidism, arthritis) that is primarily driven by emotional problems (such as domestic abuse) contributing to insomnia. The body may have as many "diseases as it pleases" (Pies, 1994), and physical and psychological difficulties frequently are found in tandem.

The primary care clinician who strictly supervises the use of addictive sleeping medications and prescribes nonpharmacologic, behavioral approaches for the treatment of insomnia is less likely to unwittingly foster addictions. Women may also be prone to overuse caffeinated beverages that disturb sleep; often their sleep difficulties can be ameliorated by decreasing or eliminating caffeine intake.

A surprising number of women find it difficult to keep the physician-recommended sleep schedule of going to bed and getting up at the same time on weekends as on weekdays. Yet this is an essential aspect of developing a regular sleep-wake rhythm.

GUIDELINES FOR TREATMENT
Relaxation and Behavioral Techniques

Relaxation and behavioral techniques produce improvement in sleep induction. Particularly when the patient is willing to *practice* the suggestions offered, sleep onset and total sleep time will improve. The clinician must *encourage* the patient as she learns any relaxation, biofeedback, or cognitive-behavioral techniques to aid sleep.

Remind the patient that, as with any new skill, mastery occurs only after sufficient practice. You may try "joining the patient" by sharing some difficult task you have undertaken in the past and the sense of accomplishment you felt after overcoming initial doubts about achieving your goal. This approach helps bridge the distance between clinician and patient, which promotes collaboration and a sense of mutual respect and affirmation.

How Relaxation Approaches Work

Relaxation techniques appear to reduce the cognitive and physiologic arousal mechanisms. They help induce sleep and decrease the number of awakenings during sleep. Relaxation is also believed to diminish the activity of the sympathetic system, permitting a more rapid and effective "deafferentation" of sleep onset at the level of the thalamus. Relaxation may also enhance parasympathetic activity, which decreases autonomic tone. In addition, alterations in cytokine activity (immune system) may play a role in insomnia and in the response to treatment (NIH Technology Assessment Panel, 1996).

Cognitive approaches (described later) appear to decrease arousal and to counter dysfunctional beliefs. Behavioral techniques, including sleep restriction and stimulus control, may help reduce physiologic arousal, reverse poor sleep habits, and shift circadian rhythms. These effects appear to involve both cortical structures and deep nuclei (e.g., locus caeruleus, suprachiasmatic nucleus).

Some women feel not only reassured but also empowered by the primary clinician who takes time to explain in nontechnical language the physiology of sleep and the rationale and potential benefits of these interventions. Individualized assessment is important because some patients want more specific information than others do. Explain to patients that qualitative and quantitative research is still needed to help understand the individual experience of insomnia and the agony it creates. You may want to underscore how science is still attempting to answer which pharmacologic, behavioral, or combined approaches to treatment yield the best outcome for each person. This nondefensive, honest approach goes a long way toward demystifying the process. In the past, women were not given full access to current knowledge—or the lack thereof—which only perpetuated their anxieties and distrust of the medical profession.

Cognitive Techniques for Office Settings

There are three main cognitive techniques that clinicians can teach their patients in the office: thought stopping, paradoxical intention, and use of imagination.

Thought Stopping. Tell the patient to force herself to think about the very thoughts that keep her awake. Then she must tell herself to stop. When the thought returns, as it invariably will, she must tell herself again and again to stop. Doing this forces an immediate shift of attention away from the preoccupying thoughts and demonstrates to the patient that she has greater control over her thoughts (and herself) than she believed. With greater self-assurance and self-acceptance, sleep is more likely to commence.

Paradoxical Intention. Instruct the patient *not* to fall asleep. Such an expectation to avoid sleep may actually induce rest. In essence, paradoxical intention addresses the problem of performance anxiety; by forcing herself to stay awake as long as possible, the patient becomes sleepy without pressuring herself.

Use of Imagination. Encourage the patient to create pictures in her mind or to imagine that she is floating or suspended in midair. Emphasize that she should reflect on the details of each of these sensory experiences—the color or setting of the pictures she creates; the softness or atmosphere she feels as she imagines herself floating above the ground. Imagining a peaceful environment or comforting bodily sensations shifts attention away from intruding thoughts or anxieties, induces the physiologic changes that result in decreased metabolic activity, and thereby promotes sleep.

Encouraging Patient Compliance

Patient compliance can be enhanced through the techniques of immediate practice, sleep restriction, and progressive relaxation.

Immediate Practice. Have the patient practice each exercise while in the office. Positive outcome is always more likely when you do more than simply explain the procedure by helping the patient anticipate and experience what to expect. In addition, this practice session allows misconceptions to be corrected more easily. Inevitably, you will get a sense of which approach works best for a particular patient. You can also especially encourage the patient to practice the particular technique that works best for her.

In the past, specific behavioral approaches were not incorporated into conventional medical care. However, meditation, progressive muscle relaxation, hypnosis, autogenic training, and relaxation techniques all have been found useful in stress management and in reducing sleep difficulties.

Having the patient repeat a word, sound, prayer, or phrase—or having her simply adopt a passive attitude toward intruding thoughts—may be enough to alter disruptive sleep patterns. When these office techniques are not enough, it may be highly beneficial to encourage the patient to learn about a behavioral or relaxation approach that fits her individual needs.

Some women have benefited greatly from yoga classes, biofeedback seminars, or meditation groups that are available through community resource centers or at local women's health cooperatives. Knowing what resources are available in your local community enables you to suggest them as part of your own medical care.

Sleep problems must be recognized for what they are—complex, multifaceted disorders that often require multidimensional evaluation and treatment. However, when even a little headway can be made toward producing greater rest in a patient with an intractable difficulty, major strides in her emotional and physical well-being occur. Nonpharmacologic approaches, in particular, help patients feel a sense of mastery in life over the chronic, unremitting problem of insomnia.

Sleep Restriction. Sleep restriction therapy, in which patients use a sleep log and then are asked to stay in bed only as long as they think they are currently sleepy, leads quickly to sleep deprivation and sleep consolidation. What usually follows is a gradual increase in the length of time in bed.

For example, when a patient complains that she is sleeping only about 6 hours a night out of an ideal 8 hours, the prescribed sleep window for the first week of treatment would be 6 hours. The patient should take 2 hours off her bedtime. If she normally goes bed at 10 p.m. and lies there for 2 hours, she should now go to bed at midnight. The patient should arise at the same time every day.

Within a few days, the patient will be in a state of relative sleep deprivation. She may feel some daytime sleepiness. She should be told that this is normal and is actually a sign that the treatment is working. She may then plan to go to bed 15 minutes earlier at night, still getting up at the same time every morning. She gradually increases her time in bed in 15-minute intervals until she is sleeping 85% of the time she spends in bed.

In essence, the main effect of sleep restriction therapy is to produce a mild sleep deprivation, which leads in turn to rapid sleep onset, improved sleep continuity, and deeper sleep. Midday naps are discouraged except for elderly patients.

Progressive Relaxation. Relaxation-based interventions share the premise that stress, anxiety, and excessive arousal interfere with sleep. A variety of relaxation methods can be used, but the one described in Table 7–3 aims at reducing muscular tension by a simple series of steps.

It is important to review the steps with the patient in the office and to follow up with a handout for review at home. The spoken and written words interact synergistically; patients take a piece of the doctor home with them in the form of guidelines and recommendations that facilitate their connection, comfort, and involvement in their own treatment.

Sometimes suggesting that the patient play relaxing music while exercising or after a warm bath adds to the effectiveness of these relaxation techniques. Psychologically speaking, you are also giving the patient permission to take time for self-care. Many women resist this "indulgence" if it is not made an explicit part of their treatment plan. Most important, these relaxation exercises are truly exercises, requiring at least 15 minutes of daily practice (Morin, 1993).

If the patient reports that insomnia is not improving after you have reviewed the techniques, ask if she is following through with your recommendations. Wonder with her whether "busyness" is getting in the way (e.g., childcare, work demands, responsibility for elderly parents) or whether she needs greater encouragement from her partner. Remind her that all of those whom she holds dear will ultimately benefit from her improved health—as will she—and that she deserves and needs time for herself if she is to stay healthy, let alone thrive. In this way, you are acknowledging the multiple islands of stress that may be getting in the way of the therapeutic strategy while confronting the reluctance many women feel when they "put themselves first," even for a few moments a day and in the interest of their health.

Sleeping Medications

Older people, particularly women, are prone to use sleep-promoting drugs (Mellinger et al., 1985). Many patients medicate their sleep problems with alcohol and over-the-counter remedies. Although the use of sedative-hypnotics has steadily declined, the use of sleeping medications on a strictly prophylactic basis is quite common for chronic insomniacs. In one study by the National Institute of Mental Health, 11% of patients with insomnia had used medications regularly for more than 1 year. Among the various prescribed sleep-promoting agents, 61% of patients received hypnotics, 27% anxiolytics, and 11% antidepressants (Mellinger et al., 1985).

Table 7–3. **Relaxation Exercise**

Goal: To work all four groups of muscles.

These instructions for the patient can be prepared and printed for home use. For best results, the physician or care extender should first have the patient work the sequence in the office at least once.

Group I

Hands, forearms, and biceps. Make a fist with left hand without lifting the arm. Tighten hand, relax it, then open it. Visualize the tension leaving the hand. Repeat once. Move on to left forearm and biceps area. Then go through same sequence with right hand, forearm, and biceps. Move on to Group II.

Group II

Head, face, neck, and shoulders. Open eyes and raise eyebrows. Notice how forehead wrinkles. Concentrate on feeling tension move to brow. Next, tense and then relax the scalp. Sequentially, tense and release eyebrows and eyelids, grip and relax, then tense and release lips, tongue, neck, and shoulders. Feel relaxation spreading over each body part. If comfortable visualizing, try to "see" the muscle move, releasing tension with each contraction.

Group III

Chest, stomach, and lower back. Fill lungs completely. Hold breath, then exhale, feeling tension leave lungs. Repeat at least three times, each exhalation draining away more tension. Move on to stomach and then to back. Focus tension in the stomach and then release it. Do same with the back. Tell yourself that the rest of your body is as relaxed as possible, with all the tension focused on the lower back.

Group IV

Thighs, buttocks, calves, and feet. Tense and relax buttocks three times. Press down on thighs and then relax, noting difference. "See" the healthy blood flow to muscles, clearing away tension. Curl toes downward, making calves tense. Again, visualize the tension and its dissipation from the body. Flex toes up toward face to create tension in shins, then relax.

Practicing this sequence for 15 minutes a day, every day, will help reduce somatic arousal (e.g., muscle tension). It is also a moderately attention-diverting procedure aimed at controlling excessive presleep cognitive activity. A side benefit is that it gives an enhanced sense of control over self and body, a feeling of resourcefulness that has been eroded by the sleep disorder.

As noted, complaints of insomnia occur twice as commonly in women as in men, possibly because of the more intricate role in women of the hypothalamic-pituitary-gonadal (HPG) axis in the secretion and regulation of gonadal hormones. More than 25% of new mothers report significant sleep disturbances (Salzarulo and Rigoard, 1987), but difficulty falling asleep and staying asleep is also reported frequently by postmenopausal women (Ballinger, 1976). Women who work night or rotating shifts, who have difficulty expressing and managing anger, or who have been victims of sexual assault have a high incidence of sleep disturbances.

For most patients, nonpharmacologic treatment of insomnia is more effective than drugs, especially over the long term (Morin, 1993; Morin et al., 1994).

However, the U.S. Food and Drug Administration has approved many drugs for insomnia, including five benzodiazepines and zolpidem (Ambien), a nonbenzodiazepine that binds to benzodiazepine receptors in the brain. Some drugs marketed for other indications, such as antihistamines, antidepressants, and antipsychotics, are also frequently used as sleeping medications in some populations (Karacan et al., 1996).

Nonprescription Sedative-Hypnotics

Antihistamines. The antihistamines diphenhydramine (Nytol, Benadryl) and doxylamine (Unisom) are two of the most commonly used over-the-counter medications. Currently approved for sale as "sleep aids" without a prescription, these medications are taken by some women chronically without reporting such use to the clinician. *Be sure to question patients with insomnia about their use of over-the-counter medications.* Because antihistamines are nonaddicting, they have a unique utility for patients with a tendency toward substance abuse. They decrease sleep latency but have not been shown to increase total sleep time. Patients should be reminded that antihistamines may cause daytime sedation and impaired performance skills (e.g., driving). Overdosage can cause delirium, psychosis, or urinary retention, especially in elderly persons.

Alcohol. Although alcohol is an ineffective hypnotic, it is frequently used by patients to initiate sleep. Tolerance and addiction develop rapidly. When an insomnia patient admits to using alcohol or any other substance to induce sleep, be sure to taper it slowly so as to avoid withdrawal and rebound insomnia.

L-Tryptophan and Melatonin. L-Tryptophan, the amino acid, gained favor in the 1980s for the treatment of insomnia because of its safety, affordability, and over-the-counter availability. This dietary supplement appeared to be helpful in correcting transient sleep disturbances by decreasing sleep latency and increasing total sleep time. Its use is currently banned in the United States because of the associated cases of eosinophilia-myalgia syndrome that were reported in 1989. Its efficacy as a sleeping agent for long-term use remains uncertain, although the soporific effects of nutritional compounds such as milk have been reported for centuries.

In the 1990s, melatonin has been touted by the popular and professional press as the ultimately safe, easily available, natural sleep aid. Secreted by the pineal gland circadially in most vertebrates, melatonin in low oral doses promotes hypnotic effects when it is administered during the evening.

The sleep-inducing properties of melatonin may differ from those of benzodiazepines by reducing deep sleep, thus negatively influencing sleep quality. Consequently, the hangover effect and daytime drowsiness, major problems with other hypnotic agents, have not been observed in the mornings after an evening administration of melatonin. Despite these promising results, the purity of the products available, as well as any adverse effects, remains unknown. Moreover, adequate clinical trials are still lacking.

Prescription Hypnotics—Benzodiazepines

Benzodiazepine sedative-hypnotics are among the most widely prescribed psychotropic drugs. Their anxiolytic action is believed to induce sleep by eliminating anxiety, which may delay the onset of sleep and cause frequent awakening. Benzodiazepines increase the inhibitory effects of gamma-aminobutyric acid (GABA), principally through interaction with the GABA-α receptor.

The most frequently prescribed benzodiazepine hypnotics are triazolam (Halcion), temazepam (Restoril), flurazepam (Dalmane), and quazepam (Doral). When used to treat acute sleep disturbances brought on by loss, illness, or other stressors, benzodiazepines can be quite helpful; however, they can produce tolerance and physical dependence (especially with higher doses) over long durations of treatment and in patients prone to addiction. The use of benzodiazepines in the elderly has been associated with increases in falls and hip fractures.

Benzodiazepines have sometimes been used to treat chronic sleep disturbances. However, some studies suggest that after 30 consecutive nights of use, these drugs lose their hypnotic efficacy owing to tolerance. Citing this fact may be useful in dealing with the patient who insists that she must have her sleeping pill every night. Occasionally, such demands can also be countered by showing the patient a textbook or journal article with the caveat that you want her to be as educated as possible about her body. Other troublesome side effects include drowsiness, dizziness, lightheadedness, impaired coordination, and anterograde amnesia (with triazolam). Alprazolam (Xanax), an intermediate-duration benzodiazepine, is not recommended for use as a hypnotic because of its high potential for rapid tolerance and abuse.

Patients must be counseled not to abruptly discontinue benzodiazepines after extended use. Not only is rebound insomnia likely to occur, but psychosis may be precipitated. Benzodiazepines should be avoided by anyone who has a sensitivity to the compounds, is pregnant (especially in the first trimester), or may be suffering from sleep apnea. However, sleep apnea is much more common in men than in women. When benzodiazepines are used, women should be cautioned about activities that require mental alertness, such as driving or caring for small children. In addition, patients must be warned about the dangers of using alcohol and other central nervous system depressants while taking benzodiazepines. Benzodiazepines are metabolized through conjugative mechanisms, and most are also metabolized through oxidation. Oxidation declines with age and liver dysfunction. Because temazepam is eliminated by conjugative mechanisms only, it is particularly useful in infirm and elderly patients with insomnia. As a general rule, half the initial dose should be prescribed for an elderly woman compared with a younger one.

Other Prescription Sedative-Hypnotics

Zolpidem (Ambien) and Zopiclone. Although chemically unrelated to the benzodiazepines, these compounds act by binding to the benzodiazepine receptors in the brain. Controlled studies have found that zolpidem offers several advantages over the benzodiazepines: lack of withdrawal symptoms, minimal effects on cognitive functioning, no daytime sedation, little or no tolerance, only occasional rebound insomnia, and no respiratory depression. Unlike the benzodiazepines, which tend to suppress stage 3 and stage 4 (deep) sleep and rapid eye movement (REM) sleep, zolpidem has little effect on the relative lengths of these sleep stages.

Zolpidem is becoming recognized as an excellent alternative to the benzodiazepine hypnotics for short-term treatment of insomnia in the United States. The usual therapeutic dosage is 5 to 10 mg/day; therapeutic action is exerted within 30 minutes. Adverse effects may include dizziness, drowsiness, headache, nausea, vomiting, and gastrointestinal pain but are usually mild and transient. This medication is considerably more expensive than other medications.

Zolpidem-induced psychotic reactions and sensory distortions have occurred in women in some rare case reports. Although most of these reactions resulted within minutes to hours after dosing (implying easy recognition) and with doses higher than 10 mg (suggesting a dose-dependent effect), extra vigilance is warranted. Women may require a smaller dose than men; a 5-mg dose is often sufficient. Recent treatment with zolpidem must also be considered in the differential diagnosis in patients, particularly women, with new-onset or unexplained psychotic symptoms (Markowitz and Brewerton, 1996).

Antipsychotics. Like most other powerful drugs, antipsychotics have multiple effects with different time frames. One of the most impressive properties of any antipsychotic is its calming action. With high-potency drugs such as haloperidol (Haldol), the effect is calming with some sedation; with low-potency drugs such as chlorpromazine (Thorazine), the overall effect may be very rapid onset of profound sedation. Advantages to using low-potency antipsychotics include sedation and calming of agitated patients and tremendous relief in staff members who must deal with agitated patients in the hospital. But the acute disadvantages of low-potency antipsychotics can be severe. They may cause substantial orthostatic hypotension when given intramuscularly. Chlorpromazine—the most commonly used low-potency antipsychotic agent—can cause severe postural hypotension that progresses rarely to shock.

Antipsychotics with sedative-hypnotic properties, such as chlorpromazine, should be used only in the treatment of insomnia in patients suffering from psychosis. Their long-term use can precipitate extrapyramidal symptoms, including tardive dyskinesia. Women are at greater risk for developing tardive dyskinesia than men. (Before the advent of safer medications, these drugs were overused in some subgroups of female patients.)

The clinician should consider administering the daily recommended dose of an antipsychotic at bedtime for its soporific effects. The anticholinergic, antihistaminic, and antiadrenergic properties of antipsychotics contribute to their sedative properties but also potentiate those side effects that contribute to patient noncompliance (e.g., akathisia, sexual dysfunction, sedation).

Antidepressants

Sedative antidepressants, including amitriptyline (Elavil), doxepin (Sinequan), maprotiline (Ludiomil), trazodone (Desyrel), and, to a lesser extent, nefazodone (Serzone), may be particularly useful in patients whose clinical depression is accompanied by insomnia. Some clinicians use low doses of the sedating tricyclic antidepressants, such as amitriptyline or doxepin, in patients who are not depressed but complain of insomnia. For the nondepressed insomniac patient, psychiatrists tend to give a trial of a low-dose antidepressant medication at night rather than a benzodiazepine, especially when there is any risk of substance abuse or self-medication with alcohol or other drugs of abuse.

As described in Chapter 2, women who are prescribed the monoamine oxidase inhibitors (MAOIs) such as phenelzine (Nardil) or the selective serotonin reuptake inhibitors (SSRIs) such as fluoxetine (Prozac) or paroxetine (Paxil) for major depression, dysthymia, or atypical depression may be at special risk for drug-induced insomnia.

When intervening with the patient with comorbid insomnia and depression, consider a trial of a sedative antidepressant to tackle both problems. Should the patient be effectively treated for depression with one agent that unpredictably induces sleep difficulties, a benzodiazepine, trazodone, or zolpidem may temporarily be added to the regimen.

Particularly when the use of multiple psychopharmacologic agents becomes necessary, the primary care clinician should consider referral to a psychiatrist. For example, some patients who take trazodone and fluoxetine report excessive sedation, nausea, dizziness, and ataxia; it is difficult, if not impossible, for any clinician to be aware of all the potential untoward or idiosyncratic side effects or the nuances of dosages in these frequently prescribed combination therapies. Specialty consultation also provides access to a broad range of new psychotropic drugs and increases the treatment options for any given patient.

Barbiturates

Barbiturates are sometimes still used in the treatment of insomnia, but their use has substantially declined because of the potential for tolerance, addiction, and death by overdose. Women, in particular, were prescribed barbiturates for a host of emotional problems in the 1950s and 1960s, leading first to psychological and then to physiologic dependence. Drowsiness, lethargy, agitation, and phobias have been observed frequently during barbiturate administration. Barbiturates are now considered of limited value in the treatment of sleep disturbance. They are habit forming, and tolerance develops rapidly; residual sedation, "hangover effect," vertigo, and lethargy are pronounced adverse reactions. Other disadvantages that contribute to their disfavor include the narrow range from therapeutic to toxic dosages, many drug interactions, and lethality in overdose.

Chloral Hydrate

This agent is an inexpensive, effective hypnotic for transient insomnia. (The beginning dose of chloral hydrate is 500 mg–1 g, not to exceed 2 g/day.) Its positive effects usually disappear within a few weeks, and physical dependence quickly develops. Disrupted sleep and nightmares are associated with its withdrawal. However, chloral hydrate may be a particularly useful agent for a stress-related problem. Because fatalities have occurred with relatively mild overdoses (e.g., 4 g), it should be avoided in the depressed, self-destructive patient.

Glutethimide, Methyprylon, and Ethchlorvynol

Glutethimide (Doridan) and methyprylon (Noludar) have been withdrawn from the market in the United States because of the potential lethality in overdose and the availability of newer, safer agents. Ethchlorvynol (Placidyl) can also cause serious side effects, which may lead to rapid habituation and tolerance, and is highly lethal in overdosage. Like chloral hydrate, it carries the same risks as the barbiturates. The current availability of safer medications is reducing its general usage, although it still plays a role in selected clinical situations such as intolerance to other classes of drugs.

SUMMARY

Insomnia affects millions of women and is a frequent complaint both in primary care and in psychiatric settings. Despite its ubiquity, patients often do not mention it to their clinician unless asked directly. Particularly at risk for chronic insomnia are victims of domestic abuse, persons balancing multiple roles of career and family, and shift workers.

Although the disorder is epidemic in our society, many patients (and their physicians) believe they cannot be helped except by taking medication. In fact, many practitioners avoid asking about sleep problems because they are afraid of confronting an intractable problem. Fortunately, despite the substantial morbidity associated with insomnia, contemporary approaches that combine counseling, cognitive-behavioral methods, sleep hygiene practices, and judicious pharmacotherapy can help the majority of patients.

After ruling out the medical and psychiatric problems that may play a role in causing insomnia, the clinician can employ a variety of simple behavioral methods and sleep hygiene practices to improve the quality of the patient's sleep and her overall physical well-being. First, however, the cause of the insomnia must be identified. Emphasis must be placed throughout treatment on encouraging the patient to empower herself through self-care, which includes finding time for periods of rest and self-restoration. In this way, the primary care provider enhances the overall mental and physical well-being of the patient.

Resources for Patients

Hauri P, Linde S: *No More Sleepless Nights*. New York, John Wiley, 1991 (paperback: 1996).
  An excellent summary for patients who want to know more about sleep and how to improve their sleeping habits. Included are a range of practical suggestions, such as bedtime relaxation techniques, the roles of diet and exercise in promoting sleep, and ways to deal with daily stress that gets in the way of good sleep. Particular sleep difficulties women encounter (e.g., due to shift work, pregnancy) are also cited. Numerous case examples and use of humor are engaging tools that involve the reader.

Morin C: *Relief from Insomnia: Getting the Sleep of Your Dreams*. New York, Doubleday, 1996 (paperback).
  Based on Dr. Morin's comprehensive work for professionals, this monograph outlines a step-by-step program for treating insomnia ("seven steps to a good night's sleep and eight strategies to beat insomnia"). Suggestions are made for keeping a sleep diary, learning to modify patterns of stress and promote relaxation, and revising attitudes about sleeplessness. The many clinical examples make for an interesting read for laypersons and professionals alike. Particularly useful are sections devoted to the hazards of sleeping pills and common myths about sleep needs with aging. Shift work, alcohol, caffeine, jet lag, and medical factors that affect the circadian rhythm are also discussed.

Resources for Clinicians

Bromfield EB: *Sleep Disturbance: A Harvard Health Letter Special Report*. Boston, Harvard Medical School Health Publication Group, 1996.

This brief overview of sleep mechanics and the range of sleep disturbances amplifies what can be found in most general medical texts. In addition to the diagnosis and treatment of insomnia, brief reviews are given of breathing disorders in sleep, movement disorders in sleep, narcolepsy, parasomnias, and disturbances of sleep timing (e.g., jet lag). Also highlighted are suggestions about how to improve sleep and those common myths that should be dispelled for optimum sleep. This monograph includes diagrams and tables for counseling patients and an appendix on sleeping medications for professional reference. A sample sleep diary to help delineate the patient's sleep patterns is found at the conclusion of the text.

Morin CM: *Insomnia: Psychological Assessment and Management.* New York, Guilford, 1993.

A thoroughly comprehensive, concise, and readable volume about all aspects of insomnia. The book covers assessment and treatment, stressing the interplay between maladaptive behavioral patterns and dysfunctional sleep. In-depth but easy-to-follow cognitive-behavioral guidelines are offered to clinicians who treat sleep problems in their practice. The book also contains outlines of structured clinical interviews for insomnia, sleep diaries, questionnaires, sample handouts and brochures, and outlines of therapy sessions that can be used in practice.

References

Ballinger CB: Subjective sleep disturbance at the menopause. *J Psychosom Res* 1976;20:509–513.

Cox JL, Connor YM, Kendell RE: Prospective study of the psychiatric disorders of childbirth. *Br J Psychiatry* 1982;140:111–117.

Gonen R, Sharf M, Lavie P: The association between mid-sleep waking episodes and hot flushes in post-menopausal women. *J Psychosom Obstet Gynaecol* 1986;5:113–117.

Hauri P, Linde S: *No More Sleepless Nights.* New York, John Wiley, 1991 (paperback: 1996).

Hobson JA: *The Chemistry of Conscious States: Toward a Unified Model of the Brain and the Mind.* Boston, Little, Brown, 1994.

Karacan I, Camuscu H, Demir B: Pharmacotherapy of insomnia. *Directions in Psychiatry* 1996;16:2–11.

Krakow B, Tandberg D, Barey M, et al.: Nightmares and sleep disturbance in sexually assaulted women. *Dreaming: Journal of the Association for the Study of Dreams* 1995;5:199–206.

Lee KA: Self-reported sleep disturbances in employed women. *Sleep* 1992;15:493–498.

Lee KA, DeJoseph JF: Sleep disturbances, vitality, and fatigue among a select group of employed childbearing women. *Birth* 1992;19:208–213.

Markowitz J, Brewerton T: Zolpidem-induced psychosis. *Ann Clin Psychiatry* 1996;8:89–91.

Mellinger GD, Balter MB, Uhlenhuth EH: Insomnia and its treatment: Prevalence and correlates. *Arch Gen Psychiatry* 1985;42:225–232.

Morin C: *Relief from Insomnia: Getting the Sleep of Your Dreams.* New York, Doubleday, 1996 (paperback).

Morin CM: *Insomnia: Psychological Assessment and Management.* New York, Guilford, 1993.

Morin CM, Culbert JP, Schwartz SM: Nonpharmacological interventions for insomnia: A meta-analysis of treatment efficacy. *Am J Psychiatry* 1994;151:1172–1180.

NIH Technology Assessment Panel on Integration of Behavioral and Relaxation Approaches into the Treatment of Chronic Pain and Insomnia. *JAMA* 1996;276:313–318.

Pies RW: *Clinical Manual of Psychiatric Diagnosis and Treatment: A Biopsychosocial Approach.* Washington, DC, American Psychiatric Press, 1994.

Salzarulo P, Rigoard MT: Long-lasting sleep disturbances in women after childbirth. *Journal of Reproductive and Infant Psychology* 1987;5:245–246.

Schramm E, Hohagen F, Kappler C, et al.: Mental comorbidity of chronic insomnia in general practice attendees using DSM-III-R. *Acta Psychiatr Scand* 1995;91:10–17.

Chapter 8

Somatization

In the classic Broadway musical, *Guys and Dolls*, the lyrics of the song "Adelaide's Lament" pose a hypothesis about what causes psychosomatic illness in women. The female lead, Adelaide, is bemoaning the case of the "average unmarried female, basically insecure," who "due to some long frustration, may react with psychosomatic symptoms, difficult to endure, affecting the upper respiratory tract!" Audiences have giggled for decades as Adelaide explains how a woman "just waiting around for that plain little band of gold can develop a cold!" Her refrains, "just wondering if the wedding is on or off, a person can develop a cough" and "a lack of community property or a feeling she is getting too old, a person can develop a bad, bad cold" both spark audience delight—because we are all intuitively aware that emotions such as sexual excitement, apprehension about beginning a new task, or suppression of anger can lead to illness. Most people have had ample opportunity to swallow or suppress emotion, only to observe how it gets released in a bout of gastrointestinal distress, a rapid pulse or elevated blood pressure, a psychogenic dermatitis, or low back pain. We assume that overpowering but unintegrated feelings cause disruption in the psychosoma that can lead to the most flagrant or subtle somatization disorders (Gallon, 1992; Smith, 1991).

What can be done to help this human tendency to become ill or to think you are ill whenever strong feelings cannot be processed? Physicians, too, are befuddled about how to help the patient who seems to have no end to a litany of physical complaints. Adelaide observes that "you can give her a shot for whatever she's got and it just won't work" and "you can feed her all day with vitamin A and Bromofizz, but medicine never gets anywhere near where the trouble is." For such people, psychosomatic symptoms become a way of functioning, a way to actually take care of themselves and to compensate for something that is missing in life (Farber, 1997). This chapter focuses on some of the reasons behind the development of psychosomatic illness and on how the primary care clinician can begin to work with the patient to promote better health.

THE PATIENT WHO WON'T GET WELL

Exaggerated physical complaints, the hallmark of somatization (Table 8–1), are the bane of the primary care clinician. By definition, no organic explanation can be found for the patient's ailments, but that does not mean these patients don't suffer. They convey their psychological distress by means of their physical complaints.

Multiple body systems are usually involved, and the patient typically undergoes numerous medical workups or surgical procedures before a psychiatric diagnosis is made (Ford, 1983, 1995a). What is especially beguiling—and

Table 8–1. **Common Somatoform Disorders Among Women and Their Treatment**

Somatization disorder

Somatization disorder is a syndrome of numerous physical complaints that are not intentionally produced or feigned. A chronic condition with onset typically before age 30, it affects women 10 times as frequently as it does men. Symptoms in several body systems must be present for the diagnosis (e.g., four pain symptoms, two gastrointestinal symptoms, one sexual/reproduction symptom, and one pseudoneurologic symptom). A familial pattern is seen in 10% to 20% of cases. Full remission is rare. Currently, no specific pharmacologic treatment is recommended unless there is a comorbid psychiatric problem. Regular visits with the primary care clinician and psychotherapy are the treatments of choice.

Conversion disorder

Conversion disorder is characterized by symptoms or deficits affecting voluntary motor or sensory functions that are not explained by a neurologic or medical condition. Conversion symptoms are very common, particularly among medically ill and postpartum women. The disorder typically begins in late childhood or early adulthood; it affects women much more frequently than men. Although individual conversion symptoms tend to remit within days or weeks, about one fourth of patients relapse within 1 year. Without prompt resolution of the conversion symptoms, there is substantial risk of recurrence or chronic disability. Treatment techniques include hypnosis, amobarbital-enhanced interviews, cognitive-behavioral therapy, psychodynamic therapy, and biofeedback. Pharmacotherapy is not recommended unless there is a comorbid psychiatric syndrome (e.g., anxiety disorder).

Hypochondriasis

Worry about having a serious disease based on a misinterpretation of bodily symptoms is known as hypochondriasis. Despite medical evaluation and reassurance, the patient continues to believe she has a serious or undiagnosed illness. The frequency is equal in men and women, more than 5% of the general medical population. Beginning in early adulthood, at least two thirds of patients have a chronic but fluctuating course. Recently, hypochondriasis has been linked to other disorders of serotonin dysregulation, namely, depression and anxiety (e.g., obsessive-compulsive spectrum disorder). Clinical improvement is seen in some cases with the SSRIs (e.g., fluoxetine, fluvoxamine), but supportive psychotherapy can also be helpful.

Pain disorder

Pain disorder occurs when there is significant distress or impairment in social and occupational functioning. It involves one or more anatomic sites. Psychological factors (financial compensation, dependency) play a significant role in etiology, but the illness is not feigned. It can occur at any age and is a dominant symptom in more than half of all general hospital admissions. Prescription of addictive drugs is associated with chronicity and should be avoided. Tricyclic antidepressants, in conjunction with nonsteroidal antiinflammatory agents (e.g., ibuprofen, naproxen) are better therapeutic options. Nonpharmacologic measures (e.g., acupuncture, massage) may be useful adjuncts for some patients.

Body dysmorphic disorder (BDD)

Body dysmorphic disorder is characterized by preoccupation with an imagined defect in appearance. This preoccupation causes significant stress or impairment in social or occupational functioning. By definition, BDD cannot be accounted for by another mental disorder (e.g., severe eating disorder). It tends to affect women much more often than men, particularly at menopause. Considered by some authorities to be part of the obsessive-compulsive spectrum, BDD responds to fluoxetine at doses recommended for obsessive-compulsive disorder (e.g., 60–80 mg rather than the 20–40 mg recommended for depression). Patients with BDD often carry the comorbid psychiatric diagnoses for anxiety or depression.

perplexing—about these patients is their reluctance to view their difficulties as psychological. It can be even more frustrating to attempt to engage them in a therapeutic relationship not based solely on diagnostic workups, requests for medication, and diagnostic procedures (Farber, 1997; Smith, 1995).

Somatization is predominantly a problem of women, with a female-to-male ratio of approximately 10:1. Among women, the lifetime prevalence has been estimated at between 0.5% and 2%, which is probably an underestimate (Martin and Yutzy, 1997). Researchers and clinicians alike tend to accept the patient's view that the reported symptoms *must* have a medical cause. It is little wonder that at least 10% (and probably more) of all medical services are provided to patients with no evidence of physical disease (Ford, 1983). Yet, in at least 30% of patients, no bona fide medical condition can be found to cause the complaints (Gise, 1998).

Patients who somatize tend to "doctor shop." In the process, they become very high utilizers of medical care, despite an absence of confirmed physical or laboratory abnormalities (Smith, 1995). Their adoption of the sick role and chronic illness carries much psychological meaning. For example, unconscious dependency needs can be met by assuming the sick role (Coen, 1992). Some young patients who go on to develop somatization or hypochondriasis as adults have a remarkable childhood history, often filled with tales of abandonment, physical or sexual abuse, or a lack of consistent affection and care (Druss, 1995; Levitan, 1982). Without adequate modeling about how to contain or modify anxiety, some patients displace it onto their body. Rather than feel tense, wound up, or even panicky, they express their emotions through a myriad of physical complaints (Walker et al., 1987).

Even though these patients are often quite bright, they do not have the capacity to name or categorize their emotions in words. Psychiatrists call this phenomena *alexithymia* (Finell, 1997; McDougall, 1989). Simply put, instead of saying, "I felt lonely, abandoned, and angry because my mother left my father when I was seven," a patient might report, "Ever since I was a little girl, I've gotten pains in my stomach almost every night when I try to go to sleep. I know I must have an ulcer. Yes, I've had lots of workups and nothing has ever been found. But you can't tell me, doctor, that my stomach pain is not real."

Indeed, the patient's pain is real. That's the problem. But what she has difficulty reckoning with is how her body expresses her long-standing emotional anguish. At the root, psychosomatic illnesses are forms of communication where the patient voices "the reasons of the heart" through her body (McDougall, 1989).

Somatizing patients have a hard time taking reasonably good care of themselves, so they look instead to you, their primary care clinician, to do it for them (Coen, 1992). It may seem as if they resist your help, even while imploring you for it. Herein lies another aspect of their dilemma. Taking care of oneself—meaning not only following through with the doctor's advice but taking responsibility for self-care through good nutrition, exercise, and adequate rest—is a developmental achievement. These behaviors actually are learned from one's parents, in the so-called psychodynamic process of internalization. When a parent is unable or unavailable—through death, narcissistic preoccupation (e.g., self-preoccupation), family discord, or innumerable work or family responsibilities—to be a source of soothing and sustenance for the youngster, the child's age-appropriate needs and wants are never met. Unconsciously, such patients look to you, their primary care clinician, to be a sort of substitute parent who will soothe their troubles away. And what is the ticket to obtain access to your receptive ear? Clearly, a physical disorder will command your full attention and medical expertise.

HOW DO I HELP THE PATIENT WHO WON'T GET WELL?

The principal treatment technique and goal when working with the somatizing patient is the formation of a long-standing, helpful relationship. Do not try to cure the patient by means of reassurance alone. Moreover, although some pharmacologic agents have been found useful in treating the comorbid depression or anxiety that often accompanies somatization, they are not the mainstay of therapy (Table 8–2). Most authorities recommend encouraging these patients to meet regularly with a single physician who can educate them about their illness (i.e., give them medical sanction for being sick) and can reassure them that no major physical problem is on the horizon (Smith, 1995; Stotland, 1997).

Meanwhile, because somatizing patients do develop real physical diseases, the primary clinician must stay vigilant for this possibility. However, what is most important is the formation of a supportive, trusting, safe relationship between patient and clinician. You can limit the number of visits or the amount of time the patient spends with you, but your continuing care of these patients can provide a great deal of satisfaction over the long term. Curbing the number of invasive tests or unnecessary medical procedures helps keep these patients from accruing additional expenses or developing an iatrogenic illness. They can instead be praised for making some positive lifestyle changes (Westberg and Jason, 1996).

Clinical Example

A rather dramatic example of the principles commonly outlined in medical and psychiatric texts occurred in the practice of one of my supervisees who consulted me about the case. A 42-year-old mother of three appeared weekly at a local emergency room in the middle of the night. Her "illnesses" fluctuated from week to week. Her complaints ranged from chest pain, palpitations, and shortness of breath to urinary retention and abdominal pain. On one occasion, she presented with such a dramatic headache that the attending staff physician ordered a full neurologic workup. On other occasions, her chronic anxiety was most notable as she begged the physician to be sure that she "only had the flu and not TB, AIDS, or herpes." Never having been sexually promiscuous, this patient had little to worry about with respect to a sexually transmitted disease. Moreover, despite her insistence on the need for treatment of an infection, she was afebrile and her workups were always negative.

Sometimes patients who present so many physical complaints without resolution over such a long period make physicians angry. This case was unique in that the entire staff, from the admissions clerk to the attending physicians, liked the patient. She had become their "emergency room pet," someone they expected to see on a regular basis. On the other hand, they gradually grew skeptical about ever being able to help her, and they realized she was diverting their attention from other patients who needed their care. She was also using the hospital's resources unnecessarily.

Table 8–2. **Strategies for Working with Patients with Physical Preoccupation and Unexplained Medical Illness**

1. Form a trusting relationship. Make regular, brief appointments. Do not underestimate the value of a helping relationship because it has been shown to be crucial in promoting change and growth.
2. Do not expect the patient to "get well," because the illness may be an entrée into an important caretaking relationship. The patient must have these dependency needs met before they can be confronted and worked through. Think care, not cure.
3. Rule out any new medical or comorbid psychiatric difficulty. Use psychotropic medications when indicated, but do not expect "cure."
4. Do expect many patients to be in the "precontemplation" stage of trying to change for a long time. Keep trying to motivate them by reassurance and through education. Avoid "high-intensity" (e.g., long-term expressive psychotherapy) interventions for these patients.
5. When you sense that the patient is ready to act for more definitive relief, do recommend psychotherapy. This intervention should help the patient deal with (1) intolerable feelings, (2) excessive dependency needs, and (3) any other underlying emotional conflicts.
6. Remember that some patients benefit from alternative healing methods. Point out this option, encouraging the patient in the safest and most researched modalities (e.g., biofeedback).
7. When you refer to a mental health professional, remain involved. Any form of psychotherapy is likely to be more successful if the patient does not feel abandoned by her primary care clinician.
8. Frequently explain and reassure the patient that there is no "real" physical damage to her body but that her anguish, nonetheless, is "real." Point out that a greater tolerance for anxiety and an increased understanding of her need for protection and care will help her over time (see Coen and Sarno, 1989).
9. Expect relapses, even in the most "successful" cases. Understand that maintaining any change is hard work. For example, the "costs" of making changes often are not realized, particularly in one's relationships to others; commitment and self-efficacy can also erode with time. Provide reassurance and help make sense of the crisis; encourage the patient to return to therapy for "booster sessions" if this makes sense.

The savvy resident decided to try to capitalize on the patient's strengths of likeability and her desire for help. She arranged to see the patient for brief, supportive therapy for 30 minutes every week. Her approach was not intended to get to the patient's core unconscious conflicts but rather to help her find new coping behaviors using cognitive-behavioral strategies. Although the resident was aware that both of these procedures have been tried with some success for a range of psychosomatic problems, she saw her role primarily as providing a safe place for the patient to talk about her worrisome physical problems.

The resident underscored to the patient that even during those weeks when she was feeling better, she needed to come for regular sessions. The doctor still wanted to meet with her as a way of staying abreast of "all the pain and misery you have been through." She empathized with the patient by saying that her problems were real, while nevertheless using the sessions to educate her about positive health practices (e.g., exercises she should do every other day). When the patient had a good week (meaning she was able to do an activity she enjoyed), the resident empathized again with the pleasure she must be feeling while reasserting the patient's need to continue their weekly visits indefinitely.

No clinician will be surprised to learn that this patient's emergency room trips soon dropped off dramatically. By establishing a sound physician-patient relationship, the resident was able to prevent unnecessary examinations, medications, and workups. Gradually, the patient was able to function better at home.

When the resident transferred to another service, she continued seeing this patient. The trusting relationship that had developed was not interrupted. Although some senior colleagues were impressed, if not amazed, by the "magic" the resident had performed, she was actually employing the most widely corroborated approach to somatization disorder. Since 1935, "reeducation, reassurance, and suggestion" have been the triadic components of the treatment (Luff and Garrod, 1935, pp. 55–57). These principles hinge on establishing a strong bond with the physician that promotes education and support.

In this case, the medical staff gained increased respect for psychiatric input—a secondary but not unwanted benefit of the young clinician's approach. Anyone able to spend time with the patient—be it a mental health professional, primary care clinician, or care extender—could probably provide the supportive nexus that seemed to work such magic.

If patients are able to accept the recommendation for more in-depth psychotherapy, it has the added benefit of helping them develop a tolerance for the "anxiety, vigilance, mistrust, rage, and destructiveness" (Coen, 1992, p. 171) that undergird the psychosomatic illness. Women learn that they must find ways to manage their conflicts, particularly their need to feel unacceptable and worthless. Even when a patient cannot at first articulate her needs or the reason for her behavior, the therapist empathizes that there are "good reasons for her behavior . . . [thereby giving] the patient a new and welcome idea about herself, one that emphasizes something good and healthy in her" (Farber, 1997, p. 102).

COMORBID PSYCHIATRIC CONDITIONS

The conditions most frequently associated with somatization are major depression (55% of patients), anxiety disorders (34%), personality disorders (61%), and panic disorders (26%) (Ford, 1995a, 1995b; Martin and Yutzy, 1997). The overlap between somatization and anxiety disorders or mood disorders is often difficult even for specialists to sort out. Specific treatments for these pathologies can be quite beneficial for the overall management of the patient.

Three general characteristics identified by Cloninger (1987) are particularly helpful. For the most part, the psychosomatic patient (1) has complaints suggestive of involvement of multiple organ systems, (2) has an early onset and chronic course without physical sequelae, and (3) has normal laboratory studies. A useful diagnostic tool is the patient's perception of her own poor health when standard measurements assessing physical, social, and emotional well-being are used. Smith (1995) opined that "patients with somatization disorder perceive themselves as 'sicker than the sick'" (p. 1724).

Patients with an acute onset of excessive somatic complaints should be asked about precipitating stressors, such as sexual abuse (Ford, 1995a; Levitan, 1982). Dissociative phenomena (see Chapter 6) are frequently associated with somatoform complaints or conversion reactions. Grief reactions (see Chapter 9) may also be accompanied by excessive somatic concerns. For example, immediately after experiencing a loss, a patient's typical complaints are throat tightness, crying, sighing, and abdominal emptiness ("Dr., I have this terrible pit in my stomach. I can't eat, and I always feel like I'm going to throw up."). A few weeks after the acute loss, the patient may tell you she feels weak, worn out, or unable to eat or sleep. Even years after a loss, it is not uncommon for patients to have "anniversary reactions" in which somatic preoccupations escalate. These reactions usually resolve after a transient relapse, especially if the patient is able to "talk through" the loss.

Finally, patients with schizophrenia or organic psychoses may have bizarre somatic complaints indicative of thought disorder. Reassurance and frequent visits to the doctor usually fail to help these patients. Some respond to long-term neuroleptic medication and to a highly structured daily activity regimen that diverts them from their physical preoccupations. Psychotherapy can also be useful for psychiatric patients with somatic delusions or preoccupations, particularly if it focuses on what the patient *can* achieve in life and offers the patient encouragement to think realistically (Karon and Teixeira, 1995).

BEWARE "REAL" ILLNESS

Although the first task in the diagnosis of somatization is ruling out other medical or psychiatric conditions, the primary clinician must be alert to those medical problems that can occur during the course of this continuum of disorders. These include multiple sclerosis, systemic lupus erythematosus, acute intermittent porphyria, certain chronic systemic infections, myopathies and neuropathies, and vasculitides (Martin and Yutzy, 1997). For example, at least one third of patients with conversion disorder are later found to have a medical or neurologic condition such as multiple sclerosis or seizure.

Clinical Example

Most practitioners will identify with the following case example from the files of a clinician who had been in practice for 40 years. This family physician knew his clientele very well; some were even close personal friends.

One 55-year-old female patient was frequently seen for a melange of physical complaints that ranged from general malaise to anxiety to sporadic myalgias to dyspepsia. One day after this woman had come to the doctor's office a couple of times for what appeared to be tension headache, the office assistant keenly observed something different about the patient that she simply could not define. In effect, she told the doctor that this time she was worried about the patient in a way she had not been before. This physician relied on the observation of his team members and had learned to appreciate their opinions, because often they were right. Although he wanted to avoid unnecessary testing, he undertook a neurologic evaluation and ordered a consultation and a cerebral angiogram (computed tomography and magnetic resonance imaging techniques were not yet available).

The patient was diagnosed with a cerebral aneurysm. After undergoing successful neurosurgical correction, she survived for another 27 years, eventually succumbing to renal failure. Interestingly, unlike many psychosomatically ill patients who mysteriously "improve" when a real disorder can be found and corrected, this patient continued to be plagued by physical complaints and afflictions for the rest of her life. However, she lived to see her children graduate from college, marry, and raise their own families, and she became the doting and beloved grandmother she had always aspired to be.

LINKING PSYCHE AND SOMA—THE ROLE OF PSYCHOTHERAPY

The Stages of Change

For the majority of patients with somatization disorder, psychotherapy plays a major role if the patient desires substantial relief. Pharmacotherapy is also indicated in some of the disorders (see Table 8–1), particularly if there is a comorbid psychiatric problem. Most of the time medication is of limited benefit in these patients; a relationship that models new modes of coping and acceptance is needed. Across many varied psychological syndromes, *a helping relationship has been found to be the most commonly emphasized factor in promoting change*. Benefits that patients describe as essential to healing include the defining characteristics of empathy, caring, trust, genuineness, and openness (DiClemente et al., 1986).

Many people with somatization do not have the energy or investment needed to move beyond a stage of precontemplation in dealing with their behavior. Prochaska and DiClemente (1986, 1992) include in this earliest point in the process of change a rationalization of behavior, reluctance to consider alternatives, and a rebellious need to hold on to old patterns. Sometimes fear of what might happen if other choices are made impedes motivation (e.g., loss of financial compensation; disruption of an important relationship). Understanding the psychology of women aids the clinician's appreciation of why some patients tend to "hang on" to somatic symptoms. They are able to form an essential relationship with the clinician who tolerates and does not condemn their expression of feelings through physical symptoms (Gise, 1998). Sometimes this is the most concern and compassion they have experienced in a lifetime. In other cases a constricted imagination, an externally oriented cognitive style, difficulty differentiating feelings and bodily sensations of emotional arousal, and inability to put feelings into words (i.e., alexithymia) place the patient at risk for intractable somatization disorders (Taylor et al., 1997).

DiClemente and Prochaska (1985) recommend that persons in this stage of change (e.g., precontemplation) be given a "low-intensity" treatment intervention. When applied to the patient with somatization disorder, this translates into regular, brief visits with the primary care clinician in which patient education is emphasized to *gradually* motivate the person to make additional change. Many "precontemplatives" do go on to make substantial changes over time, so don't be discouraged. However, more intense treatment should be reserved for patients who have made a commitment to take action with the problem. These patients have moved through the stage of thinking about changing their problem (contemplation), have resolved to address the problem (decision making), and are ready to act to implement new strategies (action) (DiClemente et al., 1986).

When "More Is Better"

Based on his work with Dr. John Sarno, a physiatrist who uses an educational-psychological treatment program for patients with low back pain at Rush Institute for Rehabilitative Medicine in New York City, psychoanalyst Stanley Coen

(1992) describes with optimism the benefits that accrue to many patients with psychosomatic problems when they are able to address psychological conflicts. Coen and Sarno (1989) found that, of more than 4,000 patients with low back pain seen over a period of 15 years, 95% had a syndrome that was not of primary structural origin but dramatically improved with psychotherapy. Their relatively brief intervention included education and explanation of the interpersonal and emotional conflicts undergirding the pain. Once the patient's tendency to be driven and/or rigid is pointed out, "the back pain usually disappears, except for a few brief recurrences" (Coen, 1992). Unnecessary medical expenditures for tests or surgeries are avoided by empathic reassurance that tissue damage has not occurred and the statement that the pain is usually totally reversible; feelings that were being avoided are made tolerable by educating the patient about underlying conflict and anxiety. These clinicians speculate that an inability to process overpowering affects inevitably leads to vascular dysfunction at the receptor level, understandably contributing to physiological dysregulation and pain. For about 5% to 10% of patients, Sarno and Coen found a more insight-oriented, expressive psychotherapy process to be essential to full and long-term recovery (Coen, 1992).

For those patients who needed and benefited from a more extensive psycho-therapy process, the illness was found to be a vehicle for obtaining caring. Such patients may actually desire to be totally dependent on others; although legiti-mate needs and desires to connect with other people must be encouraged, the patient must also learn to relinquish her sense of entitlement for special, total care. Coen uses the metaphor of the "crippled child" to interpret to his patients the wish to be rescued from the pressures of life and to unconsciously exploit their caretakers and loved ones through demands. Expressive psychotherapy or psychoanalysis then helps patients deal constructively with what is most unac-ceptable in themselves; usually this includes a deep sense of being flawed or damaged. Patients must feel safe to work through their human feelings of deprivation, anger, envy, and greed. This means forming an attachment to a therapist over time, because, "The better able patients are to tolerate what they feel, including their anxiety, vigilance, mistrust, rage and destructiveness, and depressive feelings, the less troubled they will be by psychosomatic symptoms" (Coen, 1992, pp. 171–172).

The benefits expressive psychotherapy has to offer patients across diagnostic groups was eloquently summarized by Jill Anne Kowalik. A philosophy professor, psychoanalytic research fellow, and breast cancer survivor, Dr. Kowalik speaks to the need of all patients to transcend their illnesses, real or perceived. Her resilience and inspiring approach to her own treatment for recurrent breast cancer has application to the patient who "needs" to have an illness and who must begin to bridge psyche and soma in order to live more fully, meaningfully, and productively. Psychodynamic psychotherapy and psychoanalysis are the tools Dr. Kowalik finds most valuable in her struggle to live and endure despite malignancy. The "talking cure" permitted her to separate anxieties she imagined about her illness from those that were truly derived from a life-threatening disease to arrive at a position where:

> I resolved to live hypothetically, to pretend I wasn't sick, because that might help me live longer. . . . I have decided it was in my best long-term interest not to have

time to be sick. Even though I knew I could not wish the disease away, I fantasized that I could lessen its progression with the appropriate attitude. The disease, I thought, might take my body someday, but I would not, while I waited, let it take my soul.

(Kowalik, 1998, pp. 34–35)

Clinicians and patients are faced with precisely the same dilemmas. Whether one's struggle is with psyche or soma, life forces each of us to "live hypothetically" as we meet our inner demons daily. We never really know what ultimate physical disease our bodies harbor, or what personal crisis we will be required to bear. But we can resolve to work on those oppressive and pernicious images of what might be around the next corner to strike us down. Facing our most haunting fears, and helping others to do the same, is what the essence of psychotherapy— and good doctoring—are all about.

PATIENT GUIDELINES FOR COPING WITH SOMATIZATION

1. Keep the regular schedule of outpatient visits recommended by your primary care clinician. This is sometimes difficult to do when no definite physical reason for your problem can be found. You experience having a real illness (e.g., pain, aches), and you do. But the usual treatments and diagnostic procedures are not bringing about any solid resolution to your situation. Your doctor will help find a treatment that works best for you, but you must also do your part. It is important to keep your regular appointments so that a trusting relationship can develop. You must feel that your complaints are heard and understood, and that there is a place to go to "be yourself."
2. Try to stay as active as possible. This includes practicing positive health care practices, such as exercising and learning as much as you can about your illness. Some excellent books are available to help you understand why you seem to be plagued by so many somatic complaints (see "Resources for Patients" section). Try to put into practice a routine of doing a physical workout or exercises at least four times a week instead of telling yourself what you plan to do or cannot do.
3. Take psychotropic medication if your doctor recommends it. For some patients with excessive physical complaints, an underlying depression or anxiety disorder may be found. These conditions can sometimes be greatly helped by some of the new, safer psychotropic medications, which have very few side effects.
4. Take advantage of any new adjunctive therapies that may appeal to you as an individual. For example, many patients with severe or chronic pain have found enormous relief from biofeedback therapy, hypnosis, acupuncture, or guided imagery. Your physician can refer you to a competent practitioner in your area, or you can seek one out through a women's health cooperative or your local mental health center.
5. Do all you can to sustain a positive attitude; try to take pleasure in your successes. Research demonstrates that patients who have lots of physical complaints do better if they can experience some joy. On those days when you feel better and are able to do a little bit more, try to give yourself a boost by doing something you like. This kind of diversion can not only

reduce your discomfort but can also genuinely help you function better at home and at work. Leisure time physical activity is associated with reduced mortality and improved quality of life. The more you find ways to handle life's inevitable disappointments and your anger or mistrust, the more you will be able to cope with your physical symptoms.

6. Remember that trust in your physician is essential to your care. At times you may want to have additional medical tests or ask for treatments that your physician does not believe would be wise. By all means, speak up about your symptoms or worries, but remember that a good physician will try to help you avoid unnecessary examinations, hospitalizations, or inappropriate medication.

7. Consider participating in psychotherapy when you are ready. Most people benefit from a safe place where they can share distress, be it the challenges of everyday life or worries about physical well-being. You may find it of interest to know that research has indicated that group treatment may be particularly helpful for people who have excessive somatic concerns. A group will provide you with an outlet for socialization and help you develop coping skills.

8. Remember that many women with physical problems benefit from individual psychotherapy. Sometimes people are unaware that an emotional problem actually underlies or is the basis of their physical suffering. Therapy helps some women find the links between their psychological distress and their physical aches and pains. In essence, your body is communicating that you are suffering. This suffering is real and tends to be long term. Psychotherapy helps you develop new ways (usually verbal) to express your feelings.

9. Try to master the dual problem of thinking you deserve care only when you are "good" or "sick." Face down an underlying assumption that anything negative about you makes you unlikable or unacceptable. Sometimes people hone in on physical problems or body sensations to avoid dealing with deeper interpersonal conflicts or because they have a low opinion of themselves. Therapy also helps you take a thorough look at any need you have to be self-critical and/or guarded.

10. Learn to relax your adherence to strict standards. It will help you separate your legitimate needs from what may become construed as overdependence on others (e.g., feeling that your loved ones must always put your needs first; believing that your health care team can "solve" your misery).

11. Learn to express and tolerate your feelings instead of fearing them. Some people find that the verbal therapies, such as psychodynamic or cognitive-behavioral therapy, can help them to get in touch with their emotional experiences. Others find relief in what mental health professionals call "experiential therapies." These include hypnosis, biofeedback, massage, art therapy, and music therapy. With the help of your primary care clinician, seek the right therapy for you, but by all means continue to work closely with your physician.

ADDITIONAL GUIDELINES FOR PRIMARY CARE CLINICIANS

1. Problems of excessive somatic concern (somatization disorder, chronic pain syndrome hypochondriasis, body dysmorphic disorder) tend to be long-term

problems to manage in a primary care practice. It is important to remember that even though no organic pathology can be found, these are real illnesses. It is essential for women who somatize to have a primary care clinician to whom they can turn for regular visits and who understands that each new symptom is actually a form of communicating an emotional need.

2. Be vigilant about other physical or emotional problems that can develop. A high percentage of somatizing patients also carry the diagnoses of depression and/or anxiety, which can be treated with psychotropic medication and/or psychotherapy. Because patients who somatize can be vexing to treat, physicians may understandably "turn a deaf ear" to their list of complaints. It is important to remember that these patients can also develop new, organically based illnesses.

3. Offer relatively brief, but regular, follow-up visits. To cut down on unnecessary tests or procedures, have a care extender call the patient between visits, especially if she tends to be anxious or guarded. As Brown and Walker (1987) recommend, "A general guiding principle is 'Don't just do something, sit there' " (pp. 222–223). Avoid telling the patient that the symptom is "all in your head". Although it is true that the symptom has an emotional component, the patient nonetheless experiences the illness as real or tormenting.

4. Make simple but practical suggestions. *Emphasize what the patient can do and applaud any effort to enjoy life or find ways to conquer pain or fear.* Do not be afraid to be specific. Instead of recommending, "Get some fresh air or exercise," encourage diversion away from the physical malady by saying, "Take a 30-minute walk at least every other day."

5. Remember that each patient requires an individual approach; some benefit from massage, acupuncture, breathing therapy, or biofeedback. The more the patient tries to find something that works for her, the less likely she is to be dependent on you. Emphasize that medical research continues to show the importance of leisure-time physical activity in reducing mortality and enhancing quality of life (see Kujala et al., 1998). This approach assures the patient that *you see her problems as important and medical*, which indeed they are.

6. You can help bridge the link between psyche and soma by understanding that aches and pains are a form of communication. Somatizing is the only way that some people have of conveying emotional anguish. When patients are able to tolerate their strong emotions and express them by talking or through physical outlets (e.g., exercise, dance), they are less likely to be troubled by their somatic symptoms.

7. Be aware that sexual abuse is often a precursor to somatization problems in some women. These women often deny the abuse on first interview, even if they are asked. However, it is important to keep the issue of sexual abuse an open possibility for discussion. Don't be afraid to inquire more than once or twice if you have the suspicion. This shows the patient that you care about her internal world and her past history.

8. When you believe that the patient's alliance with you is solidified, consider suggesting the additional support of a mental health professional. As noted, individual psychotherapy, group psychotherapy, and experiential therapies can be very useful, depending on the individual patient's needs and prefer-

ences. Increasingly, physicians find that patients with excessive somatic concerns need to avail themselves of more than one treatment. For example, in addition to regular visits with you, a motivated patient may benefit from attending group therapy, individual therapy, or biofeedback. The choice depends on the woman's preference and community availability. Although there can be some overlap between modalities, in general women learn new coping skills and verbal ways of expressing their emotions from individual and group therapy and enhance their psychophysiologic awareness and control through experiential therapies. They emerge from conjoint treatments such as these with a much greater capacity to care for and soothe themselves. As a result, they call you less frequently because they are less prone to psychosomatic eruptions.

9. Even with the very best of long-term care and reassurance, these patients can be frustrating to treat. Although education, reassurance, and therapy can all be very useful, there are occasions when the strongest physician-patient relationship is tested by the patient's demands for attention. Because somatizing patients make up a significant percentage of primary care practice, you must feel comfortable setting limits in regard to the amount of time, number of visits, and so forth that you are able to give. To prevent burnout, try to keep telephone calls and appointments regular but brief. When possible in your practice, use your care extenders to make routine, scheduled contacts while reassuring the patient of your availability, especially for bona fide emergencies.

10. Ask the patient how she gets support or has her emotional needs met. What one woman finds stressful, another may find supportive. Help the patient identify what she believes will be a supportive environment for her, and encourage her to try to achieve it (Mack, 1984; Sapolsky, 1997; Steptoe and Wardle, 1994; Woolf, 1996).

11. Help the patient define her goals (i.e., how you will know she is feeling better). This helps her feel ownership for the need to change. See the patient as a partner with you, especially because this counters the somatizing patient's tendency to become excessively dependent on one person, namely, the physician. Facilitate the patient's commitment to change and to achieving her goals by (1) follow-up and (2) encouragement about positive steps. Remind the patient that change for each of us is a process, rarely if ever achieved in a straight line. When backsliding occurs, you can help her identify what went wrong and alter her plan or develop a new one (DiClemente and Prochaska, 1985; Prochaska and DiClemente, 1992; Westberg and Jason, 1996).

SUMMARY

Psychosomatic complaints are among the most recalcitrant of disorders for the physician to treat. Although the tendency to have physical complaints for which an organic cause cannot be found occurs in both sexes, women appear to be afflicted with these disorders more commonly than men. In primary care, at least 10% of visits yield no evidence of any physical disease. Yet these patients' complaints are very real, and the clinician who is attuned to the emotional suffering can offer excellent medical care in the context of a solid physician-patient relationship.

Some somatization disorders (hypochondriasis, body dysmorphic disorder) have recently been shown to respond to the selective serotonin reuptake inhibitors (SSRIs). However, all patients probably can make use of a supportive relationship with the doctor, based on regular but brief visits. Over time, the clinician should also help the patient try to assess the role that physical symptoms may be playing in her life. For example, symptoms may enable her to receive attention and care from her family; they may be the result of her being the unwilling victim of past sexual trauma; or they may have developed because she is unable to express her feelings in words. In any of these circumstances, the woman is understood to be relying on her body as a medium for experiencing and expressing her psychological discomfort.

The patient's extraordinary watchfulness over her bodily functioning will not disappear until she is able to stop scrutinizing her physical symptoms. Helping her find ways to learn about and to tolerate her feelings, in addition to helping her assess her personal goals over time, enables the patient to feel better and to function better. Although somatization tends to be chronic, it is a very gratifying disorder for clinicians to treat, especially as you help the patient to become less dependent on medical intervention and more independent in her life. Those patients who find ways to overcome their conflicts and learn to self-soothe tend to have the best prognosis. Depending on the patient's needs and motivations, group or individual psychotherapy or alternative healing methods (e.g., acupuncture, massage, exercise) may be essential aspects of comprehensive treatment planning and long-term management.

Resources for Patients

Csikszentmihalyi M: *Flow: The Psychology of Optimal Experience*. New York, HarperCollins, 1990.

Dubovsky SL: *Mind-Body Deceptions: The Psychosomatics of Everyday Life*. New York, WW Norton, 1997.

Although many patients find it difficult to believe that significant physical disability can result from "deceptions" of the mind, this thoroughly researched and well-written volume provides an understanding of how this process actually occurs. The author is a professor of psychiatry and medicine at the University of Colorado School of Medicine. He includes numerous, interesting case examples to demonstrate that psychosomatic illness is "the result of pathology in the mind, not in the body" (p. 89). Dubovsky emphasizes how psychotherapy can be helpful to the patient in sorting out how the "body deceives the mind" when family conflicts or individual concerns are suppressed rather than worked through. He also explains how, why, and when antidepressants can be helpful. Clinicians will be especially intrigued by the chapter, "If Thoughts Could Kill: Fatal Mind-Body Deceptions." Intense emotional experiences and psychological vulnerability, such as anniversary reactions, loss of personal or job status, and overwhelming happiness, can sometimes herald one's demise. The psychological factors that can magnify or reduce the impact of stress on the body are thoroughly examined, so that anyone reading the book (including clinicians) can become more aware of the tendency to "set the stage for later destruction of the body" (p. 270). Although the author believes that the combination of genetic, temperamental, and early life experiences may have an impact on the final, common path toward somatization, he also demonstrates how the ability to self-reflect and garner insight can offer better everyday functioning. Emphasis is placed on how much can be saved in health care dollars by including research on the cost-effectiveness study of those medical patients who receive psychotherapy. As described in "The High Cost of Less Psychotherapy" (p. 81), the more psychotherapy medical patients receive, the less time they spend in the hospital. These patients also tend to take better care of themselves, thereby preventing illness and ultimately further reducing health care expenditures.

Levey J, Levey M: *Living in Balance: A Dynamic Approach for Creating Harmony and Wholeness in a Chaotic World.* Berkeley, CA, Conari Press, 1998.

Loehr JE, Migdow JA: *Take a Deep Breath.* New York, Villard Books, 1986.

Remen R: *Kitchen Table Wisdom: Stories That Heal.* New York, Riverhead Books, 1996.

More and more patients are interested in a holistic medicine approach. An array of possible choices is available in most bookstores. Each of these books has been selected for inclusion here because it provides practical help and encouragement for living, especially for the patient whose goal is to deal with pain, chronic disability, or somatic illness more effectively. Patients who tend to somatize need to be urged to take good care of their bodies. A holistic approach, first and foremost, promotes this kind of mind-body integration. Although each of these books approaches stress, illness, and mind-body health a bit differently, all of them contain an abundance of insights and exercises to help readers actively engage in self-care that will enable them to gain more control and have renewed energy to overcome problems. A core concept of each book is that people can be transformed to see unexpected opportunities, despite the most challenging problems or circumstances. New choices can be made to live more simply and soulfully, and with greater balance. Not all of the suggestions or clinical examples are applicable to every woman, but most readers will find an idea, a story, or a concept in one of these books that encourages them to embark on their own healing process and to choose life over illness. Clinicians can also acquire broadening perspectives by reading one or more of these books, and they can feel they are doing something for the patient by urging her to read, to grow, and to take better care of herself.

Swedo F, Leonard H: *It's Not All in Your Head: Now Women Can Discover the Real Causes of Their Most Commonly Misdiagnosed Health Problems.* New York, HarperCollins, 1996.

These authors describe the "revolution" that has taken place in women's psychiatry. As they examine the physical and psychiatric disorders that can impinge on the mind-body connection, they pay particularly careful attention to the neurobiology of illness and the available psychopharmacologic treatments. For the woman who tends to somatize, the authors have excellent sections on medical illnesses that masquerade as psychiatric disorders (e.g., metabolic, infectious, autoimmune, neurologic, and chronic fatigue disorders) and an excellent section on how stress can impinge on the body, leading to a host of mind-body difficulties. The authors empower their readers by including brief but comprehensive summaries of most of the major psychiatric disturbances (e.g., bipolar disorder, depression, trauma, anxiety and phobias, eating disorders, alcohol abuse). The patient who reads this comprehensive survey about women's mental health emerges knowing more about her particular disorder and feeling more knowledgeable about how to find help. She also feels less lonely, because Swedo and Leonard include patient examples from their own case files. Most women find concrete help by scanning the sections titled, "All This Stress Is Driving Me Crazy" (pp. 47–62), "My Hormones Are Driving Me Crazy" (pp. 63–82), and "My Doctor Thinks I'm Crazy (pp. 83–109).

Resources for Clinicians

Druss RG: *The Psychology of Illness in Sickness and in Health.* Washington, DC, American Psychiatric Press, 1995.

Most physicians are not aware that medically ill patients can also develop hypochondri- asis, meaning additional preoccupation with the body that saps their capacity to engage in life and to meet the demands of treatment. This "hypochondriasis of the medically ill" can be highly frustrating to attending physicians because there is so little they feel they can do to help such patients fixate less on their ills and more on their lives. This inspiring, insightful book describes why patients worry about every symptom and how physicians can use empathy and reassurance to counter the anxious state of their patients. Mention is also made of the beneficent effect of cognitive therapy for enhancing coping mechanisms and for underscoring the patient's personal strength and courage. Druss also gives some excellent recommendations for the primary clini- cian treating a serious, acute, or chronic illness: Encourage diversion through activities, use antianxiety agents judiciously, and understand how reassuring it can be to have even a few minutes of face-to-face talk or over-the-phone contact with the primary care clinician or care extender. These human relationships promote restoration and well-being, in part by modeling an altruistic caring for others.

Ford CV: *The Somatizing Disorders: Illness as a Way of Life.* New York, Elsevier Biomedical, 1983.

Ford CV (section ed.): *Somatoform and factitious disorders.* In: Gabbard GO (ed.): *Treatments of Psychiatric Disorders,* 2nd ed., pp. 1713–1818. Washington, DC, Ameri- can Psychiatric Press, 1995.

Patients who somatize seek out medical and surgical physicians more often than they seek out psychiatrists. In addition, somatization disorders form the bulk of the primary care clinician's practice. Both of these references are thoroughly comprehensive and contain practical summaries of a state-of-the-art understanding and treatment of the somatizing disorders (e.g., somatoform disorder, conversion disorder, pain disorder, hypochondriasis, body dysmorphic disorder). Although Ford's book is a bit dated with respect to the latest pharmacotherapy principles used in the treatment of chronic pain and hypochondriasis, it offers an in-depth understanding of the patient who takes on the sick role. Ford also shows how the doctor-patient relationship is crucial to helping the patient who somatizes. Both references review the cost to society of unnecessary medical evaluations (the socioeconomic impact of somatization) and describe why medical care delivery systems must focus more on somatizing patients. Referral of such patients for mental health care will increasingly be necessary as it is shown to be cost- effective: At least 10% (and probably much more) of all medical services are provided to patients with no evidence of medical disease.

Martin RL, Yutzy SH: *Somatoform disorders.* In: Tasman AK, Kay J, Lieberman JA (eds.): *Psychiatry,* pp. 1119–1155. Philadelphia, WB Saunders, 1997.

Another superb summary of the somatoform disorders, this chapter traces the contem- porary diagnostic understanding of the disorders and includes therapeutic guidelines for a group of patients who are uniformly challenging to treat. Up-to-date recommen- dations for pharmacotherapy are one of the strengths of the chapter. The authors again point out how patients with hypochondriasis and other somatization disorders generally present to nonpsychiatric physicians. Because of the high comorbidity with depression and anxiety and the need for such patients to undergo supportive psycho- therapy, criteria for psychiatric evaluation are reviewed.

McDougall J: *Theaters of the Body: A Psychoanalytic Approach to Psychosomatic Illness.* New York, WW Norton, 1989.

Many primary care clinicians are interested in how psychosomatic problems can be psychodynamically understood. They intuitively understand that physical problems may be a way for the psyche to protect itself from overwhelming feelings, a history of trauma, or unresolved grief. Using nontechnical language and including plenty of fascinating case material, McDougall reveals the inner world of her patients who have had heart disease, ulcerative colitis, chronic insomnia, headache, and other physical conditions. For the primary care clinician who would like a glimpse into what is actually said between patient and therapist in psychodynamic psychotherapy, this book shows a master clinician at work. By interpreting the patient's body communications and helping put strong feelings into words, McDougall demonstrates the tremendous relief many persons experience when they are finally understood and able to speak their minds openly.

References

Brown JT, Walker JI: Excessive somatic concern: diagnostic and treatment issues. In: Walker JI, Brown JT, Gallis HA (eds.): *The Complicated Medical Patient: New Approaches to Psychomedical Syndromes*, pp. 213–230. New York, Human Services Press, 1987.

Cloninger CR: Diagnosis of somatization disorders: a critique of DSM-III. In: Tischler GL (ed.): *Diagnosis and Classification in Psychiatry: A Critical Appraisal of DSM-III*, pp. 243–257. New York, Cambridge University Press, 1987.

Coen SJ: *The Misuse of Persons: Analyzing Pathological Dependency*. New York, Analytic Press, 1992.

Coen SJ, Sarno JE: Psychosomatic avoidance of conflict in back pain. *J Am Acad Psychoanal* 1989;17:359–376.

Csikszentmihalyi M: *Flow: The Psychology of Optimal Experience*. New York, HarperCollins, 1990.

DiClemente CC, Prochaska JO: Processes and stages of self-change: Coping and competence in smoking behavior change. In: Shiffman S, Wills TA (eds.): *Coping and Substance Use*, pp. 345–364. Orlando, FL, Academic Press, 1985.

DiClemente CC, McConnaughy EA, Norcross JC, et al.: Integrative dimensions for psychotherapy. *International Journal of Eclectic Psychotherapy* 1986;5:256–274.

Druss RG: *The Psychology of Illness in Sickness and in Health*. Washington, DC, American Psychiatric Press, 1995.

Dubovsky SL: *Mind-Body Deceptions: The Psychosomatics of Everyday Life*. New York, WW Norton, 1997.

Farber SK: Self-medication, traumatic reenactment, and somatic expression in bulimic and self-mutilating behavior. *Clinical Social Work Journal* 1997;25:87–106.

Finell JS: Alexithymia and mind-body problems. In: Finell JS (ed.): *Mind-Body Problems: Psychotherapy with Psychosomatic Disorders*, pp. 3–18. Northvale, NJ, Jason Aronson, 1997.

Ford CV: *The Somatizing Disorders: Illness as a Way of Life*. New York, Elsevier Biomedical, 1983.

Ford CV: Introduction: Somatoform and factitious disorders. In: Gabbard GO (ed.): *Treatments of Psychiatric Disorders*, 2nd ed., pp. 1714–1716. Washington, DC, American Psychiatric Press, 1995a.

Ford CV: Conversion disorder and somatoform disorder not otherwise specified. In: Gabbard GO (ed.): *Treatments of Psychiatric Disorders*, 2nd ed., pp. 1736–1753. Washington, DC, American Psychiatric Press, 1995b.

Gallon RL (ed.): *The Psychosomatic Approach to Illness*. New York, NY, Elsevier, 1992.

Gise LH: Medically unexplained physical symptoms. In: Wallis LA (ed.): *Textbook on Women's Health*, pp. 849–856. Philadelphia, Lippincott-Raven, 1998.

Karon BP, Teixeira MA: Psychoanalytic therapy of schizophrenia. In: Barber JP, Crits-Christoph P (eds.): *Dynamic Therapies for Psychiatric Disorders (Axis 1)*, pp. 84–130. New York, Basic Books, 1995.

Kowalik JA: Personal reflections on transference to theory. *The American Psychoanalyst* 1998;32:34–35.

Kujala UM, Kaprio J, Sarna S, et al.: Relationship of leisure-time physical activity and mortality: The Finnish twin cohort. *JAMA* 1998;279:440–444.

Levey J, Levey M: *Living in Balance: A Dynamic Approach for Creating Harmony and Wholeness in a Chaotic World*. Berkeley, CA, Conari Press, 1998.

Levitan H: Explicit incestuous motifs in psychosomatic patients. *Psychother Psychosom* 1982;37:22–25.

Loehr JE, Migdow JA: *Take a Deep Breath*. New York, Villard Books, 1986.

Luff MC, Garrod M: The after-results of psychotherapy in 500 adult cases. *Br Med J* 1935;2:54–59.

Mack RM: Lessons from living with cancer. *N Engl J Med* 1984;311:1640–1644.

Martin RL, Yutzy SH: Somatoform disorders. In: Tasman AK, Kay J, Lieberman JA (eds.): *Psychiatry*, pp. 1119–1155. Philadelphia, PA, WB Saunders, 1997.

McDougall J: *Theatres of the Body: A Psychoanalytic Approach to Psychosomatic Illness*. New York, WW Norton, 1989.

Prochaska JO, DiClemente CC: Toward a comprehensive model of change. In: Miller WR, Heather N (eds.): *Treating Addictive Behaviors: Processes of Change*, pp. 3–27. New York, Plenum, 1986.

Prochaska JO, DiClemente CC: The transtheoretical approach. In: Norcoss JC, Goldfried MR (eds.): *Handbook of Psychotherapy Integration*, pp. 300–334. New York, Basic Books, 1992.

Remen R: *Kitchen Table Wisdom: Stories that Heal*. New York, Riverhead Books, 1996.

Sapolsky RM: Requiem for an overachiever. *The Sciences* January/February 1997, pp. 15–19.

Smith GR: *Somatization Disorder in the Medical Setting*. Washington, DC, American Psychiatric Press, 1991.

Smith GR: Somatization disorder and undifferentiated somatoform disorder. In: Gabbard GO (ed.): *Treatments of Psychiatric Disorders*, 2nd ed., pp. 1718–1733. Washington, DC, American Psychiatric Press, 1995.

Steptoe A, Wardle J (eds.): *Psychosocial Processes and Health: A Reader*. Cambridge, England, Cambridge University Press, 1994.

Stotland NL: Managing patients who "want" to have a disease. *Journal Watch: Women's Health* 1997;2:55–56.

Swedo S, Leonard H: *It's Not All in Your Head: Now Women Can Discover the Real Causes of Their Most Commonly Misdiagnosed Health Problems*. San Francisco, HarperCollins, 1996.

Taylor GJ, Bagby M, Parker JD: *Disorders of Affect Regulation: Alexithymia in Medical and Psychiatric Illness*. New York, Cambridge University Press, 1997.

Walker JI, Brown JT, Gallis HA (eds.): *The Complicated Medical Patient: New Approaches to Psychomedical Syndromes*. New York, Human Sciences Press, 1987.

Westberg J, Jason H: Fostering healthy behavior: The process. In: Woolf SH, Jonas S, Lawrence RS (eds.): *Health Promotion and Disease Prevention in Clinical Practice*, pp. 145–162. Baltimore, Williams & Wilkins, 1996.

Woolf S: Functional status and mental health. In: Woolf S, Jonas S, Lawrence RS (eds.): *Health Promotion and Disease Prevention in Clinical Practice*, pp. 335–353. Baltimore, Williams & Wilkins, 1996.

Chapter 9

Catastrophic Loss and Bereavement

Death is an inevitable fact of life. Usually, clinicians can safely distance themselves from the array of maladies experienced by patients—a healthy form of denial that declares, "This is happening to my patient, not to me." Sometimes this defensive strategy serves them well, helping to maintain objectivity. But such is not the case with death. Most physicians as well as others will witness the ravages of fate when someone dear becomes ill, and ultimately, all will themselves be struck down. Few individuals have the pluck of Katherine Hepburn, who quipped, "Death will be a great relief. No more interviews." Most are more in synch with Woody Allen, who incisively observed, "It's not that I'm afraid to die. I just don't want to be there when it happens."

Physicians don't want to be there either—not for their own deaths, nor for the deaths of their patients. Perhaps this is one reason they have such a difficult time helping patients face a fatal illness or the loss of a loved one. Both experiences are such arbitrary levelers of all human beings.

Add to this observation the realization that relatively little is taught in medical school or residency training about how to actually work with dying or bereaved patients, such as the parent who has suffered an obstetric catastrophe or lost a child. Certainly, most clinicians are familiar with Kubler-Ross' (1969) classic review of the stages of death and dying, but as helpful as such guides may be in outlining the issues, they do not teach physicians what to actually *say* or *do* to facilitate the healing of those who must learn to deal with their anguish. Most important, *clinicians are not taught how to metabolize their own feelings about terminal illness, medical catastrophes, and death.* This omission not only robs them of an opportunity to learn about their own humanity but it also has a negative impact on their care for patients. Often, clinicians fail to acknowledge patients' struggles—let alone help them—to bear up through a time of profound adversity.

Fortunately, these mistakes can be rectified. This chapter aims to help the primary care clinician assist the woman who is facing a fatal illness, who has suffered a medical (particularly an obstetric) catastrophe, or who is otherwise bereaved.[1] It demonstrates how this personal involvement can teach clinicians

---

[1]Although emphasis in this chapter is placed on terminal illness and bereavement, clinicians are reminded that women who divorce also experience acute and unacknowledged losses (see Chapter 13). Because society does not generally perceive her situation as a loss, the woman receives little sympathy or support. Health care providers must attune themselves to the special burdens that divorced patients face, and many of the principles in this chapter apply generally to the divorced patient as well as the bereaved. Divorced women are particularly likely to face severe financial reversals that alter their living circumstances and affect their physical and emotional well-being. Clinicians must remember that the divorced woman loses not only a spouse but also his extended family. Moreover, important friendships are often strained or eroded.

about their own humanity, because "each time we succeed in helping someone else to face up to, and cope with, these awesome facts of life, we are also, indirectly, helping ourselves" (Parkes, 1996, p. 87).

GENDER DIFFERENCES

Women are more prone than men to develop complications of bereavement. It is unclear how much a woman's attachments to her spouse, children, and parents predispose her to this greater risk. It is assumed that the psychosocial risk factors that are implicated in the higher incidence of major depression, anxiety, and somatization disorder in women hold true also for bereavement. On the other hand, genetic or innate biologic differences may also come into play (Jacobs, 1993; Regier et al., 1988). Women also may be exposed to greater environmental stress, such as economic hardship, after sustaining a loss. Research has yet to clarify those distinct biologic and environmental vulnerabilities that, in all likelihood, are additive in predisposing women to develop complications of bereavement.

THE GRIEF PROCESS

If the grief process is blocked for any reason, the patient cannot move forward with her life. It therefore becomes an essential practice of preventive medicine to recognize the most frequent symptoms of acute grief (Table 9–1) and to take appropriate action early on. Common causes for bereavement in women include death of a spouse or child; death of a parent; death of a loved one by suicide; chronic or terminal illness in herself or in a loved one; and the special considerations of perinatal loss. Medical catastrophes, including but not limited to obstetric ones, are a source of sudden, unexpected, and traumatic bereavement. They frequently complicate the grieving process because traumatized persons will go to great lengths to avoid anything that reminds them of the loss (Parkes, 1996). In unusually traumatic circumstances, the patient who is flooded with horrific memories or images may refuse to allow friends or family to give her solace; she tends to be plagued by high levels of anxiety, recurrent dreams, nightmares, and hyperalertness.

Other kinds of traumatic bereavement, such as the death of a loved one by suicide or murder, give rise to complicated feelings of intense anger or shame, or both. Initial reactions of "I can't believe it's true; it doesn't seem real" (denial) give way to self-reproachful questioning, "What could I have done to prevent this?" (guilt). Although every person's situational response to loss is unique, some general pointers for physicians can help them steer a course that makes the process easier for the patient and her family.

Some women are troubled by continually thinking about or searching for their loved one. About 50% of the bereaved even "see" the dead person; this is not a true hallucination (i.e., the patient is not psychotic). Usually, over time, these visual or auditory images fade, particularly as the patient takes on new tasks and builds up a store of memories of life without the loved one. In other words, the grief process is actually about remodeling one's prior world—the day-to-day patterns one takes for granted. It is essential to give the patient permission to take the time she needs to grieve (see "Role of the Primary Care Clinician in

---

Table 9–1. **Symptoms of Normal and Complicated Grief**

Normal grief reaction
Time frame: usually 3–12 mo after loss
    Numbness or "damped emotions"
    Anger
    Anxiety
    Impaired concentration and short-term memory
    Turbulent mood swings
    Preoccupation with the deceased
    Vivid images of the dead person, especially when drowsy (these are not a sign of
       psychosis)
    Urge to search for the deceased
    Restless sleep
    Increased physical preoccupation, particularly in the woman who tends to somatize or
       who has preexisting medical conditions
    Self-esteem remains intact
Complicated grief reaction
Time frame: usually >12 mo after loss
Psychological trauma symptoms
    Intrusive images or thoughts, especially about the deceased
    Severe emotion (e.g., numbing, crying, startle reaction)
Depressive symptoms
    Neglect of adaptive strategies at work or at home
    Poor personal hygiene
    Low energy
    Feeling excessively alone and empty
    Diminished sense of self-esteem
    Guilt
    Excessively avoids tasks reminiscent of the deceased
    Unusual sleep disturbances

Working with Bereavement or Medical Catastrophe"), because so much of the pattern of her days was shaped around the loved one. For example:

> A widow, out of habit, will lay the table for two, then realize that there are no longer two people to eat breakfast. Every chain of thought seems to lead to a blind alley . . . . The bereaved need to seal off the blind alleys of thought and develop new and different ways of coping with life.

> (Parkes, 1996, p. 77)

With time, the patient finds solace in her memories and her newfound strength (Averill, 1997). Sometimes this process is manifested overtly by identification with the deceased. For example, more than one widow has identified with her successful husband to the extent that she was able to become an affluent entrepreneur in her own right after his death. Positive experiences and aspects of character become incorporated into the survivor, serving functions that are both "life saving and life sustaining" (Averill, 1997, p. 295).

LEARNING TO LISTEN

In helping a woman face loss, clinicians must first and foremost create an ambiance of listening. Even a few moments of your time can be enormously salutary to the patient, who experiences it as quite giving and relieving. Especially when the patient becomes tearful, angry, or nonverbal, she can benefit from a nonjudgmental, accepting demeanor. Although some authorities recommend that the primary care clinician can best help patients and families by talking about the five stages of grief (denial, anger, bargaining, depression, and acceptance) (O'Brien, 1996), what is needed most urgently is an atmosphere of acceptance and a safe place to express one's feelings (Edwards, 1997; Nadelson, 1996).

Like any procedural skill, good listening techniques can be learned. However, they also require practice, probably over the entire course of one's career. Like an experienced mason whose palms become callused over the years, the primary care clinician develops a protective emotional layer to better tolerate the pain of patients. Although this protective barrier can be useful in enhancing objectivity and preventing professional burnout caused by "feeling too much for one's patients," it takes a heavy toll on the physician-patient relationship. Clinicians may unconsciously turn off their listening, receptive ear when patients begin to talk about personal worries or losses. This silence is experienced by the patient as a need for you to distance yourself. Most women turn to other family members or friends to do this sorting out, but physicians and care extenders are also likely to be in a position to hear the story. It is a privileged and important role to play, because speaking about the loss prevents complicated (e.g., refractory) grief (see Table 9–1).

Counselors have empirically found it necessary to encourage bereaved persons to recall and recount, in great detail, all the events that led up to the loss, the circumstances surrounding it, and any experiences since then (Eells, 1995; Krigger et al., 1997). This process helps the bereaved person sort out all the feelings—including hopes, regrets, anger, and guilt—that she has about her loved one.

ANXIETY AND ANGER

Anxiety and anger are expectable companions of the grieving process (Cerney and Buskirk, 1991). Initially, you may be worried that the patient will become depressed if she expresses her feelings. However, the distinguishing feature in the person who grieves, as opposed to the person who is depressed, is that the former does not have lowered self-esteem (see Table 9–1). Moreover, grieving differs from depression primarily by the "flood of vivid memories that are part of the pining during the experience of separation or after a loss is recognized as final" (Gut, 1989, p. 63). Experts in the field of grief therapy suggest cultivating images and memories of the loved one to promote healthy adjustment. They ask the patient to "simply imagine" talking to their loved one to put to rest any unfinished business and to say goodbye.

Most patients who experience loss harbor both unrealistic and realistic anger (Cerney, 1989). Because the woman feels guilty about expressing ambivalent feelings toward the deceased, she initially needs a repository for her feelings. Clinicians are often placed in the role of "container for the anger" until the survivor is able to recognize and work through its real source.

Quite rationally, clinicians tend to dodge this anger, even to the point of avoiding the bereaved because they sense the rage, which is easily projected onto them. Helping the patient find healthy avenues to verbalize anger (e.g., through support groups or psychotherapy) or to work the anger out physically (e.g., through vigorous exercise or gardening) is a strategy that can alleviate this underbelly of the grief reaction. In their work with more than a thousand grief patients, Cerney and Buskirk (1991) found that the *resolution of grief depended, in large part, on the willingness of an individual to recognize, own, and resolve feelings of anger.*

Anxiety occurs after loss because the bereaved is separated from her loved one (Bowlby, 1982). One patient, the mother of an 18-month-old child who died in an automobile accident, experienced generalized anxiety to the point of near-panic the day after her infant's funeral. In consultation, she shared that she could not "bear to think of my baby being all alone and cold" as winter approached and the ground hardened. Imagery was used to help her visualize the infant as whole, warm, and protected, thereby reducing her separation anxiety and guilt. Her tender maternal feelings caused her to believe temporarily that she should have done something to avert the accident. Patients such as this woman typically ruminate that there is something more they could or should have done—a fantasy that must be worked through.

Some widows become anxious that they will not be able to function or that they will emotionally collapse without their husband. Indeed, grief work necessitates struggling with anxieties that are inescapable in adapting to a new life without the loved one. Psychotherapy and self-help groups for the bereaved "walk the patient through" the expectable and natural steps of life without the companion. They reduce the anxiety that accompanies loss by helping the survivor see that she is competent and worthy. Although there is no substitute for the patient's own grief work, autobiographical accounts listed at the end of this chapter can also help women recognize that others have been able to make similar transitions, however difficult. They provide excellent advice for mastering the expectable obstacles in living a full life without a mate.

PERSONAL MEMORIES: A KEY TO RESOLUTION

In attempting to give comfort, clinicians may recite euphemisms that actually cause pain. It is quite common to hear even experienced clinicians urge their patients to "keep a stiff upper lip" or to "put this behind you and get on with your life." While trying to be sympathetic, a clinician may inadvertently remark to a woman who has lost a child, "You can always have another baby" or "You should be thankful you have other children at home" (Woods, 1987).

Although such comments are intended to make strong emotions more manageable, they give the patient the message that the depth of her grief is neither understood nor appreciated. To any woman, her loss is unique, and she must deal with it individually. Her task is to recover or to restore as many positive feelings as possible about her child, husband, or other loved one. As aptly summarized in a lecture by Menninger psychiatrist Marci Bauman-Bork (1996),

> When we lose significant others in our lives, the grief is initially tremendous. The way we cope with this is by recalling things about the person that were meaningful and very specific. For example, in losing a husband, a wife may soothe herself by recalling the special way he held her hand and the funny way

he would tilt his head when he talked to her. These memories allow her to hang onto the relationship. I always cringe when I hear people coming up to someone who has just lost a loved one say, "Well, you have to let go." What they really need to do is to hang on—hang on to memories that made the relationship meaningful. The only thing they have to let go of is the hope of more memories in the future. Hopefully, they will never "let go" completely of the lost person. This is the only way they can survive a major loss in a psychologically healthy way.

ACKNOWLEDGING THE SPIRITUAL COMPONENT OF LOSS

In Western society, expressions of physical suffering are more readily accepted and addressed than are assertions of spiritual suffering. But dealing with a terminal illness or a catastrophic loss can cause the most profound spiritual anguish. For these reasons, grief therapists encourage a leave-taking ritual that enables bereaved persons to honor their loved ones by bidding farewell in a concrete manner. Clinicians should not be discouraged from attending services for their patients; family members often find this an affirming gesture that says, in effect, "You are not alone. I will not turn away from you in your time of need" (Novack et al., 1997; O'Brien, 1996).

Simply acknowledging the spiritual components of suffering can be affirming to patients who are going through their own "dark night of the soul." In addition, it can be extremely helpful to encourage counseling with clergy and with mental health professionals; to recommend outlets in artistic expressions such as painting or music; and to help quell guilt, resentment, and remorse through focusing on self-forgiveness (Edwards, 1997). Patients sometimes even seek out their primary care clinicians for "permission" to address their spiritual lives.

Finally, the terminally ill have a special need to leave a positive legacy (Cerney, 1985; Kubler-Ross, 1997; O'Brien, 1996). Concretely giving back something to life or to one's loved ones by way of family history, letters, mementos, or keepsakes provides them with sorely needed consolation (O'Brien, 1996). The clinician may also, with great humility, ask the patient to share what she has learned in her struggle with illness or with grief. In this way, the lives of both the patient and the clinician are enriched and strengthened. Ultimately, the clinician who is able to listen carefully to the patient fosters resilience for traversing the vicissitudes of life. Growth becomes possible for both through all phases of the adult life cycle, even up to the moment of death (Cerney, 1985, 1989).

PHARMACOLOGIC CONSIDERATIONS

In the early days after a major loss, benzodiazepines can be used to induce sleep and quell anxiety (see Chapter 7). Counseling the patient about the use of such medication is essential. The patient must be told that prolonged use of these compounds is neither warranted nor useful. Grief is a process that cannot be medicated away, nor should it be. Moreover, dependence on this class of drugs should be avoided. In one substance abuse clinic, bereavement "was found to be the commonest life event leading to benzodiazepine abuse" (Parkes, 1996, p. 84).

When there are signs of clear-cut depression or complicated grief (see Table 9–1), antidepressants should be used (Horowitz et al., 1997; Reynolds, 1992). Combining pharmacotherapy with psychotherapy in these situations is essential, because treatment goals are broader than symptom reduction alone. One strives to improve the patient's quality of life and her total adjustment both socially and occupationally (Jacobs, 1993).

WHAT THOSE WHO MOURN TEACH CLINICIANS

As she neared the end of her career, Dr. Elisabeth Kubler-Ross wrote that "the dying were my best teachers, but it took courage to listen to them" (1997, p. 145). When she did so, she found that she learned invaluable lessons about life from persons who "reveled in their new role as teacher" (p. 145). Over and over again, these dying patients conveyed an important message to those who gave them care and to whom they yearned to impart their own special wisdom and healing message. Kubler-Ross summarized what she gleaned from years of work with people on the verge of dying:

Live so that you don't look back and regret that you've wasted your life.
Live so you don't regret the things you have done or wish that you had acted
    differently.
Live life honestly and fully.
Live.

(Kubler-Ross, 1997, p. 146)*

This perspective stands in positive and distinct contrast from that presented by a female patient who, speaking for many others, complained to Kubler-Ross, "All my doctor wants to discuss is the size of my liver. At this point, what do I care about the size of my liver? I have five children at home who need to be taken care of. That's what's killing me. And no one will talk to me about that" (Kubler-Ross, 1997, p. 145).

Remarks such as this occur not because clinicians wish to be insensitive but because they do not know what to do when people are dying or bereaved. All they really need to do is to listen, to truly attend to their patients' suffering just by their presence and their witness. Most clinicians are aware of how their shortcomings in communicating with patients lead to needless suffering. But as they remediate their attitudes and beliefs about death, they naturally become less distant, defensive, or even hostile.

Patients inevitably respond favorably to the "humanity" of clinicians who can acknowledge their limits as healers—that they are neither omnipotent nor omniscient. Although no one knows the length of any life, clinicians can always empathize with their patients' distress and let them know that they will not be abandoned. As Kubler-Ross further revealed about working with those whose losses were substantial: "All of us [the doctors, priests, and social workers under her supervision] learned what we should have done differently in the past and

---

*Reprinted with permission of Scribner, a Division of Simon & Schuster from *The Wheel of Life* by Elisabeth Kubler-Ross. Copyright © 1997 by Dr. Elisabeth Kubler-Ross.

what we could do better in the future" (p. 146). These clinicians gave their patients an opportunity for their lives to still have purpose and to know that they had a reason to live right to the final breath. After all, they were still growing, learning, and giving to others who would carry on after them.

ROLE OF THE PRIMARY CARE CLINICIAN IN WORKING WITH BEREAVEMENT OR MEDICAL CATASTROPHE

1. Be available. Empathize with how disconcerting the loss is for the patient, even if it had been expected. Give permission to grieve. Explain that the patient may experience waves of numbness and sad, angry, or confused feelings.
2. Ask open-ended questions about the patient's experience. Avoid comments that minimize the loss or sound judgmental (e.g., "Taking care of Sam was wearing you out; you are both better off, and he is at peace.")
3. Let the patient know that every person's experience of grief is unique. Show your respect for the grief process by explaining that it takes different forms depending on the person and the relationship to the deceased. Be sure to encourage the patient to take off sufficient time from work to begin the healing process.
4. Take physical complaints seriously, but remember that they tend to be exacerbated at this time. Use psychotropic medications (e.g., benzodiazepines) to help with acute anxiety or insomnia associated with the grief. Most patients benefit from the sleep induction but do not overuse the medication.
5. Encourage the patient to find a safe place to talk about her reactions. Ambivalence toward a loved one who is lost is normal, but often patients feel very guilty in expressing any resentment or anger whatsoever. Psychotherapy can be useful to help identify and resolve any shame associated with this ambivalence.
6. Encourage the patient to make use of rituals. This also gives her permission to grieve and is a concrete, socially sanctioned time for friends and loved ones to formally "say goodbye." By all means, attend the funeral if you can, even in cases of medical catastrophe. Patients and families experience your presence as reassuring and comforting, and this in turn builds their positive alliance with you. Particularly in cases of perinatal death, encourage parents to hold and/or name the baby, in order to facilitate the internalization that will aid them in the grieving process.
7. Ask about suicidal thoughts. Contrary to myth, patients are not offended when you do this. Most bereaved persons briefly entertain thoughts of suicide but then quickly discard them. The seriously depressed patient, however, may have developed a suicide plan that should be taken very seriously.
8. Encourage self-care. Patients and their family members need time for resting, eating, and diversion. Following a steady routine can also be helpful, particularly in the first few weeks, when the natural tendency is to feel torpid and "suspended in pain" (Rosof, 1994, p. 131).
9. The patient may feel confused or worry that she is "going crazy" because she thinks about or perceives that she "hears" or even "sees" the deceased.

This psychological reaction is based on an urge to recover or restore the lost person in one's life. When the beloved is internalized—living on in one's memory—these intrusive thoughts will probably diminish, although they may never go away completely (Parkes, 1996).

10. Acute grief can be a time of exacerbation of any medical or psychiatric problems. A history of depression, substance abuse, or posttraumatic stress disorder can complicate grief and certainly deserves specific treatment (Prigerson et al., 1995). Refer the patient with any signs of pathologic grief to a mental health specialist, and be on the lookout for a recurrence of emotional difficulties in patients with a history of psychiatric problems.

11. Remind the patient that a pang of grief can come on suddenly, even years after the event. This normal reaction can be triggered by an anniversary, a photograph, or even an odor—anything that brings the loved one to mind.

PATIENT GUIDELINES FOR COPING WITH CATASTROPHIC LOSS AND BEREAVEMENT

1. Take the time you need to grieve. In our busy, competitive, work-oriented society, women tend to take less time than they should for themselves. The hard work of grief uses psychological energy. Resolution of the "numb state" that occurs after loss requires a few weeks at least, but to discover what loss means takes much longer. A minimum of 1 year, to cover all the birthdays, anniversaries, and other important dates without your loved one (Cerney and Buskirk, 1991), is required before you can "learn to live" with your loss.

2. Express your feelings. Remember that anger, anxiety, loneliness, and even guilt are normal reactions and that everyone needs a safe place to express them. Tell your personal story of loss as many times as you need to—this repetition is a helpful and necessary part of the grieving process.

3. Make a daily structure and stick to it. Although it is hard to do, keeping to some semblance of structure makes the first few weeks after a loss easier. Getting through each day helps restore the confidence you need to accept the reality of loss.

4. Don't feel that you have to answer all the questions asked of you. Although most people try to be kind, they may be unaware of their insensitivity. Down the road, you may want to read books about how others have dealt with similar circumstances. They often have helpful suggestions for a person in your situation.

5. As hard as it is, try to take good care of yourself. Eat well, talk with friends, get plenty of rest. Be sure to let your primary care clinician know if you are having trouble eating or sleeping. Make use of exercise. It can help you let out pent-up frustrations. If you are losing weight, sleeping excessively or intermittently, or still experiencing deep depression after 3 months, be sure to seek professional assistance.

6. Expect the unexpected. You may begin to feel a bit better, only to have a brief "emotional collapse." These are expectable reactions. Moreover, you may find that you dream, visualize, think about, or search for your loved one. This, too, is a part of the grief process.

7. Give yourself time. Don't feel that you have to resume all of life's duties right away.
8. Make use of rituals. Those who take the time to "say goodbye" at a funeral or a viewing tend to find it helps the bereavement process.
9. If you do not begin to feel better within a few weeks, at least for a few hours every day, be sure to tell your doctor. At this point, it may be wise for you to seek out a mental health professional to talk with about your loss, especially if you have had an emotional problem in the past (e.g., depression, substance abuse). Be sure to get the additional support you need, because losing a loved one puts you at higher risk for relapse of these disorders.

ADDITIONAL GUIDELINES FOR PRIMARY CARE CLINICIANS
Practice Good Communication Skills

1. Take time to listen. All patients have expectable reactions to grief. Express empathy or sympathy for what they are going through (Nadelson, 1996). Above all, do not skirt the issue that their loss is uniquely painful to them.
2. Carefully review the circumstances that led to the loss and respond to questions about the medical treatment. This is often a sticky point, because physicians (mistakenly) think they are more likely to be sued if they discuss what happened; in fact, physicians who are better communicators tend to have fewer malpractice suits (Whitman et al., 1996).
3. "Bad news" should be conveyed with a heavy heart and great compassion. Face-to-face personal contact is always better than talking over the phone. Nonverbal communication skills (e.g., speaking with unfolded arms, putting a hand on the shoulder) can also be useful. Remember that communicating good news is easy for doctors, but conveying caring and empathy when giving bad news is also your duty.
4. Try to avoid body language that indicates nonreceptiveness, such as folding arms and crossing legs, turning away, or moving away from the patient while she is talking. Lean forward to indicate interest. Try not to interrupt while the patient is speaking or, if you must do so, preface your comments with an apology.
5. Remember that working with any kind of grief or loss is "labor intensive." It demands that the physician spend unhurried time with the patient and her family. Of particular helpfulness are consoling statements such as, "This must be very difficult for you. I don't think that anything else would have changed the outcome."
6. Try to withstand the human tendency to minimize or rationalize loss. Women who have experienced the death of a parent or husband (after a long illness) feel deep pangs of loss, even if they anticipated the outcome. Try to be particularly attuned to the woman's feelings after the loss of a child, saying something like, "Nothing can ever replace this particular child." Convey your understanding that no one fully gets over a loss. We simply learn to adjust.
7. Avoid statements that close off expressions of grief, such as, "The best thing to do is to go on with your life." This encourages the suppression of feelings, which can then foster depression, anxiety, and complicated grief.

Encourage Tension Release

1. Try not to feel overwhelmed by the emotional outpourings of your patient. Listening, giving reassurance, and providing clear and understandable explanations at such times are useful strategies. Instead of damaging the relationship between patient and caregiver, permitting intense emotional reactions to unfold often clears the air and strengthens the therapeutic relationship.
2. Be straightforward, especially about medical issues. Physicians may avoid being direct or giving bad news to patients because they believe that doing so leaves the door open for litigation. Sometimes they do not even hear the patient's questions because they are already on the defensive (Whitman et al., 1996). A better tactic that actually facilitates care is to listen, console, support, and provide as many answers as possible.
3. Realize that in the heat of the moment (e.g., on hearing bad news, learning of a death), the patient or her family members want to hold someone responsible. Irrational anger may be projected onto you. This is more likely to dissipate when you listen carefully despite the patient's highly charged emotions. It is actually a prudent and compassionate course of action.

Be Hopeful about the Patient's Capacity to Cope

1. Be sure to give clear and understandable explanations. Attend carefully to the patient's choices, and demonstrate positive regard. Tell the woman that, although she now feels unable to "bear any more suffering," with time she can be helped to endure.
2. Help the patient tolerate or manage with an altered physical appearance (e.g., spinal cord injury) or a life-threatening medical condition (e.g., renal failure) by referral to the appropriate specialists and/or self-help groups. Problem-solving and emotion-focused strategies have both been associated with a lessening of the stress that accompanies illness (Dewar and Morse, 1995). These techniques are particularly helpful because they teach disabled or disfigured patients how to manage difficult interpersonal situations (e.g., by deflecting embarrassment with humor).
3. Ask the patient about what she learns in these groups. Patients learn coping behaviors from each other and feel empowered when others inquire about their experience. In one instance, new spinal cord injury patients who could not bear the stares of strangers while attempting to maneuver their wheelchairs in the shopping mall, wore T-shirts inscribed with the message "What the f . . . are you looking at?" to deflect the gazes and intrusiveness of strangers (Laskiwski and Morse, 1993).

Know When to Refer to a Mental Health Professional

1. Expect the grieving process to require at least a year, and usually longer. It takes a minimum of 1 year to cover all the birthdays, anniversaries, and important dates without the loved one. Give your patients permission to take

the time it takes to grieve and to be angry. Encourage them to seek out additional modes of support, particularly if they convey to you that their friends or family members, while helpful, do not seem to be able to "hear" their misery. This is a particularly important concern for women who seek to "protect" loved ones by "staying strong."

2. Use resources within your community, and have their phone numbers and addresses readily available to give patients. Support groups can be enormously helpful. For survivors of the death of a child, Compassionate Friends is an invaluable resource. Many churches or mental health centers have support groups, especially for widows or bereaved parents. Healthy expression can be given to one's anger or resentment toward a spouse who is no longer available, and the individual can take advantage of adult companionship. Sometimes these groups strategically meet at mealtime, when the individual is likely to feel most lonely and unable to sustain the self by eating.

3. Be on the lookout for stress-induced physical illnesses occurring after loss. The literature is peppered with case studies of patients who acquired an illness that was the same as or similar to that of their deceased loved one. Such illnesses may be an expression of unresolved grief or unresolved anger that responds to grief counseling or psychotherapy.

4. Recognize that pathologic grief reactions (complicated grief reaction, see Table 9–1) occur even among the healthiest persons (Horowitz et al., 1997). Some women derive secondary gain after loss; an example is the woman who holds onto her grief in order to continue receiving sympathy from friends, children, and even her doctor. Despite the authenticity of their love for the deceased, these patients often harbor unconscious angry feelings and have a difficult time acknowledging their dependence on others. Their psychological needs require more time than a primary care clinician can usually spend; they require a skilled therapist to help them examine their underlying feelings of guilt, need to suffer, and need to stay pathologically dependent on others.

SPECIAL CONSIDERATIONS WITH THE WOMAN WHO HAS HAD A MISCARRIAGE OR OBSTETRIC CATASTROPHE

1. Maintain a high degree of awareness that women who experience a reproductive loss, particularly those who are childless or who have a history of major depressive disorder, are likely to suffer depressive symptoms after that loss (Neugebauer et al., 1997). Because motherly attachment increases with the length of pregnancy, grief intensity can be predicted by the length of time that the prospective mother carries the fetus (Janssen et al., 1997).

2. Recognize that women who miscarry have definite psychological needs, particularly the need to mourn the life that will never be. As writer Elizabeth Cohen remarked regarding her own miscarriage (1997), "No one can tell you what it feels like to hear silence where the fetal heartbeat is supposed to be . . . . To become the mother I hope to become, I must say goodbye to the mother I will never be" (p. 84). To help the mother through the initial stages of grief, be sure to acknowledge explicitly her loss and emotional pain. Keep an ongoing attitude of interest and availability (Bauman-Bork, 1996; Woods, 1987).

3. Refrain from comments that are critical or gratuitous, or that gloss over the loss. Women have fantasies about their babies very early; that is, they develop a psychological relationship with the child long before it is born. They also tend to blame themselves if something goes wrong, and they wonder about "what might have been." Although you may feel better temporarily by reassuring the patient that "you can always have another baby" or "you weren't far enough along to be attached," statements of this kind only prolong grief. Moreover, they compromise the physician-patient alliance. At least 50% of women who experience a lost pregnancy subsequently seek a different physician because their doctor did not seem to understand their emotional needs during the crisis (Bauman-Bork, 1996).

4. If the infant is far enough along so that it can be wrapped and cradled, encourage parents to do so. The grief process is actually facilitated by having a tangible relationship with the child or fetus. A religious service can also be helpful. As painful as perinatal or neonatal loss can be, viewing and holding the baby "allows the parents to have some memories of the child, which allows them to hold onto the child psychologically" (Bauman-Bork, 1996). The chance to internalize is particularly important to help the parents grieve the loss of a continued relationship with the child, which facilitates their eventual internalization of the relationship. As in all losses, grief is surmounted by "hanging onto the memories that made the relationship meaningful. The only thing that must be let go of is the hope of more memories in the future" (Bauman-Bork, 1996).

SUMMARY

As one grows older, loss becomes a principal ingredient of life, but it is never easy to master. Clinicians tend to neglect the grief reactions of their patients because they share common vulnerabilities with them. These include the loss of bodily integrity through acute or chronic (terminal) disease, death of a loved one, and sequelae of medical catastrophes. Women, in particular, tend to stifle their grief reactions because they do not wish to burden their family members or clinicians. Consequently, their emotions may become "frozen," leading to complicated grief reactions, depression, psychophysiologic reactions, and medical illness.

Practical suggestions can help the practitioner deal with the various unsettling emotions that arise after loss. The emphasis in this chapter has been on helping the primary care clinician to provide the patient with a "safe haven" for experiencing and working through inevitable change, and to know when to refer to a mental health professional for additional support. As clinicians are able to help their patients deal with loss (and the accompanying guilt and anger), they are strengthened to face subsequent adversity in their own lives. Moreover, the clinician's "humanity" at these precarious times inevitably buttresses the doctor-patient relationship. On the other hand, when the clinician ignores or fails to help patients with their losses, the doctor-patient relationship is weakened and a reservoir of pain and resentment builds up, disrupting even the most stable of therapeutic alliances.

Many patients develop illnesses when they are not able to work through grief and the often-repressed anger and rage that accompany it. The process of psychotherapy for grief frequently lessens or completely alleviates these physical complaints. Most important, it allows patients to understand and eventually let go of their own remorse, that "gnawing sense of guilt that they should behave differently and are responsible for some grievous happening" (Cerney, 1988, p. 245).

To help an individual face loss, the clinician must first listen. Research demonstrates that significant predictors of overall patient satisfaction (and well-being) include caring, communication, reliability, empathy, and responsiveness—all of which have a listening component. Developing those skills that help patients bear "bad news" and endure even the most traumatic events or catastrophes (e.g., perinatal loss) inevitably enhances the doctor-patient relationship. Therefore it is wise to include leave-taking rituals, to allow the patient time to internalize the loved one and then to say goodbye and let go, and to use ancillary support systems.

Grief work necessitates that both clinician and patient accept their essential humanity with all its imperfections, recognizing but then letting go of anger and any unrealistic expectations of perfection. Grieving persons must come to grips with the ambivalence inherent in all relationships. Love and care can thrive only in an atmosphere where we can acknowledge both the positive and the negative facets of our loved ones. Acknowledging ambivalence enables bereaved persons to work through loss in a healthier way, allowing them access to a fuller life that is less encumbered with anguish and resentment about unmet or unfulfilled expectations.

When women have the opportunity to handle unfinished business by the resolution of their grief, they are more likely to be and to stay healthy. Even brief contact on the part of the clinician can facilitate the process of working through grief, thereby decreasing the woman's guilt, self-blame, and isolation. Empathy exhibited by the clinician at these most painful times is never forgotten.

Resources for Patients

Most bookstores and libraries have a large section devoted to the subjects of coping with terminal illness, bereavement, and grief. Their scope ranges from personal memoirs to workbooks that outline the grieving process and actions or steps that individuals can take to move through it. Clinicians will find helpful perspectives in these books that are rarely taught or mastered in training. Most patients can readily find a book that answers their individual questions and gives them solace. This partial list of some easily acquired resources can guide the practitioner to suggest a particular reading that will touch the patient's unique grief issue.

For Patients with a Terminally Ill Family Member

Callanan M, Kelley P: *Final Gifts: Understanding the Special Awareness, Needs, and Communications of the Dying.* New York, Poseidon, 1992 (paperback: New York, Bantam Books, 1997).
  This compendium of individual experiences with the dying was written by two hospice nurses. Their purpose is to help family members understand the human reactions, needs, and perceptions of their loved one as death approaches. Also useful for the terminally ill patient herself are the stories of men and women who, as they near death, communicate their feelings, find reconciliation, and move through the leave-taking process with growth and dignity. This book has particularly moving descriptions

of some of the less scientifically understood phenomena that occur around the time of death (e.g., seeing loved ones who have long since died).

Coughlin R: *Grieving: A Love Story.* New York, Random House, 1993.
   Although this book is billed as a widow's story of her own grief process, it also tells the tale of a loving couple's struggle with terminal illness. Full of wisdom and laced with humor, it cannot help but touch readers through Coughlin's very human responses to her husband's life—and death.

For Survivors of Suicide

Chance S: *Stronger Than Death.* New York, WW Norton, 1992.
   Dr. Chance, a writer and psychiatrist in private practice, poignantly tells the story of her own reactions after her son's suicide. Those who experience this kind of loss may feel particularly bereft and lonely, because they often cannot acknowledge, even to those most dear, their deepest questions about what went wrong or what they could have done differently. Frequently recommended by the self-help groups Survivors of Suicide and Compassionate Friends, Dr. Chance's humane and honest account of her torturous ordeal ends with a statement about healing, growth, and hope for all who experience this tragedy.

For Widows

Brothers J: *Widowed.* New York, Ballantine, 1990.
   When Dr. Joyce Brothers' husband of more than 30 years died, she found herself riveted by her pain and the chasm his death created in her life. In this account, the prominent psychologist shares her personal story of loss in a manner that every woman who has survived the death of a partner can identify with and understand. Virtually all patients will find this readable, first-person account filled with important tips on how to survive the myriad emotions that bombard every widow. For example, at the end of the book, Brothers has brief sections on how to fight loneliness; face important anniversaries, holidays, and weekends; and deal with the tendency to brood or "let things slide." There are additional tips for friends and relatives of the bereaved; some are real gems. For example, Brothers urges us to avoid asking "the impossible question," that is, how the widow is doing or how she is bearing up. Instead, she advises the use of concrete questions such as, "How has your sleep been?" or "Is there something that I could do that would be helpful or useful?" This focus is just as important for clinicians to remember, too.

Caine L: *Being a Widow.* New York, Penguin Books, 1988.
   When Lynn Caine's husband died, she experienced "impeccable ignorance about death and dying" (p. 8). Her writings became an effort to help others face the realities of death with greater openness and more knowledge. This book is essentially an update of the author's best-selling book, Widow (1974). What is particularly engaging about this volume is how it addresses the many unspeakable issues faced by widows. They includes the stages of widowhood; denial and angry feelings; dreams about the deceased; the need to express pent-up emotions; dating and sexuality; rebuilding self-confidence; and how to help children when you yourself are wrought with feelings of loss. The author includes a number of letters that widows have written to her and gives straightforward answers to their questions. Final sections on resources—those places widows can get help—and suggestions for friends and loved ones cap off this comforting, sensible guide.

Ginsberg J: *Widow: Rebuilding your Life.* Tucson, AZ, Fisher Books, 1995.
   Written from the author's own experience as a widow, this book confronts the issues that new widows struggle with most (e.g., What do you do about "the dumb things people say"? How do you handle your guilt and crying when emptying closets or

drawers?). She recommends that women play an active part in rebuilding their own lives. She also tackles sensitive issues such as whether or not to wear a wedding ring, dating and sex, traveling, and starting a support group. A particularly useful chapter addresses what to do when you feel lonely during the holiday season.

For Bereaved Parents

Rosof BD: *The Worst Loss: How Families Heal from the Death of a Child.* New York, Henry Holt, 1994.

According to the author, parents who lose a child endure "a loss like no other." This book helps patients understand and begin the hard work of grieving what is experienced as an insurmountable tragedy. Sections for spouses and for children emphasize how much each person in the family loses when a child dies. A particularly wrenching, but important, section draws on the experiences of other families who have faced the death of a child yet found ways to prevail. Special topics include stillbirth, infant death, terminal illness, AIDS, sudden death, murder, and suicide.

Schiff HS: *The Bereaved Parent.* New York, Crown, 1977 (paperback: New York, Penguin Books, 1978).

This classic text helps the parent from the time of the funeral through the inevitable and seemingly endless aftermath of guilt, powerlessness, sorrow, and despair that follows the death of a child. The special challenges of being a parent to surviving offspring (e.g., how to be helpful to them) and rebuilding one's marriage, as well as the essential but agonizing task of going on with life after the child's death, are described with genuine emotion and compassionate advice. Schiff knows her subject and her audience—her own son died at age 10. She believes that parents "have a great need to know that others have experienced the emotions they are feeling and that these others are dealing with both their bereavement and life . . . . You are not alone in knowing you can and must learn to carry on despite the most unnatural of disasters" (p. xiv). Patients who have lost a child will feel heard and comforted by this author whose own loss colors her message.

For Children

Lionni L: *Little Blue and Little Yellow.* New York, Astor-Honor, 1959 (paperback: New York, Mulberry, 1995).

This classic picture story was routinely used by the late Dr. Mary Cerney, a psychologist and pioneer in the study of grief psychotherapy at The Menninger Clinic, to help persons of all ages deal with loss. The fable of the best friends Little Blue and Little Yellow captures how others change our lives; they are a part of us even after a painful separation. This book can be used to help families, particularly children, understand how individual people "add color and life to our existence, which can never be taken away, even through death" (Cerney, 1989, p. 117).

For Those Who Have Lost a Loved One

Kelley P: *Companion to Grief: Finding Consolation When Someone You Love Has Died.* New York, Simon & Schuster, 1997.

This general text about the intense and unpredictable emotions that can erupt after a death normalizes the grief process. Although a number of books are available for widows, this one is applicable for women who have endured the loss of anyone close. Emphasis is placed on how bereavement is unique for each person—we all grieve differently and for different lengths of time. The work is broad: Special sections on AIDS, losing a coworker, and encouragement for self-care are samples of the topics included. To assist someone who is grieving, Kelley emphasizes the importance of listening "with concern and patience and without judging, explaining, or advising" (p. 123). Pointing out progress, keeping in touch, and paying attention to danger signs such as poor hygiene or weight loss are insightful points for friends of the bereaved and for the clinician to remember.

Kubler-Ross E: *The Wheel of Life: A Memoir of Living and Dying.* New York, Scribner, 1997.

The author of the profoundly influential On Death and Dying *(1969) now tells the story of her own life and terminal illness. Many will disagree with some of Kubler-Ross' spiritual beliefs (e.g., channeling, communication with the deceased after death), but they cannot help but be moved by her profound conviction that every life has a purpose and that, as long as we are alive, we must devote ourselves to truly living. For Kubler-Ross, living fully is a matter of faith that allows one to "handle anything that God would send, that no matter how painful and agonizing, I would be able to see it through" (p. 220). Any patient who has experienced a major illness or loss and is trying to come to grips with life's purpose will find much comfort and hope in this fascinating, final autobiographical statement.*

Lewis CS: *A Grief Observed.* New York, Bantam Books, 1961/1976.

This memoir by theologian C.S. Lewis describes the anxiety, anger, personal angst, and spiritual doubt that the author felt after the death of his wife. It is widely available and frequently read by people experiencing grief and/or remorse. Deeply probing and spiritual in tone, this book is frequently recommended by grief therapists and religious counselors.

Resources for Primary Care Clinicians

Bowlby J: *The Making and Breaking of Affectional Bonds.* Suffolk, Great Britain, Tavistock/Routledge, 1979/1989.

This brief summary by a psychoanalytic pioneer on attachment theory takes its title from a special section about loss (Lecture 7). Intuitively, everyone knows that loss wreaks havoc on individuals, particularly children, but Bowlby's research demonstrates how facets of psychological growth and development can be stunted by bereavement. In this lecture for physicians, he also describes those conditions that can aid in the process of healthy mourning. Highlighted is the principle of providing a reliable and empathetic human relationship for anyone at any age who undergoes trauma or major loss. Because primary care clinicians are often in the pivotal role of knowing the family over a period of years, axiomatically they can supply a sense of safety or "a secure base" for their patients. In times of travail, this aspect of the doctor-patient relationship particularly helps the family to traverse anxiety, helplessness, and despair.

Parkes CM, Laungani P, Young B: *Death and Bereavement Across Cultures.* London, Routledge, 1997.

All societies and cultures have their own customs and unique beliefs surrounding death. In order to understand a culturally diverse patient population's reactions to mourning, this handbook explains the rituals and beliefs of the world's major faiths. A final section on the practical implications of maintaining a cross-cultural perspective is invaluable for clinicians involved in the care of the dying. The summaries are easy to read and full of tips about how to provide comfort and support to bereaved adults and children.

Viorst J: *Necessary Losses: The Loves, Illusions, Dependencies, and Impossible Expectations That All of Us Have to Give Up in Order to Grow.* New York, Simon & Schuster, 1986.

Loss may be a necessary fact of life and growth, but that doesn't mean it is easy. Judith Viorst explains how each stage of life, from childhood to death, is filled with lessons about "loving, losing, leaving, letting go." Although the particular sections devoted to growing older, facing severe or fatal illness, and dying are most applicable to the management of bereavement, this text (now available in paperback) should be read by everyone who is interested in better understanding themselves and mastering life's inevitable transitions. Because clinicians are also profoundly affected when their patients are stricken with incurable illness or die, Viorst's compassion and illumination provide balm for their own grievous aches and pains.

References

Averill SC: Recovery of the lost good object. *Bull Menninger Clin* 1997;61:288–296.

Bauman-Bork M: Psychosocial needs for a woman enduring an obstetrical catastrophe. Unpublished manuscript presented to the Shawnee County (KS) Medical Society, May 1996.

Bowlby J: *The Making and Breaking of Affectional Bonds.* Suffolk, Great Britain, Tavistock/Routledge, 1979/1989.

Bowlby J: *Attachment and Loss III: Loss, Sadness and Depression.* New York, Basic Books, 1982.

Brothers J: *Widowed.* New York, Ballantine, 1990.

Caine L: *Being a Widow.* New York, Penguin Books, 1988.

Callanan M, Kelley P: *Final Gifts: Understanding the Special Awareness, Needs, and Communications of the Dying.* New York, Poseidon, 1992 (paperback: New York, Bantam Books, 1997).

Cerney MS: Imagery and grief work. In: Stern EM (ed.): *Psychotherapy and the Grieving Patient,* pp. 35–43. New York, Haworth, 1985.

Cerney MS: "If only . . . ": Remorse in grief therapy. *Psychotherapy-Patient* 1988;5:235–248.

Cerney MS: Use of imagery in grief therapy. In: Shorr JE, Robin P, Connella JA, et al. (eds.): *Imagery,* pp. 105–119. New York, Plenum, 1989.

Cerney MS, Buskirk J: Anger: the hidden part of grief. *Bull Menninger Clin* 1991;55:228–237.

Chance S: *Stronger than Death: When Suicide Touches Your Life.* New York, WW Norton, 1992.

Cohen E: The ghost baby [editorial], p. 84. *New York Times Magazine,* May 4, 1997.

Coughlin R: *Grieving: A Love Story.* New York, Random House, 1993.

Dewar AL, Morse JM: Unbearable incidents: failure to endure the experience of illness. *J Adv Nurs* 1995;22:957–964.

Eells T: Relational therapy of grief disorders. In: Barber JP, Crits-Christoph P (eds.): *Dynamic Therapies for Psychiatric Disorders (Axis I),* pp. 386–419. New York, Basic Books, 1995.

Edwards MJ: Doctors and patients: facing life-threatening illnesses. *Pharos* 1997;60:19–21.

Ginsberg JD: *Widow: Rebuilding Your Life.* Tucson, AZ, Fisher Books, 1995.

Gut E: *Productive and Unproductive Depression: Success or Failure of a Vital Process.* New York, Basic Books, 1989.

Horowitz MJ, Siegel B, Holen A, et al: Diagnostic criteria for complicated grief disorder. *Am J Psychiatry* 1997;154:904–910.

Janssen HJ, Cuisinier MC, de Graauw KP, et al.: A prospective study of the risk factors predicting grief intensity following pregnancy loss. *Arch Gen Psychiatry* 1997;54:56–61.

Kelley P: *Companion to Grief: Finding Consolation When Someone You Love Has Died.* New York, Simon & Schuster, 1997.

Krigger KW, McNeeley JD, Lippmann SB: Dying, death, and grief: Helping patients and their families through the process. *Postgrad Med* 1997;101:263–270.

Kubler-Ross E: *On Death and Dying.* New York, Macmillan, 1969.

Kubler-Ross E: *The Wheel of Life: A Memoir of Living and Dying.* New York, Scribner, 1997.

Laskiwski S, Morse JM: The patient with spinal cord injury: the modification of hope and expressions of despair. *Can J Rehabilitation* 1993;6:143–153.

Lewis CS: *A Grief Observed.* New York, Bantam Books, 1961/1976.

Lionni L: *Little Blue and Little Yellow.* New York, Astor-Honor, 1959 (paperback: New York, Mulberry, 1995).

Nadelson CC: Ethics and empathy in a changing health care system. *Pharos* 1996;59:29–32.

Neugebauer R, Kline J, Shrout P: Major depressive disorder in the six months after miscarriage. *JAMA* 1997;277:383–388.

Novack DH, Suchman AL, Clark W, et al.: Calibrating the physician: personal awareness and effective patient care. *JAMA* 1997;278:502–509.

O'Brien M: Relief of suffering: where the art and science of medicine meet. *Postgrad Med* 1996;99:189–208.

Parkes CM: Bereavement. In: Kendrick T, Tylee A, Freeling P (eds.): *The Prevention of Mental Illness in Primary Care,* pp. 74–87. New York, Cambridge University Press, 1996.

Parkes CM, Laungani P, Young B: *Death and Bereavement Across Cultures*. London, Routledge, 1997.

Prigerson HG, Franke E, Kasl SV, et al.: Complicated grief and bereavement-related depression as distinct disorders: preliminary empirical validation in elderly bereaved spouses. *Am J Psychiatry* 1995;152:22–30.

Regier DA, Boyd JH, Burke JD, et al.: One month prevalence of mental disorders in the United States. *Arch Gen Psychiatry* 1988;45:977–986.

Reynolds CF: Treatment of depression in special populations. *J Clin Psychiatry* 1992;9(Suppl):45–53.

Rosof BD: *The Worst Loss: How Families Heal from the Death of a Child*. New York, Henry Holt, 1994.

Schiff S: *The Bereaved Parent*. New York, Crown, 1977 (paperback: New York, Penguin Books, 1997).

Viorst J: *Necessary Losses: The Loves, Illusions, Dependencies, and Impossible Expectations That All of Us Have to Give Up in Order to Grow*. New York, Simon & Schuster, 1986.

Whitman AB, Park DM, Hardin SB: How do patients want physicians to handle mistakes? A survey of internal medicine patients in an academic setting. *Arch Gen Med* 1996;156:2565–2569.

Woods JR (ed.): *Pregnancy Loss: Medical Therapeutics and Practical Considerations*. Baltimore, Williams & Wilkins, 1987.

Chapter 10

Major Medical Illness

When poet Audre Lorde was diagnosed with breast cancer, she refused to handle her crisis "with a blanket of business as usual" approach, keeping her "feelings forever undercover, but expressed elsewhere" (1980, p. 9). Instead, she made a conscious decision to join the battle for physical integrity and against personal despair. In *The Cancer Journals* (1980), Lorde urges women who face a serious illness to eschew their tendency to remain silent and instead to speak out, particularly about their medical and personal needs.

Women who have faced the multiple challenges inherent in a severe, potentially life-threatening illness have embraced the message and wisdom of Lorde and others who have witnessed about their own treatment and recovery. Their determination to have more input—and more choices—in their health care is changing the face of contemporary medical practice. One consequence is the desire to be more open about personal needs, including psychological concerns. These women make a conscious commitment to increase their odds of survival or to face down the ravages of a chronic condition by finding ways to choose life over death. For Lorde, it took breast cancer to come to grips with "my mortality . . . what I wished and wanted for my life, however short it might be" (p. 20) and to "own my feelings . . . my sorrow and my joy" (p. 77). Every patient must likewise take command of her body and her mind in order to find new sources of power within herself to sustain health and fight disease.

The psychological approach to medical illness helps women speak out rather than remain silent. When the female patient finds new avenues of caring for herself and for those she loves, she is more apt to bear up against disease and to be sustained during the treatment process. She also learns lessons about "living a self-conscious life . . . with the consciousness of death at my shoulders" (Lorde, 1980, p. 16), which can, among other things, have a profoundly positive impact on her overall health and well-being.

How can the primary care clinician engage the patient, who is now more likely to ask questions, look at all the treatment options, and desire opportunities to speak her own personal truths (e.g., what can be learned) about her illness? Much interest in alternative medicine has been spawned by men and women who were dissatisfied with the answers of traditional medicine. However, technologic advances and a humanistic approach need not be antagonists. But the contemporary physician must certainly "move beyond polarized, dualistic conceptualizations which so often pit one against another" (Parks, 1997, p. 91).

Even the most seriously ill medical patient can benefit from the strategies, tools, medications, and techniques that modern psychiatry has to offer. It would be wise for primary clinicians to invest some time to carefully consider these options. But it does require a shift in how clinicians think about their role. They must return to their sense of themselves as healers, not simply as health care professionals. Moreover, what clinicians learn about caring for the psychological needs of patients ultimately benefits them as well. Almost everyone will be a patient at some point, and it is often said that the best physicians have themselves been seriously ill at some time and therefore have experienced the process of being navigated through a stormy recovery. As a result, these clinicians have an intuitive understanding of, and empathic resonance for, what their patients are going through. They have also learned that illness can be a grim but great teacher.

This chapter outlines some basic principles to help primary clinicians meet the psychological needs of their patients. Clinicians do not have to keep in mind a variety of gender-specific questions to enhance the relationship with a patient. In most cases, all that is required is the capacity to listen well and to make suggestions about available tools or strategies the patient might find useful for improving her quality of life. Both men and women who face a routine evaluation vary in their level of emotional stress. Their worry naturally skyrockets if a specific problem is uncovered. Possible disfigurement, disrupted relationships, long-term disability, and pain are the most frequent concerns women must face. In such circumstances, social support is crucial. Many patients are alone—or feel they are alone—in dealing with their problem, but the primary clinician may not be aware of this situation. For example, one patient, a research fellow and mother of two, was abandoned by her husband after she was diagnosed with severe cardiomyopathy. Heart transplantation was being considered, and the husband thought his wife might be "too much of a financial burden."

Clearly, patients who face this degree of travail need a particular kind of emotional support that allows them to face their burdens without censure or fear of judgment. But other medical patients also have a need to discuss how the illness is affecting all areas of their life and to find new modes of coping. For these medical and surgical patients, psychotherapy can be extremely beneficial. In fact, appropriate psychotherapy for the medically ill patient reduces overall health care costs, as a number of succinct reviews have underscored (Gabbard et al., 1997; Spiegel and Lazar, 1997).

The stress inherent in having a serious illness creates the need to be heard and understood as an individual, placing one's life and personal situation in its unique context. Psychotherapy not only provides that support but also, in many situations, enhances compliance with overall medical care, thus improving well-being and longevity (Druss, 1986; Lamberg, 1996; Spiegel, 1990, 1993; Steptoe and Wardle, 1994). Primary care clinicians are all too aware of the intangible toll of medical illness, which is difficult to quantify by even the most sophisticated cost-benefit analysis. Still, as the cost-offset argument goes, adequate psychotherapeutic support results in fewer lost workdays, substantial reductions in morbidity and mortality, and less use of medical care and expensive diagnostic tests (Gabbard et al., 1997).

THE HEALING POWER OF HEARING THE PATIENT'S STORY

As children, most of us at one time or another clamored for an adult to "tell me a story." We didn't care whether we had heard it a thousand times before—or even what the content was. It could be a familiar fairy tale, a cherished fact of family history, a long and complicated riddle or joke, or a reminiscence about our own babyhood. We attended to every nuance and detail of the narrative. Sometimes a parent or grandparent would mischievously introduce a new feature or reverse a sequence in the beloved tale—only to be chided for "not telling it right." A good laugh would erupt, indicative of the relationship between audience and storyteller and of the need for each person to "be heard."

Human beings are mesmerized by good storytelling from the cradle to the grave, not merely for its entertainment value alone. We also learn from stories—ours and those of others—about all facets of living, and particularly about the value of relationships, which thrive in the mutually created ambiance of give and take. *Hearing a good story reminds us that we are not alone, because it occurs within a relationship and is often about a relationship.*

As much as we enjoy listening to stories, physicians in a busy practice often find it a difficult, time-consuming, almost impossible task. We want to listen but feel conflicted because there is so much to do and to find out from each patient. Beckman and Frankel's classic study (1984) demonstrated that physicians interrupt each patient after an average of only 18 seconds. They found that if patients are allowed to respond to an open-ended question, they speak on average only about 90 seconds; the answers of most patients in this study took less than 2 minutes. Although we clinicians intuitively know that a central aspect of communication is providing time for the patient to tell her story, we tend to rush in with a question, a procedure, or a medicine because of our own anxiety. A better approach, recommended by the late Dr. Jack Ross, a training and supervising psychoanalyst at The Menninger Clinic, is to "bring buckets" or Kleenex. By that, he meant that we should be present and emotionally available to absorb the patient's tears and anguish. For women in particular, the physician's receptiveness helps to ferret out the social context of her problem, why she seeks care now, and clues to what additional supportive measures she may need in order to carry out your recommendations. Encouraging the patient to ask questions and helping her to organize information are other important healing functions of the initial interview (Carlson and Skochelak, 1998).

Simply put, patients bring their personal stories, and they need to have them heard. The telling itself is balm for the wounded spirit, and the technical procedure for carrying it out is relatively simple. Goldberg (1997) recalled a moving example of one patient's story to a young intern. Before he died, this patient simply wanted to have his doctor listen to the story of his own derailed career in medicine. He asked for nothing except human responsiveness. Interviewing strategies and active listening techniques have been developed to improve medical communication. But getting to the heart of the patient's worries about the illness can usually be pinpointed by using two simple phrases: "Tell me about . . . " and "What else?"

An excellent medical interviewer is endowed with the same characteristics as those of the best conversationalists—interest in the other person and the ability to listen well. Physicians can more easily understand the essence of a patient's concerns and expectations of treatment when they avoid interrupting her narrative. Some simple advice by communications expert Sam Horn is as applicable to the medical interview as it is to personal relationships and daily conversations:

Would you like to learn two simple words that are the key to kicking off conversations? They are the simple words, "Tell me." Most people ask closed questions that already contain the answer. This relegates the other person to confirming or denying what you have just said. "Did you have fun at the dance?" "Yeah." "Did you enjoy the ball game?" "It was okay." End of conversation. "Tell me . . . " as in "Tell me about the dance" gives people a hook on which to hang a conversation.

(Horn, 1997, p. 41)

This approach also shifts the traditional power dynamic in the physician-patient relationship. Greater importance is placed on the woman's autonomy and capacity to make central choices about her treatment and her life (Carlson and Skochelak, 1998; Silverstein and Blumenthal, 1997). Employing a feminist model, patient and physician form a partnership that is less hierarchic, more egalitarian, and based on the woman's need to voice her questions, concerns, and goals. This approach emphasizes the actual context of her situation, her interpersonal relationships, and her pivotal role in treatment decisions that affect her body and her life.

THE HEALING POWER OF PROVIDING "A SAFE PLACE" FOR THE PATIENT

For just a moment, forget you are reading a medical textbook. Consider this anxiety-riddled fantasy: This morning, on the way to the hospital or office, you were run off the road by an individual afflicted with society's new malady, "road rage." You emerged unscathed, grateful your spouse and youngsters were not with you. Still quite shaken, you manage to gather your belongings, and your fortitude, enough to get to work after the wrecker has hoisted your overturned car and towed it away to the automotive shop for major body and engine repairs. What do you do when you see the first familiar face, be it a secretary, colleague, housekeeper, friend, or patient? *You tell them about the incident*—often in great detail and with palpable emotion—in order to master what has happened to you and to go on with the rest of your day! In the telling, you also rid yourself of the immediate anlage of visceral turmoil that has set your heart racing, your blood pressure skyrocketing, and your anger erupting. (More than once, I have commented only half in jest to my secretary that if she heard any more of my minor daily calamities and brushes with disaster, she would need to be licensed as a psychotherapist by the Kansas Board of Healing Arts.)

The point, of course, is that human beings need each other, and they make use of each other every day as they talk through all the problems and irritations that befall them. One need not be a psychotherapist or a psychoanalyst to be helpful to most people, most of the time. Merely being a trusted confidant with a reasonable amount of good sense and a little bit of time does the trick.

But what happens when the going gets tougher—as when one receives the confirmed diagnosis of cancer or heart disease, or has to deal with the longer-term disability of a collagen, vascular, or neurologic disorder? Is there a special role for psychotherapy in helping to improve the quality of life? Can patients, by talking to someone, be assisted in mastering illness much as they master daily traumas? What evidence is there, if any, that "the talking cure" has more value than simply emotional release? Can psychotherapy actually improve not only the quality of life but also the length of life itself?

A surprising and growing amount of literature answers these questions in the affirmative. This is important information for primary care clinicians who work with patients and families who might not seek psychological assistance without their physician's guidance. Ways must be found to help them take advantage of the psychotherapeutic and psychopharmacologic assistance that is available in their communities. In addition, psychotherapy can actually reduce overall health care costs and therefore may increasingly be viewed as a "managed-care-friendly" modality. Putting politics and policy aside, it behooves the primary clinician to be fully aware of the actual data describing the benefits of psychotherapy for patients with medical conditions, not only because it is cost-effective but also because it is personally effective and improves overall quality of life.

THE HEALING POWER OF PSYCHOTHERAPY: NEW RESEARCH INFORMING PRIMARY CARE

Over the past 15 years, a series of outcome studies of medically ill patients have reported physiologic and psychological improvements with the use of psychotherapy. Patients are themselves becoming aware of these facts, which are reported on radio and television and in women's magazines. Simply summarized, these reports document that both individual and group therapy can have a positive impact on the depression, anxiety, adjustment problems, fatigue, and pain that accompany the diagnosis of many physical diseases (Fawzy et al., 1990, 1993; Druss, 1986; Goldstein and Niaura, 1995; Niaura and Goldstein, 1995; Spiegel, 1991; Spiegel and Lazar, 1997; Spiegel et al., 1989).

The most extensive studies have examined heart disease and cancer, but positive health outcomes have also been shown when psychotherapy is given to patients with arthritis, hypertension, diabetes, gastrointestinal disturbances, and renal dialysis. Psychotherapy techniques include cognitive-behavioral, psychodynamic, experiential (e.g., hypnosis, biofeedback, massage), and individual and group modalities (Borenstein, 1996; Butler and Wing, 1995; Severino, 1980; Shumaker and Smith, 1995). There are few clues about the final common pathways for the effectiveness of this diverse set of procedures, because understanding the specific "interrelatedness of mental, emotional, and physiological processes" (Parks, 1997, p. 109) is still in its infancy. Nevertheless, it would be unfortunate, if not unethical, if patients who could be helped were not offered therapy that could be particularly useful to them. Even susceptibility to the common cold appears to be lessened through a buttressing of supportive social ties (Cohen et al., 1997). Psychotherapy can provide one crucial tie to help women increase their repertoire of available supports.

Cancer

Women with breast cancer who participated in weekly group psychotherapy for 1 year experienced a reduction in anxiety and depression and an enhanced quality of life. Moreover, their survival time increased by 18 months, compared with patients not given group therapy (Spiegel, 1995; Spiegel et al., 1981, 1989).

Spiegel and Kato (1996) hypothesized that *permission to express anger in the group* is one of the most important factors for increasing survival. Hypothetically, patients find that "safe place" described previously in this volume, a place where they can express their strong emotions, including fear of death, frustration with treatment, and a sense that their bodies have betrayed them. Patients learn coping techniques from each other, but primarily they have a place where it is permissible to let down pretenses and feel bad.

These women reorient their priorities and redirect their attention away from physical and emotional pain. This camaraderie in the group appears to help control pain (e.g., medication use is reduced) and may enhance compliance with chemotherapy or other treatments and procedures. Overall, self-care improves because the women find a reprieve from stress and loneliness and use this natural championing to "make a conscious commitment to survival" (Lorde, 1980, p. 73).

Other studies found that patients with malignant melanoma who were involved in 6 weeks of structured psychiatric group therapy exhibited more vigor, less depression, increased hopefulness, and more energy than controls; at 6-year follow-up, the patients who participated in the group had a lower rate of death and a trend toward less recurrence (Fawzy et al., 1990, 1993).

Diabetes and Coronary Heart Disease

Several studies have reported the positive effects of psychosocial interventions on glucose control in diabetic patients (Butler and Wing, 1995). As in the development of cardiovascular disease, stress may be a key variable. In fact, hostility, anger, and interpersonal conflicts have been linked to coronary risk in women (Weidner, 1994).

Hypothetically, the rates of coronary heart disease among women can be reduced through behavioral interventions analogous to those used for patients with malignancy, but as yet no long-term studies have proved that dealing with role conflicts, job stress, and interpersonal struggles influences the risk of coronary heart disease in women. For both genders, emotional stress has been linked to myocardial ischemia (Gullette et al., 1997). It is likely that techniques that enable both genders to deal constructively with depression and anxiety will improve longevity (Frankenhaeuser, 1994; Levin et al., 1998). Depression is strongly associated with more frequent and more malignant cardiovascular disease (Glassman and Shapiro, 1998) and is likely to be involved in all other vascular diseases (e.g., stroke). Relaxation techniques, biofeedback, and individual and group psychotherapy have a modest effect on hypertension (Niaura and Goldstein, 1995).

WHAT PATIENTS "LEARN" FROM SERIOUS ILLNESS

Audre Lorde (1980) spoke for many men and women when she explained how her illness became a path for growth and renewed investment in life. She wrote that the hard lessons of breast cancer led her to embrace "my life and my love and my work" (p. 17). "I would never have chosen this path, but I am very glad to be who I am, here" (p. 77). Like most people, including physicians who have faced a long recovery after an accident or malady, she would have preferred not to become sick, but her illness taught her to be more passionate and assertive about the value and meaning of every day.

Druss (1995), writing from the perspective of 40 years' experience in consultation-liaison psychiatry, described on a case-by-case basis the benefit of psychotherapy for a wide array of patients who have traveled a similar path. Clinicians of every specialty have observed what Druss voices quite eloquently: A serious medical illness can be a turning point when individuals are forced to take stock, self-reflect, and find new and better ways of coping. The question becomes: What factors let some people accomplish this while others do not? The more clinicians understand the factors that enable many patients to be resilient, the more they can make these factors available to others (Zerbe, 1997).

Apparently, those patients who are able to take advantage of the healing modalities they are offered and who do not tend to view themselves as passive victims fare better than those who complain or blame others for their travail (Table 10–1). Druss (1986, 1995) found that the therapist's perseverance and flexibility assist the patient on the road to recovery. These patients "need one place they can go and speak their minds about disease, its care, and what it means to them" (Druss, 1995, p. 57). Personal crises are surmounted, pain is assuaged, and resiliency is discovered. Druss also believes that an essential feature of these progressive healers is their hopefulness and confidence. They prod their patients to choose life over death. Especially in the face of debilitating or terminal illness, psychotherapy helps women have an enhanced quality of life because the therapist stays optimistic, "not about the patient's course or ultimate prognosis, which no one knows, but about the patient's courage, no matter what the outcome" (p. 65).

This salubrious prescription actually reflects a core value of all psychotherapy—that is, that growth occurs and quality of life improves when the individual transforms "adversity into challenge" (Druss, 1995, p. 103). The psychotherapist's task is to enter into the subjective world of the medically ill

---

Table 10–1. **Characteristics of Good Copers**

Optimistic attitude
Capacity for endurance despite suffering
Capacity for "healthy denial"
Ability to actively seek and use information
Assertiveness and inquisitiveness
Courage in the face of adversity
Capacity to reevaluate life and to take stock (e.g., tendency to "see the glass half full rather than half empty")
Capacity to integrate bodily changes into overall body schema (e.g., not narcissistically invested in having "a perfect body")
Ability to seek out and benefit from social supports (e.g., support groups, friendships, psychotherapy)
Capacity to retain belief in integrity of body despite illness
Relative freedom from self-pity, anger, envy, and guilt about "having caused" illness

person to help the patient put the illness in context and to encourage self-discovery. In this way, sanction is given to the patient's inner life, which promotes endurance, courage, and resiliency, even in the face of despair (Zerbe, 1997).

Expanding on the seminal contributions of Alyce and Elmer Green, two pioneers in biofeedback and psychopharmacologic therapy at The Menninger Clinic, Dr. Peter Parks summarized the goal of the contemporary therapist who promotes health. Parks believes that to heal body and spirit it is essential to bridge disciplines:

> If we are to move beyond polarized, dualistic conceptualizations, which so often pit one against another, we must become self aware of our culturally driven tendency to view life through dualistic binoculars. We must learn to reevaluate our own presuppositions if we are to make genuine contributions to the reconceptualization of our Western scientific tradition. . . . The unfolding of this multisensorial experiential journey can lead to discovery of an emergent self, a self with access to inner resources that previously remained below the level of conscious awareness.
>
> (Parks, 1997, pp. 91, 107)

MODERN TOOLS FOR HELPING WOMEN MANAGE STRESS

As women move out of the home and into the marketplace, they appear to exhibit the same reactivity patterns as men, leading to chronically higher physiologic arousal levels with probable and possible deleterious long-term health consequences (Frankenhaeuser, 1994; Steptoe and Wardle, 1994). Stress research has identified those factors in the environment that can increase or dampen physiologic responses, affecting the neuroendocrine functions that ultimately mediate stress. Increased neuroendocrine and glucocorticoid reactivity have been linked with numerous diseases, including stroke, heart disease, ulcer, and colitis, to name a few. Although both sexes are likely to benefit from new ways of modulating responses that help the individual adapt to stress and promote healthy behaviors (Frankenhaeuser, 1994), the present discussion of these new insights is particularly targeted to female patients.

Women must increasingly negotiate the multiple demands of family, career, and self. Women in the "sandwich generation" feel compelled to sustain both hearth and health, spouse and children, and, more and more commonly, aging parents. How can one simultaneously meet the demands of job and family and have any energy left over for oneself? Usually the woman places herself last on the list of needs. Over time, this is not only physically and emotionally exhausting but it also makes her feel frustrated and angry. She looks for a way out. She may even develop physical illness. Although she may turn to her social supports (e.g., friends, significant other), she is also likely to seek comfort from you, her primary clinician.

Consider the additional burdens of the woman who has been diagnosed with a significant medical problem. Even in the most fortuitous of circumstances (e.g., solid financial resources, a caring and committed significant other), the patient must find a way to care for herself, contain the anxiety she naturally has about the disease, and still manage her home and occupational responsibilities.

Herein lie many of the "women-specific" problems facing a patient (Hensley and Reichman, 1998). She wonders how she will go for treatment when her children need to be chauffeured to games, music lessons, or daycare. She worries about whether changes in her physical appearance will alienate her spouse (Table 10–2) or whether she will lose the capacity to become pregnant if she chooses. If she has young children or aging parents, she will especially ruminate about how to care for those dependent on her. Physicians can be an enormous resource simply by empathizing and showing concern for the woman bedeviled by personal demands such as these.

Physicians demonstrate an understanding of the context of a female patient's life by asking how she is meeting her multiple responsibilities and by taking seriously her embarrassment about any physical and emotional changes brought on by the illness. It is helpful to remind her that stresses that promote the disease process may be ameliorated by interpersonal connections. Because social support and a sense of personal control have been found to help women buffer the effects of stress, they should be mentioned in any routine treatment plan. When working with a woman facing a serious medical illness or occupational problem, I routinely write out on a prescription pad "Seek social support by _____" and "Today I am going to feel more in control by _____." I then ask the patient to fill in the blank with a specific activity.

Emphasize to the patient the importance of maintaining friendships and of engaging in activities she enjoys. Because social support and personal control have such positive health benefits, attune yourself in the interview to the patient's unique ways of finding these in her environment. She may turn to a network of friends, benefit from daily exercise or a walk, or find that her spouse is more than willing to sit down and talk more frequently. Some of her health patterns may have slipped over the years, but your verbal advice, combined with a directive to learn about stress management in appropriate books (see "Resources for Patients"), makes a huge difference in pointing her in a positive direction.

You might begin by reminding the woman who is trying to cope with illness of the classic work of University of Pennsylvania psychologist Martin Seligman (Hiroto and Seligman, 1975; Seligman, 1991). In his pioneering studies about learned helplessness, Seligman found that when animals are exposed to shocks, noises, or other stressors that they can neither predict nor control, they become apathetic, stop paying attention, and generally fail to perceive even those events they would otherwise attempt to control or master. Analogizing these findings to

---

Table 10–2. **Specific Sensitivities of Women Undergoing Medical Treatment**

Body image concerns (e.g., scarring after mastectomy or bypass surgery, amputation)
Weight gain associated with pharmacotherapy (e.g., chemotherapy, corticosteroids)
Alopecia associated with chemotherapy
Loss of childbearing potential
Early menopause
Concern about childcare arrangements during treatment
Concern about family responsibilities (e.g., fatigue, sexual functioning)

humans, he concluded that depression results when we experience predicaments from which there appears to be "no exit" (Sapolsky, 1994). Seligman is now studying "learned optimism"; that is, the capacity in hardy individuals to deal successfully with either good or bad news.

Optimists hear good news with the expectation that history will repeat itself and that their positive efforts to take charge will continue to pay off. Pessimists, on the other hand, repeatedly "see the glass as half empty rather than half full." Good copers have a healthy quotient of "learned optimism." They are not sanguine about getting bad news, but neither are they devastated by it. They begin to help themselves by taking charge. They use modalities such as prayer, meditation, dancing, psychotherapy, and exercise to actively handle external stressors, including illness.

Relationships with other women have been found to be protective of not only of men's health but also of women's (Spiegel, 1995). Women should therefore seek out and rely on female friends and support groups, in addition to any formal psychotherapy. Women who are good copers tend not to blame themselves for events or situations they cannot control (see Table 10–1). Another facet of their active coping is the tendency to learn about their condition in various media. They ask their health care practitioners many questions, because getting accurate information helps them feel empowered to do what they can for themselves.

Another feature of good copers is the tendency to make the clinician aware of new treatments on the horizon. They read from many sources that the physician may not be familiar with (e.g., women's magazines are offering increasingly sophisticated information, Internet sites update women's health information continually). Well-informed patients are not afraid to write down their questions and concerns. The physician should encourage this practice—even though it increases the time spent with the patient—because it lends itself to that sense of mastery that bodes well for recovery.

Some women confront adversity with "healthy denial" (Druss, 1995), meaning that they do not disavow the fact that they must deal with the malady, but they refuse to see it as an impediment to living a full and fulfilling life. In essence, they view a severe disability "almost as an enviable asset" or face a diagnosis of cancer or diabetes, "not as a narcissistic injury but as an opportunity for growth" (Druss, 1995, pp. 73–74). These inspirational patients are as much a pleasure to have in one's practice as they are to know in one's life. Clinicians may count them as their friends because they teach their treaters much about maintaining a generous spirit "free of self-pity, anger, and envy towards those who are whole and well" (Druss, 1995, p. 74).

The clinician will still find there are personal costs involved when working in a holistic, humanistic manner. Even the most appreciative and compliant patient feels ambivalent about her doctor (Dreifuss-Kattan, 1990). No one relishes a reminder of one's own mortality. Clinicians can expect to be hated as well as loved by patients, because ultimately they do inflict pain and suffering. They cannot stem terminal illness, let alone answer existential questions about life's ultimate purpose. Journeying with patients through serious illnesses means that clinicians must also come to grips with their own mortality. To avoid burnout, physicians must take time for personal restoration and employ the same restorative aids (e.g., rest, exercise) that they suggest to their patients (Grosh and Olsen, 1994; Kash and Breitbart, 1993; Nouwen 1972).

MEDICAL ILLNESS AND DEPRESSION

Numerous studies are garnering support for the hypothesis that treating depression may play a significant role in improving the prognosis and quality of life of those enduring a medical illness.

Coronary Heart Disease

Depression is a risk factor for coronary mortality and morbidity in women. Women also have more anxiety and depression than men after a myocardial infarction. They are less likely than men to participate in cardiac rehabilitation programs. The specific reasons are unknown, but it may be that physicians are less apt to encourage their female patients to participate. However, when they do, they gain the same benefits as men (Shumaker and Smith, 1995; Weidner, 1994).

Some investigators have suggested that a woman's caregiving roles and family responsibilities limit her attendance in rehabilitation programs. Although data are still limited, it behooves the physician to be aware of role conflicts and cultural biases that may negatively affect treatment and recovery. The physician should also use those treatments that have been found effective for depression in patients with ischemic heart disease. For example, although tricyclic antidepressants (TCAs) and selective serotonin reuptake inhibitors (SSRIs) may have equal efficacy in countering depression, nortriptyline has been associated with a higher rate of serious adverse cardiac events, compared with paroxetine (Roose et al., 1998). The clinician who treats women with primary diagnoses of coronary heart disease and depression must stay aware of this rapidly evolving literature base to render state-of-the-art treatment or to involve a psychiatrist in the treatment.

Chronic Fatigue Syndrome and Fibromyalgia

Other illnesses garnering interest in the women's health agenda are diabetes, chronic fatigue, fibromyalgia, and cancer. Throughout this chapter, cancer is cited as a "model disorder" to which modern psychological and psychopharmacologic modalities have been employed (Temoshok and Dreher, 1991). However, the primary clinician must remain vigilant about the co-occurrence of depression with any underlying medical disorder (see Chapter 2).

Between 50% and 70% of patients with chronic fatigue syndrome meet the diagnostic criteria for depression. Their clinical course is improved by small doses of a TCA (which may particularly help their sleep disturbances) or an SSRI. An essential therapeutic task is to "listen to the patient, taking seriously her recounting of her illness and explaining honestly what is known and not known" (Komaroff, 1997, p. 1183; see also Fuller and Morrison, 1998).

A diagnosis of depression concomitant with these illnesses is always complicated: Clinicians wonder whether depression occurs primarily because of underlying neurobiologic substrates associated with the disorder, or whether the medical illness causes depression. Women are more prone than men to develop musculoskeletal disorders, including osteoarthritis, rheumatoid arthritis, lupus, and fibromyalgia. Although TCAs and SSRIs are not panaceas, they can be useful treatment adjuncts.

Cognitive-behavioral therapy has been shown to be an acceptable, effective treatment in some randomized, controlled trials. It may work by helping patients avoid heightened physical or emotional stressors by pacing themselves. This form of therapy may also counter the tendency toward self-blame while it promotes the health benefits of a regular routine (Canoso, 1997; Komaroff, 1997). The patient finds herself to be in greater control than she otherwise thought. Regular exercise and staying as active and involved as possible may also promote health via the endorphin system. Deconditioning and further physical deterioration increase the chance of a downward spiral into physical restriction—and depression. As always, in any disease process, mind and body are inevitably and inextricably linked.

Diabetes

Many women diabetics appear to suffer from and experience disease differently from men. Women with diabetes can experience a plethora of sexual problems and family issues. A question that research has not yet answered definitively is why female diabetics are prone to more depressive relapses and a greater number of diabetic complications. However, the SSRIs (particularly sertraline) have been found to reduce insulin resistance, leading to a lessening of depression and hemoglobin A1c levels.

Women with diabetes are also prone to develop overt and subclinical eating disorders (see Chapter 5) and to have difficulties with weight management if they are obese. Dietary restraint and weight gain with insulin therapy appear to place diabetic women at greater risk for development of anorexia or bulimia. The primary clinician must be vigilant that some diabetics will even manipulate their insulin to lose weight, worsening their glycemia control and ultimately increasing their physical jeopardy (Butler and Wing, 1995; Zerbe, 1993/1995). Interventions that encourage appropriate weight loss for diabetic women have been found to be more effective when a spouse or significant other is involved in the total program. Calorie intake, goals for target weight, and exercise programs improve when patient and loved one participate together and are taught social supports (see Butler and Wing, 1995). The central point again underscores that women's health appears to be mediated by social and relationship support when initiating and maintaining positive health practices.

Chronic Pain

It is always wise for the clinician to wonder what role pain may play in the life of the individual woman and why it persists in some persons and not in others. Although personality factors may be influential, many women can be helped to cope more effectively with their pain without resorting to surgery or becoming addicted to narcotic agents. Pain may trigger depression, exacerbating a loss of functioning and of one's sense of control over life. When the depression is treated effectively, pain is ameliorated in a significant percentage of patients.

The treatment of pain syndromes is a model for helping women with other medical treatments: Encourage empowerment by learning as much as you can about the illness. Stress an active lifestyle to help the woman overcome the tendency to remain passive or to avoid activities. Include some "holistic" strategies. Although the specific treatment of every disorder is beyond the scope of this chapter, the "laying on of hands" during massage therapy or therapeutic touch can help some women's physical and emotional states. For example, psychotherapist Ilana Rubenfeld combines traditional psychotherapy, education, and touch for a variety of psychological and physical problems. Her Rubenfeld Synergy Method (Rubenfeld, 1988; Simon, 1997) is not a replacement for traditional medicines or the pharmacotherapies for depression and anxiety; instead, it is aimed at helping the patient observe and listen to her body to promote relaxation and physical restoration.

HELPING THE PATIENT FACE PHYSICAL CHANGES RESULTING FROM ILLNESS

With rare exceptions, women who undergo treatment for a life-threatening or chronic illness must deal with distressing physical side effects and changes in their body image (see Table 10–2). For example, although a colostomy for ulcerative colitis or carcinoma of the colon may be lifesaving, the patient must not only learn techniques for managing her stoma but also face lifelong consequences to her physical appearance and in her relationships. Unless the physician asks, these fears usually remain unspoken. Does the patient worry about whether she will still be attractive to her partner? Will her own sexual interest wane? Sometimes friends can be supportive, but in their curiosity they can also be cruel. The patient worries that she will be embarrassed by questions about her treatment and physical changes.

The physician must take these "woman-specific problems" seriously and make them as discussible as possible (Carlson and Skochelak, 1998; Hensley and Reichman, 1998). The failure to do so perpetuates repression or nondisclosure of distress that may impede any medical treatment (Druss, 1986; Spiegel, 1990). By all means, consider referral to an appropriate patient support group. You may know another patient who has undergone a similar ordeal and would be willing to visit or talk. Millions of women have been helped by the camaraderie of other survivors who openly share their techniques for learning to deal with appliances or prostheses; they also can help the patient respond to well-intended but probing or embarrassing questions. Women who have previously traveled the same path are the best resources for helping the patient establish appropriate boundaries regarding intrusive questions (e.g., "Are you wearing a wig because you lost all your hair from the chemotherapy?"). Many patients feel great relief when you express permission and encouragement to seek out these supports. Nor should you be afraid to say that you do not have all the answers to some very real concerns.

The important point to remember is that any woman has many questions about the consequences of treatment that she may be reluctant to share with you directly. Addressing these questions enhances compliance with overall care and furthers psychosocial adjustment. Consider the magnitude of nonadherence to treatment or follow-up care among cancer patients alone. In one study, 23% of patients did not keep their chemotherapy appointment. In another study, more than one fourth withdrew from the recommended treatment protocol. In still another study, more than one fourth of patients with an abnormal Pap smear did not return for follow-up. *Improving survival rates for any disease necessitates not only finding new treatments but also helping patients take advantage of treatments that are already available. Many patients do not return because they are afraid.* When we help them face their fears by increasing their knowledge and reducing their anxiety, compliance is improved and emotional anguish is diminished (Hensley and Reichman, 1998; Ott and Levy, 1994; Spiegel, 1995; Spiegel et al., 1989; Surbone and Zwitter, 1997).

Oncologist Carolyn Runowicz, a breast cancer survivor, knows that her patients abhor hair loss from chemotherapy; she persistently reminds them that it will grow back—just as hers did—but that survival is the first order of business (Runowicz and Haupt, 1995). Runowicz acknowledges that chemotherapy has some temporarily negative effects, but she focuses on the value of a fighting spirit and on ways patients can buttress self-esteem in the face of a life-threatening illness. Runowicz also emphasizes the importance of both psychotherapy and pharmacotherapy should a patient become depressed.

Maintaining a sense of humor, learning to pace oneself, and developing a plan for self-care are essential, because "staying alive is just the initial challenge; living with the consequences of the disease and therapy becomes a lifelong responsibility" (Runowicz and Haupt, 1995, p. 9). Care extenders in your office can intervene effectively by making frequent but brief calls, a "reminder" of your concern, availability, and desire to see your patients through their fight. Telephone counseling has been shown to increase adherence to treatment for low-income women at risk for cervical cancer (see Ott and Levy, 1994; Meyerowitz and Hart, 1995). Incorporating this kind of support improves compliance because it is a reminder of your caring presence and because it helps patients answer those hidden but essential questions they have about their illness.

WHAT CAN I TELL MY PATIENTS ABOUT THE BENEFITS OF PSYCHOLOGICAL THERAPIES?

This question has sparked heated controversy among practitioners over the past three decades. There is increasing evidence that psychotherapy affects not only adjustment to medical illness but also survival time. The beneficial effects appear to be mediated via the endocrine and immune systems; a hyperactive hypothalamic-pituitary-adrenal axis can influence the rate of disease progression by differential effects on glucocorticoid production (Sapolsky, 1994; Spiegel and Kato, 1996) or on immunosuppression, or both.

To date several randomized, prospective studies have found that cancer patients in psychosocial treatments survived longer than did controls, whereas only one matching and one randomized study did not show such a difference (Spiegel and Kato, 1996; Spiegel and Lazar, 1997). Psychotherapy has also been shown to improve immune functioning in patients with the acquired immunodeficiency syndrome or malignant melanoma (Fawzy et al., 1990, 1993; Spiegel and Lazar, 1997). More research is necessary, but current findings have shown the cost-effectiveness of psychotherapy in improving overall health outcomes among the medically ill.

How is survival time enhanced by emotional expression and social support? The possible explanations are limitless, but current speculation suggests that positive connections with other people promote improved body maintenance activities (e.g., diet, sleep, exercise), leading to enhanced endocrine and immune functioning. Some believe that even a seemingly poor prognosis "enriches life" by helping patients focus on what most of us fail to do during our daily round; that is, "live with our own mortality" (Bartholome, 1997, p. 47). William Bartholome, a professor of pediatrics and a medical ethicist, finds that his "terminal" adenocarcinoma of the esophagus has forced him to "live life in the present . . . living in the light of death, living as fully and richly as possible regardless of how much time I have left . . . powerfully shaped by joy and caring and loving" (Bartholome, 1997, p. 44). The capacity to accept one's condition, write about it, and find one's own inner truths may be powerful forces in sustaining survival.

What Is the "Best Therapy" for the Medically Ill Patient?

Determining which particular kind of psychological help will work for an individual patient is a more difficult issue. Because at least 30% of seriously medically ill patients also have depression or an anxiety disorder, pharmacotherapy should be used liberally, sometimes in consultation with a psychiatrist (see Chapters 1 and 2). Even if patients choose not to participate in formal psychotherapy, they can benefit by "confessing" their anxieties in writing. This technique has repeatedly been shown to help people weather emotional storms, master traumas, and find a sense of meaning and purpose in difficult circumstances (Pennebaker, 1991, 1997; Pennebaker and Beall, 1986).

"Prescribing" the most appropriate form of psychotherapy for a patient is as challenging to the physician as planning any medicinal or surgical treatment. Individual factors such as age, motivation, the comorbid problems of anxiety and depression, and the capacity for insight all need to be taken into consideration. Usually a psychiatrist or other mental health professional experienced in working with the medically ill can join the treatment team to offer a truly multidisciplinary and multimodal approach (Powers et al., 1986). The goal is to enhance the patient's capacity to engage in treatment and to have greater resiliency. Adapting to changes brought about by diagnosis and treatment is hard psychological work (Breitbart and Holland, 1993; Stoudemire, 1995). Beneficial psychotherapy approaches include: (1) cognitive-behavioral psychotherapy; (2) guided imagery, biofeedback, and hypnosis; and (3) psychodynamic psychotherapy.

Cognitive-Behavioral Psychotherapy

Some women benefit most from a cognitive-behavioral approach. They are taught that it is not the disease itself but the thoughts about it that causes their distress. Once they understand the link between their negative thoughts and their emotions, they are encouraged to keep a record of their thoughts in a diary. The therapist then uses various techniques based on questioning, guided imagery, and actual behavioral tasks to examine their thoughts (Moorey, 1991) and to reduce their tendency to expect the bleakest outcome.

Guided Imagery, Biofeedback, and Hypnosis

Other patients can enhance their pain tolerance, diminish anxiety, and increase feelings of self-awareness and physical control through psychophysiology self-awareness training (e.g., biofeedback, hypnosis, acupressure, acupuncture, or even just becoming absorbed in a new or favorite activity) (Csikszentmihalyi, 1990/1991; Green and Green, 1977/1989). Clinicians unfamiliar with these techniques can learn some basic imagery scripts, for example, to help soothe their patients.

Repeating the phrase "you are in a safe place" or performing a relaxation exercise (see Chapter 7) creates an experience of solace or "oneness" that paradoxically focuses attention away from the source of pain and onto new modes of control and reliable self-regulation. Most people find that it takes little effort "to improve control of their attention" so that even when "objective circumstances are brutish and nasty" (Csikszentmihalyi, 1990/1991, pp. 211–213), they can learn to enjoy the immediate experience, set new goals, and find more joy, thus diverting their attention away from bodily threats or pain.

Psychodynamic Psychotherapy

Still other women benefit from exploratory or psychodynamic psychotherapy or even psychoanalysis when they have a serious medical illness. These patients glean much from the opportunity to examine their lives, coming to view their illness as a crisis time that enables them to reevaluate themselves and take stock (Druss, 1986, 1995). A common thread of the psychotherapies, and of the healing relationship itself, is the therapist's capacity to walk shoulder-to-shoulder with the woman during her time of need. The clinician becomes another witness or companion who is privileged to see the patient through adversity in order to "heal old wounds and permit reconciliation to a new life trajectory" (Druss, 1995, p. 54).

A Key to Successful Treatment: The Personality of the Healer

Primary physicians and psychotherapists share common goals and some common attributes. Through their human connections with their patients, both hope to reduce patients' suffering and promote their well-being. The healing relationship is filled with intangible subtleties that defy even the most meticulous of quantitative research studies. But when people get sick—and this eventually includes everyone—they want more than an expert technician at the bedside.

It is understandable to wonder which physicians have the best track record—and why. Does achieving good "outcome" truly boil down to which practitioner uses the latest pharmacologic algorithm or validated protocol? Or will true healing always be permeated with a tincture of mystery? To achieve the kind of psychological well-being described in this chapter, spirit as well as body must be taken into account. "Who *really* makes the best doctor, and how can I model myself after him or her?"

There actually has been some savvy research on the personality patterns of successful psychic healers (Appelbaum, 1993) which may enhance the traditional clinician's approach to the patient. This research helps treaters call into question their most cherished assumptions about "what heals" and what facilitates the treatment of their patients. According to this research, the core ingredient of these healers' success was *their confidence in their capability as an effective caregiver and healer*. Small wonder patients sought out these successful healers. They tended to have original, creative responses to stimuli and enjoyed taking on tasks with an odd, imaginative, or even oppositional point of view. They were not put off by seemingly hopeless situations. Their intuitive and original responses to questions were not readily categorized, which made them difficult for even an experienced psychologist and psychoanalyst to interview! Appelbaum (1993) makes the case that the effectiveness of these healers was an actual expression of love modeled after the original relationship between mother and child. He goes on to suggest that those who help and those who are helped (e.g., patients) may have much in common:

> Just as the mother-child relationship begins in symbiosis, so, too, does healing. . . . Perhaps those persons who benefit most from such healing may have similar or complementary personalities. They, too, may be people who tend to suspend disbelief, who submit easily to awe and admiration of others, who are oriented toward having their needs met by others, and who are confident that others have the power to help them. Healing may indeed be a temporary, symbiotic return to a time when love between mother and child conquered all, when mother often did, through the laying on of hands, make it "all right.". . . *All healing comes about, ultimately, through the patient's willingness to take advantage of whatever healing measures are offered.*
>
> (Appelbaum, 1993, pp. 39–40, emphasis added)

Resilient caregivers who are themselves good copers give their patients permission to be so also. Over time, a companionable partnership (i.e., the doctor-patient relationship) enables the woman to find her true self, even in the most difficult of circumstances. This partnership encompasses an easier oscillation between feelings of legitimate loss, anger, and frustration and willingness to move forward and to grow. Inevitably, those clinicians who are open to stories of their patients' healing are also transformed by the experience of facing illness. Effectively and compassionately addressing the psychological needs of the medically ill also provides a rare opportunity for the clinician's personal self-discovery.

PATIENT AND FAMILY GUIDELINES FOR COPING WITH MAJOR MEDICAL ILLNESS

1. Learn all you can about your illness. Increased knowledge reduces anxiety. By keeping your anxiety about your illness at manageable levels, you will be more likely to adhere to treatment recommendations. Many patients who can be helped with modern treatment do not receive it because they are fearful.
2. Avoid the temptation to blame yourself for your illness. A modern myth that must be faced down is that people control their bodies. If they get sick, it

is perceived as a failure. Although those who cope best with illness tend to maintain an optimistic attitude and confront the news head on, they know where to draw the line between what is and is not within their control.

3. Practice healthy behaviors. Although good nutrition, adequate amounts of sleep, and routine exercise are always recommended to maintain a healthy lifestyle, this advice becomes all the more important when dealing with a medical illness. All but the most frail can find a way to be active. Exercise promotes a generally positive state of well-being. Develop a program that you can do despite your physical limitations. Practice good sleep hygiene and tell your doctor about any problems. Sleep disturbances are associated with increased pain, irritability, and fatigue. Sustained sleep deprivation is life-threatening and can impair your resistance to disease.

4. Enhance your personal social supports, such as friendships. Women who have at least one positive relationship tend to survive cancer longer (Spiegel, 1993). Contact with other people appears to reduce mortality risk from cancer and other diseases (Frankenhaeuser, 1994). When you feel less isolated and frightened, you will be more inclined to practice healthy behaviors, such as exercising or remaining vigilant about your prescribed treatment.

5. Take advantage of support groups. In addition to providing a social outlet, a support group that focuses on your particular medical problem will help you meet and learn from others who have been in similar circumstances. Other women can give you not only emotional support but also practical advice. More than one woman has coped with the hair loss associated with chemotherapy, learned how to manage a stoma after a colostomy, or dealt with change in body image after extensive surgery or an amputation. Sometimes even the most well-meaning people can ask insensitive questions. In a support group, you will meet others who want to share how they have handled difficult interpersonal situations or embarrassing questions. You will be helping them by listening attentively and appreciating their hard-won wisdom.

6. Consider entering psychotherapy. There is growing evidence that psychotherapy helps patients to endure medical illness. Benefits may include less pain, better coping skills, and even longer survival in some situations. Some patients can use their illness as a time of finding new meaning and direction. Depending on your needs, a particular kind of psychotherapy may be most helpful (e.g., hypnosis, guided imagery, biofeedback for pain control or relaxation). Psychotherapy can also help you deal with the emotional and life changes that occur with severe illness or disability. *Cognitive-behavioral therapy* emphasizes the opportunity to find better ways of coping with your emotions. It also encourages you to challenge catastrophic thinking (e.g., the idea that having cancer is an inevitable death sentence). We all have a tendency to waver between minimizing and magnifying problems; cognitive-behavioral therapy lets you sort out those events that are important from those that are less essential for living. *Psychodynamic psychotherapy* helps you put your illness into an overall life perspective and can guide you on a path of self-discovery. Although an illness is certainly nothing to be coveted, those patients who maintain an optimistic and resilient attitude may eventually learn to view their illness as an opportunity for personal growth.

7. Find a way to express your feelings. Put your worries into words. Try not to be negative, full of blame, or envious of others who are "well." Remember that many studies have examined the profound healing power of putting upsetting experiences into words. Writing down your deepest concerns helps you come to terms with your problems and learn about yourself in the process (Dreher, 1992; Francis and Pennebaker, 1992; Pennebaker, 1991). Acknowledging your thoughts and feelings also helps your nervous system relax.

8. Try to "look at the glass half full, not half empty" (Druss, 1995, p. 73). Studies of good copers show that they experience joy, even in the face of adversity; they also tend to feel good about their bodies and themselves despite the physical changes brought on by illness or treatment. In other words, they are self-reliant, non-self-critical, and able to reach out both to those more fortunate and to those less fortunate than they are. In this way, they exhibit empathy and the capacity for concern, two hallmarks of good psychological health.

9. Seek additional help if you become depressed, demoralized, anxious, or panicky or have unremitting pain. A high percentage of medically ill patients do develop these psychiatric symptoms, which can often be alleviated with medication. Your physician may not be aware of changes in your mood or level of physical pain unless you acknowledge it. New approaches for pain management (e.g., acupuncture, acupressure, biofeedback) are enabling many patients to control their physiologic responses and thereby reduce the need for high doses of medication.

10. If you are a caregiver, do not neglect your own self-care. Take time for rest and restoration, remembering that should you become emotionally or physically exhausted you will be unable to give the support and care to your loved one that you desire. Even the most generous and well-meaning person cannot give what she does not have in her power or person to give.

11. Choose life. Even though your treatment will inevitably confront you with some difficult moments—and difficult choices—try to remember that there is still meaning in living and learning in your situation. Novelist Reynolds Price, himself a long-term cancer survivor, writes in his memoir, *A Whole New Life* (1994), about the daunting courage it took to keep living in the face of extreme pain and poor odds. Nevertheless, by relying on a deep religious faith, an excellent health care team, and a circle of friends and loved ones who helped him through the worst times, he did so. In your darkest days, consider his words for the needed push to get you through: "Such a reach for life is another tall order, especially for a human in agonized straits. . . . The visible laws of nature are willing you to last as long as you can. Down at the core, you almost certainly want to survive. . . . Never give death a serious hearing until its ripeness forces your final attention and dignified nod" (Price, 1994, pp. 185–186).

12. Find a creative outlet. The experience of writing poetry or prose, painting or making collages, playing an instrument or singing can be enriching and uplifting. These activities can help you feel more whole, and they are powerful tools in working on the fear, anger, and loss that are stirred by illness (see Dreifuss-Kattan, 1990).

ADDITIONAL GUIDELINES FOR PRIMARY CARE CLINICIANS

1. Listen to your patients. Spending even a little time can be the necessary balm for healing wounded spirits. In the face of suffering, many patients show notable courage, resilience, and a desire to tell what they have learned about life from their illness. By all means, learn as much as you can from them. It is perhaps the greatest challenge and the greatest reward of a physician to sit at the bedside and accompany a patient on her journey through an illness and its healing.

2. Help the patient take advantage of psychotherapy. The evidence for its beneficial effects on morbidity and longevity are briefly reviewed in this chapter. Share this notable research with the patient and be prepared to support your referral to managed care gatekeepers. They are often unaware of the overall cost savings of therapy. Help the patient face down stigma ("I don't want to talk to a shrink; do you think I'm crazy?") by emphasizing the medical gains that can be accrued from "talking through" the situation.

3. Review the available therapy options, and consider using judicious pharmacotherapy as an adjunct in treatment. Let the patient know about new strategies for coping with illness (e.g., cognitive-behavioral therapy) or dealing with pain (e.g., visualization, hypnosis, biofeedback). For the patient who can benefit from reviewing her life and who would like the opportunity to put the illness in context through self-reflection, suggest psychodynamic psychotherapy. Its effectiveness with the medically ill has been well established (Druss, 1995; Spiegel, 1993). Several studies of depressed medical and surgical patients have demonstrated the clinical efficacy and the cost savings resulting from a brief psychotherapeutic intervention (Katzelnick et al., 1997). Compared with a matched control group of depressed medical and surgical patients, one treated group spent 31.8 days less in the hospital, with a cost savings of $25,405 per patient (Verbosky et al., 1993).

4. Encourage the patient to ask questions about treatment. Open discussion with the treater helps the patient to feel empowered. Those patients who face their illness head on with a sense that they can actively master it tend to have a better outcome.

5. Be vigilant about the diagnosis and treatment of anxiety disorders and depression in the medically ill (see Chapters 1 and 2). There is a high prevalence of psychiatric disorders among medical and surgical patients. Secondarily, medical illness causes inherent stresses that can potentiate depression and anxiety. For example, almost half of all cancer patients have a diagnosable psychiatric disorder (Derogatis et al., 1983). New psychotropic agents with few side effects (e.g., SSRIs) can rapidly help a large percentage of patients. Refer to standard texts for dosages and medication profiles, but seek specialty consultation if the patient does not improve quickly.

6. Respect your own needs as a caregiver. Even under the best of external circumstances, clinicians are prone to burnout. Treating patients can be uniquely gratifying and life enhancing, but few people outside the profession actually recognize the physician's personal sacrifice. Collegial support is essential, but it is being eroded in the current zeitgeist of extraordinary financial and bureaucratic pressures. Healers benefit from the same prescrip-

tions they advise their patients to follow; this promotes optimism and resiliency in the face of the increasingly restrictive, punitive environment in which they practice (Zerbe, 1997). Social supports, daily exercise, personal time and space for reflection, a sense of humor, finding joy and purpose in the work, and personal faith enable the "wounded healer" to confront the exigencies of contemporary practice (Grosch and Olsen, 1994; Nouwen, 1972).

SUMMARY

Several controlled outcome studies of medically ill patients who received psychological treatment have found robust and striking medical, mental health, and longevity benefits. Although further research is necessary to clarify the precise psychosocial and organic factors involved, current studies show a marked decrease in overall medical costs among patients with certain diseases (e.g., breast cancer, melanoma, lymphoma, leukemia). It appears that appropriate pharmacotherapy and psychosocial treatment for the medically ill are cost-effective and inspire compliance with overall medical treatment. The opportunity to disclose a full range of feelings (e.g., anger, guilt) appears to have a positive impact on health and in many cases lengthens life.

The ways in which emotional expression and psychosocial support decrease the morbidity and mortality associated with medical illness are not well understood. However, there is good reason to believe that the neuroendocrine and immune systems are intimately involved. Psychosocial support via group therapy or individual therapy positively improves medical outcome by buffering the stress of social isolation and psychoneuroimmunologic response, possibly via glucocorticoids or a neuroendocrine effect on helper T-lymphocytes. Body maintenance activities recommended in this chapter (diet, sleep, exercise, creative expression) may also enhance immune and endocrine functioning. These activities definitely promote an overall feeling of well-being and engagement in the healing process.

In practical terms, women with medical illnesses who are helped to deal with "negative emotions" such as anger, fear, and depression tend to be better copers overall and to survive longer. Those who learn how to express anger appropriately—without blaming others, acting destructively, or becoming bitter—and who find at least one avenue for social affiliation and support face their illness more effectively. Their psychological fortitude permits them to hear even "bad news" as a challenge and not necessarily as a betrayal or a foreshadowing of their demise. They are able to live fully, and often creatively, even in the face of death, because they see themselves as whole. They are confident of their capacity to mourn what has been lost while taking full advantage of what life continues to give (Dreifuss-Kattan, 1990).

The woman who is medically ill needs a physician who understands the context of her life. Each situation is unique, but the patient is reassured when the physician asks open-ended questions about her fears, hopes, and what might hinder effective treatment. For example, some women delay life-saving surgery because of anxiety about their physical appearance. Acknowledging this realistic concern and referring the patient to an appropriate support group can go a long way toward ameliorating resistance to treatment and helping the patient feel heard.

Some mothers cannot take full advantage of health care opportunities because they worry about childcare. Clarifying local opportunities for this resource is as important as providing information about treatment choices. It encourages active patient involvement, blending the best aspects of technical science and psychological sensitivity to enhance the physician-patient interaction and personal autonomy.

Special effort must be made to eschew the tendency to make the patient feel guilty or remorseful about her condition. Some women have a tendency to blame themselves for their illness, the so-called "tyranny of positive attitude" mentality (Spiegel, 1990, 1993). Although the patient should be encouraged to do all she can to live fully and to "take control" of her treatment (e.g., to be autonomous), she should not be protected from recognizing the reality that she may die. Expressing a full range of emotions and learning to adapt to the sequelae of the illness are essential components of any comprehensive treatment plan.

Individual and group psychotherapies are appropriate avenues of support to disclose distress and find comfort. The full range of feelings that inevitably accompany an illness can be openly acknowledged. Group members help the patient to problem solve as she has the cathartic experience of relating her personal story. Decreasing her sense of isolation strengthens self-worth, defends against depression and demoralization, and aids the patient in creatively tackling her conscious and unconscious reactions to the diagnosis. The patient who learns to live fully and richly in spite of severe illness also imparts invaluable lessons about the value and meaning of life to her physicians.

Resources for the Patient

Brand P, Yancey P: *Pain: The Gift Nobody Wants*. New York, HarperCollins/Zondervan, 1993.
  Whether the patient has an acute or a chronic illness, is experiencing emotional or physical travail, or simply appears to be suffering from a languishing spirit in confronting daily life, this book teaches active techniques to increase endurance and mastery. By describing his experiences as a hand surgeon and leprosy specialist in the Third World, Dr. Paul Brand demonstrates how pain is actually both beneficial and lifesaving. While offering practical advice about the strategies that deintensify pain (e.g., distraction, meditation, prayer, concentration on projects or hobbies and productive work), Dr. Brand shows how patients are restored only when they have a renewed sense of "personal destiny over their bodies" (p. 225). These are the people who refuse to be victimized by their illness but see in each circumstance the daily challenge to live as fully as possible. This physician's half-century of practice treating the ravages of leprosy is humbling and inspiring. Allowing himself to be touched and taught when ministering to the suffering, he found that "each of our patients was acting out a lead role in a personal drama of recovery. Our mechanical rearrangement of muscles, tendons, and bones was but one step in rebuilding a damaged life" (p. 159). Every clinician and patient knows this intuitively, but the individual case examples provide a welcome reminder of how life can be reclaimed despite devastating circumstances. Stressing individual responsibility for making slow, wise changes in lifestyle, the authors document how healing and adaptation to illness is a job that the patient can—and must—do in order to survive and thrive. Those psychological "intensifiers

of pain—fear, anger, guilt, loneliness, and the tendency for most of us to feel victimized by reversals of fortune" (p. 262) must be met straight on. The felicitous bottom-line message of this straightforward book for clinicians working daily with the medically ill is this: Adversity, whether physiologic or psychological, can act as a transforming experience that increases overall well-being and happiness.

Meldin M: *The Tender Bud: A Physician's Journey Through Breast Cancer.* Hillsdale, NJ, Analytic Press, 1993.

The author is a senior psychiatrist who writes under a pseudonym about her personal journey in facing disease and the threat of death. In poignant detail, she retraces her path from the initial discovery of her cancer through surgeries and chemotherapy to her eventual return to everyday life and her clinical practice. She believes that in order to go on living fully, it is essential for the patient to "make peace" with the possibility of dying. Patients will find Dr. Meldin a sympathetic and appealing companion through their own journey as they, too, must try to gain hope, solace, and maturity to meet the challenges of reckoning with major illness. For this author, cancer has been a way to tackle her mortality head on and to arrive at a new joy in living daily, even in the face of suffering. For Meldin, the experience of living with cancer has "taught me a lesson in humility. . . . I had learned, in my very flesh, about my own mortality and that of other human beings. . . . I had discovered that we can get so immersed in our daily lives that we forget how precious life is. . . . All things, big and small, count, every smile and every tear. Simply to appreciate what is there now is what life is about. Simply to appreciate the riches in the temporal stream of our personal lives may be the deepest act of thanksgiving we can offer to the Giver of all Life" (pp. 202–203).

Price R: *A Whole New Life: An Illness and a Healing.* New York, Plume, 1994.

Reynolds Price, winner of the National Book Critics Circle Award for Fiction and professor of English at Duke University, recounts his agonizing battle and extraordinary recovery from cancer. This memoir is full of vignettes about the value of personal relationships and spiritual faith in overcoming the despair that must be surmounted when encountering any potentially life-threatening malady. There are plenty of practical suggestions about how to manage disease, withstand long-term rehabilitation, and endure a permanent disability, but Price is at his most eloquent when he exhorts others to "choose life" over death. Even in the most lamentable or pessimistic of circumstances, "down at the core, you [the patient] almost certainly want to live" (pp. 185–186). Patients will empathize—and sympathize—with Price's tale of his encounters with modern health care, laced as it is with well-intentioned but awkward professionals and the seemingly unending schedule of consultations, operations, and medical therapies. But the author also gives credit where credit is due. He minces no words in sharing his gratitude for the tenacious and compassionate care he received from physicians and nurses who did all in their power to help him survive. Interspersed are lessons for others about the merits of hypnosis, biofeedback, and alternative therapies in helping the patient endure physical agony and tap the deepest wellsprings of spirit, mind, and body. Most of all, Price believes that the ultimate "rescue from any despair" associated with illness lies in letting go of one's old self to develop "a whole new life" (p. 188). Thus Price stands firmly in the tradition of those who believe that good can come out of the most wrenching, frustrating, frightening life experience—including illness—if one is only willing to let go to learn the formidable lessons it has to teach.

Runowicz CD, Haupt D: *To Be Alive: A Woman's Guide to a Full Life After Cancer.* New York, Henry Holt, 1995.

Dr. Carolyn Runowicz is a breast cancer survivor. Although her book is written principally to help the cancer patient cope with a host of physical and psychological sequelae (e.g., need for follow-up care, cancer's effects on family life), it can also be read and appreciated by anyone dealing with a severe medical illness. For example, her chapters on managing stress and loneliness, diet and nutrition, and job and insurance discrimination are readily applicable to diseases other than cancer. Dr. Runowicz speaks with special authority to the survivor who must live with the continual specter of recurrence. She believes everyone must face down denial by having routine checkups, maintaining positive health practices, and developing a strategy "to gain control of our fears, and move on with life" (p. 200). She also deals straightforwardly with a woman's anxiety about physical and emotional changes brought on by disease (e.g., scars and attractiveness, effects on the patient's family, menopause, sex after cancer). Her sensitivity to the emotional side of physical illness leads her to recommend psychotherapy and pharmacotherapy when appropriate. A list of resources, including various support groups for specific problems and/or cancers (e.g., National Lymphedema Network, United Ostomy Association), is included in a comprehensive appendix.

Resources for Spouses and Family Members

Horowitz KE, Lanes DN: *Witness to Illness: Strategies of Caregiving and Coping.* Reading, MA, Addison-Wesley, 1992.

The majority of adults will eventually be called on to care for a loved one facing a significant illness; we must find consolation and accept useful strategies to be effective caregivers and advocates for those we hold most dear. This highly recommended resource reaches out to those who are often left behind to struggle with their questions and anxiety about how to be helpful and supportive without burning out. Emphasis is placed on helping the caregiver develop a capacity to self-nurture; even the most well-adjusted person must take time for self-replenishment and self-renewal when faced with the challenge of giving so much of one's self on a daily basis. In the context of numerous, poignant case vignettes, the authors tackle everything from hearing the initial diagnosis to the inevitable changes that occur in the family system. The pivotal importance of building a network of support and sharing the reward of caregiving with others so afflicted (e.g., going to a support group) is underscored. Chronic illness, acute illness, cancer, AIDS, heart disease, and rheumatologic illnesses are addressed. The authors emphasize the process of introspection and self-analysis for helping the caregiver (or "witness") deal with emotions such as frustration and anger. In their view, maintaining hope is as crucial to the caregiver as it is for the patient. Finding healthy and creative outlets for emotions, building a sustaining support network, and setting limits with others ("Do I really have to visit my mother in the nursing home every day?") are emphasized.

Resources for Clinicians

Druss RG: *The Psychology of Illness in Sickness and in Health.* Washington, DC, American Psychiatric Press, 1995.

Based on his years of practice as a psychoanalyst and consultation-liaison psychiatrist, Dr. Druss now reaches out to primary clinicians as well as mental health professionals to address the psychological tolls inherent in being medically ill and the various psychotherapy approaches that can be useful in recovery. This brief, beautifully written book deserves a place on every clinician's bookshelf. Topics include the courage patients must have when coping with chronic illness, the value of psychodynamic or cognitive-behavioral psychotherapy for those with a serious medical illness, the role of healthy denial in illness, and the value of self-care to promote restoration and well-being. Druss acknowledges that the scientific literature has failed to address the inner life of the patient, and this omission has imperiled physicians' appreciation of the essential personhood of the patient. By objectifying the individual, physicians miss opportunities to address the patient's underlying worries and preoccupations with illness (e.g., "Will anyone understand how betrayed I feel not to see my children grow up? Will anyone find me attractive after the amputation?"). He goes on to discuss how illness can conjure up many different psychological meanings, depending on the patient, and can be an avenue for self-discovery. Courage and optimism are essential in developing endurance and resiliency when facing illness or pain. According to Druss, people who have these attributes can navigate even the most harrowing experiences. They see them as opportunities for growth, not for surrender. To nurture this capacity for robustness, self-reliance, and exuberance, he believes that "medically sick patients need one place they can go and speak their minds about the disease, its care, and what it all means to them" (p. 57) (e.g., psychotherapy).

Gabbard GO, Lazar SG, Hornberger J, et al.: The economic impact of psychotherapy: a review. *Am J Psychiatry* 1997;154:147–155.

For clinicians interested in a thorough yet brief summary of the extant literature documenting the benefits of psychotherapy for the medically ill, either of these articles is ideal. The authors review the evidence that psychotherapy improves not just adjustment to medical illness but also actual survival time via the enhanced functioning of the endocrine and immune systems. They also document the cost-effectiveness of psychotherapy. Whether your purpose is to help your patient take advantage of group or individual therapy or to have a ready reference for managed care personnel when you suggest a referral, these articles will help you make your case.

Sapolsky RM: *Why Zebras Don't Get Ulcers: A Guide to Stress, Stress Related Diseases, and Coping.* New York, WH Freeman, 1994.

Most patients—and most physicians—can benefit from a primer on managing stress. This crossover text has a superb chapter on what is known and what is yet to be learned about how to flourish despite this modern malady. In lively prose, Sapolsky writes for a sophisticated lay and professional audience about the links between stress and depression, aging, reproduction, and disease. A research physiologist by training, he makes some clinical recommendations based on his immersion in the neuroscience of stress. These include finding sources of social affiliation and support and learning when to mobilize one's "healthy denial" when faced with terrible news. Once again, the importance of maintaining a sense of hopefulness or optimism appears to be corroborated by the most comprehensive of research studies, which the author describes with a rare blend of humor, personal anecdote, and scientifically accurate information.

Spiegel D: *Living Beyond Limits.* New York, Random House, 1993 (also New York, Ballantine Fawcett, 1994).

This book is based on the work of the author, a noted clinician-researcher, with breast cancer survivors. It describes psychosocial treatments that have been found to increase survival after the diagnosis of a serious illness. It is highly recommended for the clinician or patient who wants to learn more about strategies for enhancing quality of life and controlling pain, with an emphasis on "fortifying families" and "detoxifying death." Spiegel takes special issue with the "wish your illness away" pundits. Although he offers advice about how patients can improve their quality of life, particularly through group therapy or psychophysiologic modalities, he also believes that "the will of positive thinking" has made many patients feel guilty when they are facing death. No one "wills" himself or herself to get cancer; life is limited for everyone. Spiegel believes that death anxiety is best confronted by taking control of the time one has left, handling any unfinished business, and experiencing the refreshing "authenticity that comes from a confrontation with the fragility of life" (p. 154).

Spiegel D, Lazar SG: The need for psychotherapy in the medically ill. *Psychoanalytic Inquiry* 1997;154:45–50.

References

Appelbaum SA: The laying on of health: personality patterns of psychic healers. *Bull Menninger Clin* 1993;57:33–40.

Bartholome W: Are you still terminal? *Kansas University Medical School Bulletin* 1997;3:44.

Beckman HB, Frankel RM: The effect of physician behavior on the collection of data. *Ann Intern Med* 1984;101:692–696.

Borenstein DB: Does managed care permit appropriate use of psychotherapy? *Psychiatr Serv* 1996;47:971–974.

Breitbart W, Holland JC: *Psychiatric Aspects of Symptom Management in Cancer Patients.* Washington, DC, American Psychiatric Press, 1993.

Brand P, Yancey P: *Pain: The Gift Nobody Wants.* New York, HarperCollins/Zondervan, 1993.

Butler BA, Wing RR: Women with diabetes: A lifestyle perspective focusing on eating disorders, pregnancy, and weight control. In: Stanton AL, Gallant SJ (eds.): *The Psychology of Women's Health: Progress and Challenges in Research and Application,* pp. 85–116. Washington, DC, American Psychological Association, 1995.

Canoso JJ: *Rheumatology in Primary Care.* Philadelphia, Saunders, 1997.

Carlson KJ, Skochelak SE: What do women want in a doctor? Communication issues between women and physicians. In: Wallis LA (ed.): *Textbook of Women's Health,* pp. 33–38. Philadelphia, Lippincott-Raven, 1998.

Cohen S, Doyle WJ, Skoner DP, et al.: Social ties and susceptibility to the common cold. *JAMA* 1997;277:1940–1944.

Csikszentmihalyi M: *Flow: The Psychology of Optimal Experience.* New York, Harper, 1990/1991.

Derogatis L, Morrow G, Fetting J: The prevalence of psychiatric disorders among cancer patients. *JAMA* 1983;249:751–757.

Dreher H: The healing power of confession. *Natural Health* July/August 1992, pp. 74–80.

Dreifuss-Kattan E: *Cancer Stories: Creativity and Self-Repair.* Hillsdale, NJ, Analytic Press, 1990.

Druss RG: Psychotherapy of patients with serious intercurrent medical illness (cancer). *J Am Acad Psychoanal* 1986;14:459–472.

Druss RG: *The Psychology of Illness in Sickness and in Health.* Washington, DC, American Psychiatric Press, 1995.

Fawzy FI, Fawzy NW, Hyun CS, et al.: Malignant melanoma: effects of an early structured psychiatric intervention, coping, and affective states on recurrence and survival six years later. *Arch Gen Psychiatry* 1993;50:681–689.

Fawzy FI, Kemeny ME, Fawzy NW, et al.: A structured psychiatric intervention for cancer patients: II. Changes over time in immunological measures. *Arch Gen Psychiatry* 1990;47:729–735.

Francis ME, Pennebaker JF: Putting stress into words: The impact of writing on physiological, absentee, and self-reported emotional well-being measures. *Am J Health Promotion* 1992;6:280–287.

Frankenhaeuser M: A biopsychosocial approach to stress in women and men. In: Adesso VJ, Reddy DM, Fleming R (eds.): *Psychological Perspectives on Women's Health,* pp. 39–56. Washington, DC, Taylor & Francis, 1994.

Fuller NS, Morrison RE: Chronic fatigue syndrome: helping patients cope with this enigmatic illness. *Postgrad Med* 1998;103:175–184.

Gabbard GO, Lazar SG, Hornberger J, et al.: The economic impact of psychotherapy: a review. *Am J Psychiatry* 1997;154:147–155.

Glassman AH, Shapiro PA: Depression and the course of coronary artery disease. *Am J Psychiatry* 1998;155:4–11.

Goldberg M: An old man's story. *Pharos* 1997;60;28–29.

Goldstein MG, Niaura R: Cardiovascular disease: Part I. Coronary artery disease and sudden death. In: Stoudemire A (ed.): *Psychological Factors Affecting Medical Conditions,* pp. 19–37. Washington, DC, American Psychiatric Press, 1995.

Green E, Green A: *Beyond Biofeedback.* Fort Wayne, IN, Knoll, 1977/1989.

Grosh WN, Olsen DC: *When Healing Starts to Hurt: A New Look at Burnout Among Psychotherapists.* New York, Norton, 1994.

Gullette ECD, Blumenthal JA, Babyak M, et al.: Effects of mental stress on myocardial ischemia during daily life. *JAMA* 1997;277:1521–1526.

Hensley ML, Reichman BS: Women-specific problems with chemotherapy. In: Wallis LA (ed.): *Textbook of Women's Health,* pp. 505–514. Philadelphia, Lippincott-Raven, 1998.

Hiroto D, Seligman M: Generality of learned helplessness in man. *J Pers Soc Psychol* 1975;31:311–327.

Horn S: *Concrete Confidence: A 30-Day Program for an Unshakable Foundation of Self-Assurance.* New York, St. Martin's Press, 1997.

Horowitz KE, Lanes DN: *Witness to Illness: Strategies of Caregiving and Coping.* Reading, MA, Addison-Wesley, 1993.

Kash KM, Breitbart W: The stress of caring for cancer patients. In: Breitbart W, Holland JC (eds.): *Psychiatric Aspects of Symptom Management in Cancer Patients*, pp. 243–260. Washington, DC, American Psychiatric Press, 1993.

Katzelnick DJ, Kobak KA, Greist JH, et al.: Effect of primary care treatment of depression on service use by patients with high medical expenditures. *Psychiatr Serv* 1997;48:59–64.

Komaroff AL: A 56-year-old woman with chronic fatigue syndrome. *JAMA* 1997;278:1179–1185.

Lamberg L: Treating depression in medical conditions may improve quality of life. *JAMA* 1996;275:857–858.

Levin RW, Janes RG, Pearson MR, et al.: Prinzmetal's angina and emotions: a neglected psychosomatic entity. *Bull Menninger Clin* 1998;62:96–111.

Lorde A: *The Cancer Journals.* San Francisco, Spinsters Ink, 1980.

Meyerowitz BE, Hart S: Women and cancer: Have assumptions about women limited our research agenda? In: Stanton AJ, Gallant SJ (eds.): *The Psychology of Women's Health*, pp. 51–84. Washington DC, American Psychological Association, 1995.

Meldin M: *The Tender Bud: A Physician's Journey Through Breast Cancer.* Hillsdale, NJ, Analytic Press, 1993.

Moorey S: Adjuvant psychological therapy: A cognitive-behaviour therapy for cancer. In: ten-Have-de Labije J, Balner H (eds.): *Coping with Cancer and Beyond: Cancer Treatment and Mental Health*, pp. 55–63. Amsterdam, Netherlands, Swets & Zeitlinger, 1991.

Niaura R, Goldstein MG: Cardiovascular disease: Part II. Coronary artery disease and sudden death and hypertension. In: Stoudemire A (ed.): *Psychological Factors Affecting Medical Conditions*, pp. 39–56. Washington, DC, American Psychiatric Press, 1995.

Nouwen HJ: *The Wounded Healer.* Garden City, NY, Doubleday, 1972.

Ott P, Levy SM: Cancer in women. In: Adesso VJ, Reddy DM, Fleming R (eds.): *Psychological Perspectives on Women's Health*, pp. 83–96. Washington, DC, Taylor & Francis, 1994.

Parks P: Psychophysiologic self-awareness training: The integration of scientific and humanistic principles. *Journal of Humanistic Psychology* 1997;37:67–113.

Pennebaker J: *Opening Up: The Healing Power of Confiding in Others.* New York, Avon, 1991.

Pennebaker JW: Writing about emotional experiences as a therapeutic process. *Psychological Science* 1997;8:162–166.

Pennebaker JW, Beall SK: Confronting a traumatic event: toward an understanding of inhibition and disease. *J Abnorm Psychol* 1986;95:274–281.

Powers PS, Maher M, Helm MD, et al.: Impact of a disaster on a burn unit. *Psychosomatics* 1986;27:553–557,561.

Price R: *A Whole New Life: An Illness and a Healing.* New York, Plume, 1994.

Roose SP, Laghrissi-Thode F, Kennedy J, et al.: Comparison of paroxetine and nortriptyline in depressed patients with ischemic heart disease. *JAMA* 1998;279:287–291.

Rubenfeld I: Beginner's hands: twenty-five years of simple Rubenfeld synergy—the birth of a therapy. *Somatics* Spring/Summer 1988; pp. 3–8.

Runowicz CD, Haupt D: *To Be Alive: A Woman's Guide to a Full Life After Cancer.* New York, Henry Holt, 1995.

Sapolsky RM: *Why Zebras Don't Get Ulcers: A Guide to Stress, Stress Related Diseases, and Coping.* New York, WH Freeman, 1994.

Seligman M: *Learned Optimism.* New York, Knopf, 1991.

Severino S: Body image changes in hemodialysis and renal transplant. *Psychosomatics* 1980;21:509–510.

Shumaker SA, Smith TR: Women and coronary heart disease: a psychological perspective. In: Stanton AL, Gallant SJ (eds.): *The Psychology of Women's Health: Progress and Challenges in Research and Application*, pp. 25–49. Washington, DC, American Psychological Association, 1995.

Silverstein B, Blumenthal E: Depression mixed with anxiety, somatization, and disordered eating: relationship with gender-role-related limitations experienced by females. *Sex Roles* 1997;36:709–724.

Simon R: Listening hands: an interview with Ilana Rubenfeld. *Family Therapy Networker* 1997;21:62–73.

Spiegel D: Can psychotherapy prolong cancer survival? *Psychosomatics* 1990;31:361–366.

Spiegel D: Effects of group support for metastatic breast cancer patients on coping, mood, pain, and survival. In: ten-Have-de Labije J, Balner H (eds.): *Coping with Cancer and Beyond: Cancer Treatment and Mental Health*, pp. 11–29. Amsterdam, Netherlands, Swets & Zeitlinger, 1991.

Spiegel D: *Living Beyond Limits*. New York, Random House, 1993 (also New York, Ballantine/ Fawcett, 1994).

Spiegel D: Essentials of psychotherapeutic intervention for cancer patients. *Support Care Cancer* 1995;3:252–256.

Spiegel D, Bloom JR, Kraemer HC, et al.: Effect of psychosocial treatment on survival of patients with metastatic breast cancer. *Lancet* 1989;2:888–891. [Reprinted in: Steptoe A, Wardle J (eds.): *Psychosocial Processes and Health: A Reader,* pp. 456–477. Cambridge, England, Cambridge University Press, 1995.]

Spiegel D, Bloom JR, Yalom ID: Group support for patients with metastatic cancer: a randomized prospective outcome study. *Arch Gen Psychiatry* 1981;38:527–533.

Spiegel D, Kato PM: Psychosocial influences on cancer incidence and progression. *Harv Rev Psychiatry* 1996;4:10–26.

Spiegel D, Kraemer H, Gottheil E: Effect of psychosocial treatment on survival of patients with metastatic breast cancer. *Lancet* 1989;2:888–891.

Spiegel D, Lazar SG: The need for psychotherapy in the medically ill. *Psychoanalytic Inquiry* 1997;17(Suppl):45–50.

Steptoe A, Wardle J (eds.): *Psychosocial Processes and Health: A Reader*. Cambridge, MA, Cambridge University Press, 1994.

Stoudemire A (ed.): *Psychological Factors Affecting Medical Conditions*. Washington, DC, American Psychiatric Press, 1995.

Surbone A, Zwitter M (eds.): *Communication with the Cancer Patient: Information and Truth*. New York, New York Academy of Sciences, 1997.

Temoshok L, Dreher H: Recognizing and changing Type C behaviour. In: ten-Have-de Labije J, Balner H (eds.): *Coping with Cancer and Beyond: Cancer Treatment and Mental Health*, pp. 81–102. Amsterdam, Netherlands, Swets & Zeitlinger, 1991.

Verbosky LA, Franco KN, Zrull JP: The relationship between depression and length of stay in the general hospital patient. *J Clin Psychiatry* 1993;54:177–181.

Weidner G: Coronary risk in women. In: Adesso VJ, Reddy DM, Fleming R (eds.): *Psychological Perspectives on Women's Health*, pp. 57–81. Washington, DC, Taylor & Francis, 1994.

Zerbe K: *The Body Betrayed: Women, Eating Disorders, and Treatment*. Washington, DC, American Psychiatric Press, 1993. (*The Body Betrayed: A Deeper Understanding of Women, Eating Disorders, and Treatment*. Carlsbad, CA, Gürze Books, 1995).

Zerbe K: [Book review of Druss R: *The Psychology of Illness in Sickness and in Health*.] *Bull Menninger Clin* 1997;61:269–271.

Chapter 11

Menstruation, Pregnancy, and Menopause

The psychological similarities between women and men far exceed the differences. By and large, both sexes strive to lead emotionally satisfying and physically healthy lives. A stable home life, fulfilling career, meaningful friendships, and opportunities for fun and "letting go" are sought-after goals, regardless of gender, culture, or socioeconomic status. Although some psychiatric syndromes occur with greater frequency and tenacity in females (e.g., anxiety, depression), almost every disorder discussed in this text can also beset a man (e.g., bereavement, traumatic stress and violence, eating disorders). Clearly, psychiatric problems are not a province of one sex.

In the future, mental health professionals may be able to employ lessons learned about gender differences to help men and women overcome an emotional or a relationship difficulty, prescribe psychotropic medication based on gender-specific findings, or use particular psychotherapeutic techniques in such a way as to take biologic sex into account. For the most part, this cannot be done as yet because theoretical knowledge has outpaced therapeutic application.

This chapter discusses the one area that is unique and distinct to women—the capacity to bear children. There are several times in a woman's life, notably when substantial hormonal changes occur, that emotional disorders are observed at a particularly high rate. Adolescence, young adulthood, the postpartum period, and menopause are associated with an amalgam of symptoms, most notably anxiety and depression. The mechanisms by which gonadal hormones participate in the pathobiology of reproduction-related syndromes have yet to be determined. Effective treatments have outpaced our understanding of the causes of these disorders and the interplay between cultural, biologic, and psychological factors. Most likely, a complex interaction of hormonal, neurotransmitter, and psychosocial disruptions comes into play in the development of a particular woman's difficulty.

All women have basically similar hormonal changes when these life cycle events occur. Medical science has yet to solve the mystery of why some women develop mood, cognition, or behavioral problems and others do not. An increasing number of treatment options are available for women who have emotional difficulties associated with reproductive functioning; these range from hormonal supplements to the selective serotonin reuptake inhibitors (SSRIs) and environmental manipulations (shifts in lifestyle, stress reduction), depending on the particular problem and symptom complex.

This chapter describes the most commonly encountered problems in a primary care practice—premenstrual syndrome (PMS), postpartum depression and anxiety disorders, and menopause-related dysphoria. After a brief review of the major psychiatric aspects of each, clinical management options are emphasized and suggestions are made as to when more intensive mental health consultation is warranted. Also described are some of the psychological consequences of spontaneous and planned abortions. Because many women take psychotropic drugs during their reproductive years, the general safety of these drugs in regard to the fetus and lactation is briefly reviewed.

Although some generalizations can be made about psychiatric treatment in these areas, each woman is an individual with a unique personal history, social situation, and psychobiologic matrix. Treatment must be individualized, in part because it empowers the patient to make her own decisions and to become a partner with you in her care. Psychiatric consultation is especially encouraged in the area of reproduction-related syndromes, because the number of available therapies is rapidly expanding. The risks and benefits must be carefully considered for both mother and child, but comprehensive intervention may stop the pernicious effects on the patient and her loved ones.

MENSTRUATION

Approach to the Patient with Premenstrual Syndrome

The term PMS refers to significant distress and impairment of normal functioning during the luteal phase of the menstrual cycle (Block et al., 1997; Brown, 1997; Steiner and Wilkins, 1996; Yonkers, 1997; Yonkers et al., 1997) (Table 11–1). Hormone treatment (e.g., progesterone, contraceptive pills) was widely used in the past, on both empirical and theoretical grounds. But PMS does not appear to be caused by a disturbance of reproductive or endocrine function, and the notion that PMS results from simple hormone excess or deficiency has been abandoned. Research reveals that PMS mood disorders occur within the context

---

Table 11–1. **Symptoms of Premenstrual Syndrome**

Affective symptoms

Anxiety and tension
Irritability
Mood lability (anger outbursts, oversensitivity, crying spells)
Social withdrawal
Difficulty concentrating and forgetfulness

Somatic symptoms

Breast tenderness
Abdominal bloating
Swollen extremities
Fatigue
Headache
Carbohydrate craving

Table 11–2. **Summary of Pharmacologic Approaches to Premenstrual Syndrome**

Treatment Modality	Effect
Tricyclic antidepressants	Generally unhelpful unless serotonin reuptake is blocked (i.e., clomipramine); other agents have lower than expected placebo response
SSRIs (e.g., fluoxetine, sertraline, paroxetine)	Effective in 50%–75% of women
Venlafaxine, Nefazodone	Highly effective in studies to date, but more trials are needed
Alprazolam	Significantly more effective than placebo, but has the potential of causing addiction and physical dependence; in 25% of women who do not respond to SSRIs, alprazolam is an option
Gonadotropin-releasing hormone agonists	Helpful to patients with severe symptoms and those who do not improve with or cannot tolerate SSRIs; because of increased risk of osteoporosis, consider a regimen that includes estrogen-progestin replacement to protect against bone loss if these agents are used

of normal rather than dysregulated endocrine function and that other biologic factors probably explain why some women experience mood changes in association with overtly normal reproductive endocrine functioning (Block and Schmidt, 1997; Freeman et al., 1995; Severino, 1993; Severino et al., 1989) (Table 11–2).

Only 3% to 8% of women of reproductive age have dysphoric PMS severe enough to warrant treatment (Brown, 1996a, 1997; Gold, 1997; Munjiza and Ljubomirovic, 1997). Although a myriad of genetic and biologic abnormalities have been implicated in the cause of PMS, learned attitudes undoubtedly contribute to the reporting and experiencing of the syndrome (Block, 1997; Klebanov and Ruble, 1994; Koeske, 1987). However, the demonstration that SSRIs specifically, rapidly, and powerfully relieve severe PMS symptoms in most patients underscores the biologic reality of this condition (Brown, 1996b; Freeman et al., 1996; Steiner et al., 1995; Wood et al., 1992). Women who do not respond to this treatment may respond to alprazolam or to psychosocial intervention (Harrison et al., 1990; Smith et al., 1987; Yonkers and Brown, 1996).

The effectiveness of the SSRIs—in contrast to nonserotonin antidepressants—suggests that increasing the amount of serotonin at the synapse is a mechanism of action. In a number of carefully conducted studies, hundreds of women in different countries have benefited from SSRIs, with almost immediate relief of PMS symptoms (Erickson et al., 1997; Gold, 1994; Rubinow and Schmidt, 1995; Stotland and Harwood, 1994). Mood, behavioral, and somatic symptoms are best relieved consistently with SSRIs but not with tricyclic antidepressants or monoamine oxidase inhibitors.

Many women with PMS never receive effective treatment, in part because of the long-standing societal notion that menstruation is "bad" or "evil," as indicated by references to it as "the curse" or "falling off the roof," and because physicians do not view PMS as a bona fide medical disorder warranting treatment. Certainly, the fact that cultures that hold negative beliefs about menstruation has a negative impact on a woman's experience of her symptoms (Klebanov and Ruble, 1994; Koeske, 1987) and contributes to her reluctance to seek help. A woman's psychological expectations about menstrual cycle symptoms probably also play a key role in what she anticipates about her own period. In the now classic study of 44 Princeton undergraduates, premenstrual symptoms of pain, water retention, and eating habit changes were reported when the investigator suggested to the women that they were in a premenstrual phase (1 to 2 days before their periods), when in fact they were intermenstrual (due in 7 to 10 days) (Ruble, 1977). For many women, their own beliefs about discomfort and debilitation play an important role in how they experience premenstrual symptoms.

A statistical association has been reported between PMS and some other hormone-related disorders, including postpartum depression, adverse emotional effects of some contraceptive medications, and dysphoric mood during sequential hormone replacement therapy (HRT). Dysphoric PMS has been associated with major depressive disorder and seasonal affective disorder (SAD) (see Chapter 2). It appears that women with PMS may be particularly vulnerable to depressive episodes over their life cycle; 25% of depressed women are vulnerable to premenstrual exacerbation of depression, anxiety, irritability, and fatigue. Alternatively, the primary care clinician should be aware that PMS can be experienced for the first time after the patient has a baby, particularly if she develops bona fide postpartum depression.

With respect to treatment, ovarian suppression (e.g., with gonadotropin-releasing hormone agonists) has been effective for PMS (Mortola et al., 1991), but the cost is high and the treatment has not yet been recognized as standard medical practice by most third-party payers. Because PMS has been assumed to be caused by an excess or a deficit of one or more ovarian hormones, clinical trials have evaluated the use of progesterone, synthetic progestin, and oral contraceptive agents. In most of these studies, the treatments were not found to be effective. Likewise, trials of lithium carbonate, diuretics, vitamins, and tricyclic antidepressants have given mixed or disappointing results (Kravitz, 1998; Yonkers et al., 1997).

In contrast, a number of newer antidepressants have led to substantial improvements over placebo: the 5-HT reuptake inhibitors clomipramine, fluoxetine, paroxetine, sertraline; the reuptake and serotonin (5-HT 2) antagonist nefazodone; the 5-HT agonist fenfluramine; and the dual reuptake inhibitor venlafaxine (Freeman, 1998; Klein-Stern, 1998; Rickels et al., 1990; Stone et al., 1991) (see Table 11–2). Most of these trials have evaluated treatment for only a few cycles; controlled, definitive, long-term studies are lacking.

PMS is an intermittent disorder that may respond to unique dosing patterns, such as treatment limited to the luteal phase. If luteal phase treatment proves equivalent to continuous treatment, women may be spared the side effects and costs associated with continuous dosing. Not all agents may be effective in luteal phase dosing; moreover, it may be only a small subgroup of women who experience symptomatic improvement with intermittent administration. Future studies are needed to test which subpopulations can benefit from continuous or intermittent therapy (Gold, 1997; Harrison et al., 1990).

These psychotropic agents have largely relegated oophorectomy to the past, although suppression of ovulation by medication may be the only option in some severe cases. With respect to SSRIs, it is still not known how long treatment should continue, nor is it firmly established that treatment beyond 6 months remains beneficial. Because women with PMS typically are young and potentially fertile, the risks and benefits of long-term psychotropic management must be weighed. At this point, primary care clinicians who target the serotonin system with one of the newer antidepressants are practicing the most conservative but also state-of-the-art care.

What is the Role for Nonpharmacologic Treatment of PMS?

Although nonpharmacologic treatments have been less systematically studied than medications, lifestyle modifications and psychotherapy have proved helpful in some subgroups (Table 11–3) (Pearlstein, 1996; Rivera-Tovar et al., 1994). Moreover, many women prefer dietary modifications, vitamin or herbal remedies, and exercise to pharmacologic therapy. Some women with strong feelings that the pharmaceutical industry advocates for medicinal remedies for fiduciary reasons turn to alternative healing methods to control their symptoms (Astin, 1998; Doress-Worters and Siegal, 1994).

Nonpharmacologic treatments of PMS have centered on (1) dietary modifications, (2) exercise, (3) over-the-counter dietary and vitamin supplements, (4) biofeedback and/or relaxation therapy, and (5) group and individual psychotherapy (Severino and Gold 1994; Yonkers and Brown, 1996; Yonkers et al., 1997). Each of these modalities may benefit a particular woman or subgroup of women. An individualized treatment program that meets the needs of each patient is essential. Because women in general tend to associate their periods with negative images, physicians can begin by challenging these stereotypes. "Premenstrual tension" can be reframed to include a fuller appreciation of one's power and wisdom as a woman with the capacity to bear new life and engage in other life-affirming activities. In this way, a woman may begin to experience her body not as "a burden or a nuisance" and realize "that negative moods and behaviors are not inevitable during the premenstrum" (Koeske, 1987, p. 143).

Table 11–3. **Nonpharmacologic Approaches to Premenstrual Syndrome**

High-carbohydrate diet and beverages
Exercise
Good sleep hygiene (see Chapter 7)
Group or individual psychotherapy
Biofeedback, relaxation training
Cognitive-behavioral therapy (e.g., anger/anxiety management)
Reframe negative images of menstruation into positive ones about one's body as
    powerful, helpful, wise, womanly
Encourage efficacy and self-understanding

Is There Anything to Recommend for Premenstrual Food Cravings?

As many women avow, premenstrual food cravings are very real. Consumption of additional carbohydrates improves the mood of some women with PMS, supposedly by increasing dietary tryptophan. The suspected mechanism is that serotonin synthesis is also increased. This mechanism may account for increased appetite and carbohydrate cravings in a variety of disorders, including depression, SAD, bulimia, smoking withdrawal, and PMS.

By eating more sweets (carbohydrate-rich foods), women may be replenishing the brain serotonin, which can become depleted during the luteal phase. In a sense, homeostasis is restored when the woman increases her carbohydrate intake. The physician may wish to recommend a carbohydrate-rich beverage (available over the counter) that is being studied specifically in women with PMS. Controlled studies are still needed to confirm the benefits of specific dietary recommendations, but primary care clinicians can safely urge a trial-and-error approach of increased carbohydrate consumption in women with PMS.

What Is the Role of Exercise and Psychotherapy in Treatment of PMS?

Increased exercise has been found to lessen fluid retention, breast discomfort, and premenstrual depression. Although aerobic exercise and strength training are in general beneficial to women's health, you may want to emphasize their value in improving mood states and lowering physical symptoms across all menstrual cycle phases. Cognitive behavioral techniques, including anger and anxiety management and targeting of negative cognitions, have also benefited some women in controlled trials. Relaxation training appears to be a useful addition to a comprehensive treatment package for premenstrual symptoms. Psychosocial treatments may be all that is necessary for some patients, but most women with significant PMS symptoms are likely to need adjunctive treatment (i.e., pharmacotherapy).

Patient Guidelines for Coping with Premenstrual Syndrome

1. Premenstrual syndrome (PMS) is characterized by tension, irritability, and moodiness that begin a few days before menstruation and end a few days after its onset. Depression, headache, craving for carbohydrate foods, work impairment, and physical discomfort (e.g., fatigue, breast tenderness) also occur in a significant proportion of women. Although the exact cause of PMS remains unknown, there is increasing evidence that the neurotransmitter serotonin plays a role. Women with PMS have normal circulating estrogen and progesterone, but for unknown reasons they appear to also be hypersensitive to changes in the concentration of those hormones.
2. Learn as much as you can about the biology of PMS. For many years, PMS and its more severe cousin, premenstrual dysphoria disorder (PMDD), have been controversial subjects. Some feminists, including physicians, believe that a diagnosis of PMS or PMDD pathologizes menstruation and stigmatizes

women. However, there is increasing evidence that 5% to 10% of women have significant PMS or PMDD, and for them cyclic changes associated with the menstrual cycle present a real problem.

3. If you have a mild form of PMS, it may be sufficient for you to make dietary changes, to exercise, and to practice relaxation therapy. For more severe forms of PMS, the new serotonin reuptake inhibitors (SSRIs) have been found to be highly effective.

4. If your doctor recommends a trial of an SSRI (e.g., fluoxetine, sertraline, paroxetine), you can expect a rapid onset of action. In the treatment of depression, SSRIs usually take several weeks to be effective. In contrast, PMS improves with an SSRI within a matter of days. This quick response time gives additional proof that the condition is biologic in origin. Furthermore, as many as 90% of women with even the most severe forms of PMS improve with one of the drugs that enhances serotonin activity.

5. In addition to taking any prescribed medication, make use of available psychosocial supports (e.g., group or individual therapy, daily exercise, adequate diet, moderate or no alcohol use), which have also been shown to be helpful to women with PMS. These activities can help you change any negative images you have about menstruation and can help you reconceive thoughts about your body, even during the premenstrual time, as you consider yourself as being wise, strong, and capable (Koeske, 1987; Northrup, 1994/1998).

Additional Guidelines for Primary Care Clinicians

1. Institute a trial of treatment with one of the SSRIs (see Table 11–2), which usually are highly effective. Also, encourage the patient to take advantage of psychosocial supports and to practice positive health care measures (see Table 11–3).

2. A diet high in carbohydrates may help alleviate PMS symptoms because it provides additional amounts of the amino acid tryptophan, which makes serotonin. Fenfluramine, a drug that is not an SSRI, powerfully stimulates production of serotonin. Both a high-carbohydrate diet and fenfluramine reduce symptoms in many cases; a trial of a high-carbohydrate diet or an over-the-counter carbohydrate beverage can be conservatively recommended.

3. Other medications used for premenstrual disorder include venlafaxine (25 mg twice daily to start; increase by 25 to 37.5 mg/day until remission is achieved or to a maximum of 450 mg/day); nefazodone (200 to 500 mg daily), and buspirone (10 to 20 mg two or three times daily) or alprazolam (0.25 mg two or three times daily). Consider their use in patients who do not improve with an SSRI or psychosocial supports.

4. If the patient prefers to avoid pharmacologic strategies altogether, recommend dietary changes, increased exercise, and relaxation training. Cognitive-behavioral modalities have also been used successfully in some patients. A meal high in complex carbohydrates theoretically enhances cerebral uptake of tryptophan, making more serotonin available. More frequent meals high in complex carbohydrates are effective in many patients.

5. Pharmacologic dosage and timing must be individualized. It is not yet clear whether medication should be given at the onset of symptoms, during the premenstrual week, or for longer periods (i.e., continuous treatment over the month and year).

6. Be aware of the phenomenon of premenstrual magnification in those women who meet the criteria for PMS or PMDD and have a current major psychiatric disorder or unstable medical condition. Their psychiatric difficulties (e.g., depression) typically worsen premenstrually. This situation frequently calls for referral to a psychiatrist for additional assessment, pharmacologic management, and psychotherapy.

PREGNANCY

Psychological Consequences of Abortion

Both spontaneous abortion (i.e., miscarriage) and planned abortion have psychological significance to women. How a woman is affected by an interrupted pregnancy depends on her conscious and unconscious wishes to give birth, her past and current relationships, and the support (or lack of support) that she receives from her immediate environment. Psychoanalysis and long-term psychodynamic psychotherapy of women have demonstrated by the case study method that everyone's response is unique; some are able to move on, seemingly untouched by the loss, whereas others have a prolonged period of grief and unresolved mourning (Eigen, 1997; Pines, 1994; Stotland, 1998a, 1998b). This anecdotal evidence has been corroborated by studies examining the psychological consequences associated with recurrent spontaneous abortion and pregnancy loss (Janssen et al., 1996; Klock et al., 1997). The majority of women who experience an abortion or a pregnancy loss are almost never referred, nor do they seek psychiatric care. These studies of volunteers who filled out questionnaires and other psychological instruments confirmed the anxiety, grief, sadness, self-blame, anger, diminished libido, poor sleep quality, and general lack of well-being in a significant proportion of an otherwise healthy group of women. For example, in a study of 100 women at the Recurrent Miscarriage Clinic at Brigham and Women's Hospital in Boston, 32% of those who completed a questionnaire had significant depression; they also reported acute and chronic anxiety, sleep alterations, and impairments of appetite and libido (Klock et al., 1997).

Part of the reason for distress is the early attachment women have to their babies, which begins long before birth. Women begin to note changes in their bodies and establish a relationship to the fetus very early. Psychoanalytic psychotherapy and psychoanalysis with pregnant women demonstrate how, even in the first trimester, women begin to have fantasies and dreams about their baby. In a sense, the child is a psychological reality long before it is a physical actuality.

For women who very much want to have a child, miscarriage in particular can be an excruciating loss. If they do not have an opportunity to grieve the loss, unresolved mourning sets in with the possibility of depression, physical illness, and numerous other consequences to the quality of life of the patient and her loved ones (see Chapter 9). In cases of both spontaneous and planned abortions, the primary care clinician must remain vigilant for emotional reactions that may not be readily apparent.

For example, Stotland (1998b) described a woman who had two miscarriages during psychoanalysis. The patient and her husband very much wanted a child and were demoralized by the events. At the beginning of the treatment, the analyst was not aware that the patient had had an abortion 10 years previously;

it had not been one of the patient's psychological concerns during the initial interviews. Because the analyst was decidedly "pro-choice," she acknowledged that she would "not necessarily have identified the abortion as a potential problem even if the patient had revealed it" (p. 967). Psychoanalytic treatment provided a safe haven for the patient to investigate a number of conflicts related to her personal life and inhibitions in the workplace. She also uncovered that she was still troubled by her decision to have an abortion in her late teens. Stotland suggests that the unconscious guilt, shame, and anger the patient harbored for many years about the abortion was one factor that may have contributed to her inability to experience contentment and to give birth even though she now had a loving and supportive partner and social support she did not have as a teen.

Other emotional conflicts that interfered with the patient's sense of self-worth were revealed in the psychoanalytic treatment, but the opportunity the patient had to struggle with the meaning of and feelings about her abortion appeared to be particularly salutary. As Stotland wrote, "A single case such as this is a vehicle to illustrate the psychological consequences of abortion [which demonstrate] a woman's authentic, multilayered emotional experience" (p. 967). Whatever one's personal beliefs about the legal and medical issues surrounding abortion, physicians must recognize that it can be "experienced by that woman as both the mastery of a difficult life situation and as the loss of a potential life" (p. 967). It behooves the primary care clinician to be aware that feelings about spontaneous or planned abortion may not be readily apparent. The patient may uncover them only in an extended psychotherapy or psychoanalytic process, or they may be triggered by a story the patient hears, reads, or sees on television.

Medical history demonstrates that abortion is far from a late 20th-century trend to deal with problem pregnancy but has ancient roots (Bilge, 1998; Cosmar, 1998; Riddle, 1997). For at least two millennia, women have used herbal remedies and other abortifacients to curtail pregnancy. These ancient and contemporary methods reflect a woman's desire to take control of her body; the decision to terminate pregnancy is then understood "as the least destructive alternative to bad situations" (Stotland, 1998b, p. 967).

Although the majority of women recover from pregnancy loss without psychiatric treatment or overt psychological difficulties in about 1 year, they are nonetheless more likely to suffer from submerged depression or anxiety and to have a tendency to somatize than those who give birth to living babies (Janssen et al., 1996). What can be learned from these more global psychological research inventories does not capture the unique history or inner life of the patient in your office, who may not readily admit or even be aware of the residual effects of an interrupted pregnancy. The primary care clinician should therefore be vigilant about the often unspoken but far-reaching consequences of spontaneous or planned abortion in the life of an individual patient.

Approach to the Patient with Postpartum Depression and Anxiety

Many primary care clinicians are unaware that pregnancy and the postpartum period are high-risk times for psychiatric illness (Sharp, 1996). During and immediately after pregnancy, the clinician must be vigilant about emotional symptoms in the patient that might be taken for granted or considered "normal." The emotional disturbances during the puerperium occur on a continuum, with about 50% of women experiencing transient and mild "postpartum blues" and 10% suffering full-blown depression. Postpartum depression is associated with infanticide and suicide, making early psychiatric intervention essential (Lenhart and Bernstein, 1993). Because of this potential for substantial morbidity and even mortality, most attention has been paid to the onset and treatment of postpartum depression, but postpartum psychosis and postpartum anxiety disorders can be very serious illnesses as well (Kendell et al., 1987; McNeil et al., 1989; Sichel et al., 1993a, 1993b). Research has revealed that the months surrounding birth are the time at which women face their greatest lifetime risk for development of a mental illness (Kendell et al., 1987; Robinson and Stewart, 1993).

Postpartum blues occur in about 50% of women, with onset at 3 to 7 days after birth; postpartum depression occurs in about 10% to 15% of mothers in the first 6 months. Both postpartum blues and postpartum depression are believed to be hormonally driven, although psychosocial stressors play a factor. Any stressor in a woman's life that occurs at about the time of birth increases the risk of postpartum illness, particularly affective illness (Righetti-Veltema et al., 1998; Sharp, 1996). A subgroup of patients who experience severe affective symptoms quickly after delivery were previously well or only mildly depressed.

Mothers who become psychiatrically disturbed after the birth of a child may have no history of an emotional disorder. Usually, there are few prior psychosocial triggers and no affective warning signs. Soon after delivery, the patient may begin to tell you that she feels odd or peculiar. Her sleep habits may change; she may become restless and anxious; she may become observably tearful, confused, agitated, or listless. To some degree, these symptoms are common in many women who do not develop full-blown postpartum depression or postpartum anxiety. But because of the toll that untreated illness takes on the developing mother-child bond, clinicians must be alert to early manifestations of postpartum illness. Major depression, bipolar disorder, psychosis, and bona fide anxiety disorder may appear for the first time after the birth of the baby (Brockington, 1992; Sharp, 1996).

Primary care clinicians who treat the entire family must also be aware of the possibility of depression in the postpartum period in fathers as well as in mothers. These men, who commonly have a history of depression themselves, are unable to provide support or to be emotionally available to the baby or the new mother (Areias et al., 1996). The effects of parenthood on men with major mental illness are not well understood; nevertheless, they usually value their children and derive great happiness from them. The primary care clinician should understand that both mothers and fathers have reactions to pregnancy and parenting and make efforts to help both in their new roles. Education about child rearing, respite care, early intervention programs, psychotherapy and psychopharmacy, and adequate housing and financial help may be key supports in helping the new parents to cope and adapt. In many cases, the father's role is to buffer the mother's depressive or anxious reactions (Apfel and Handel, 1993). Contemporary psychiatry and psychoanalysis are placing more emphasis on the importance of fathers in the development of children and the role they play in sustaining the mother. Their healthy functioning becomes even more important when the mothers are incapacitated by a physical or emotional problem. If neither parent is able to be the primary caregiver because of mental illness, other options such as a 24-hour available social network or supportive contact may be the necessary "extra ego" to monitor well-being and assist in rearing the child (see Apfel and Handel, 1993, pp. 147–166).

A history of postpartum depression places a woman at greater risk for development of a similar puerperal episode. Moreover, difficulties during pregnancy predispose a woman to the development of other varieties of reproduction-related depression after birth (Apfel and Handel, 1993; Parry, 1989). Mother-infant bonding can be disrupted. Offspring of depressed caregivers are at increased risk for maladaptive behavior and emotional difficulties, but the risk to the child may also be mitigated by social supports. Early intervention in families with a depressed caregiver is therefore warranted, and referral to a mental health professional who is skilled in family and marital issues may be essential to the child's well-being (Cicchetti et al., 1997, 1998). At times, the patient's autonomy may be impaired, and she may be unable to care for her child. In such cases, psychiatric opinion should be sought to help the patient make an informed decision about treatment. Psychotherapy, psychopharmacology, and electroconvulsive therapy (ECT) are safe and effective treatments that enable most mothers to continue in their parenting role (Coverdale et al., 1997).

Guidelines for Primary Care Clinicians

1. Provide women during pregnancy with information about normal and abnormal psychological reactions to childbirth. Without instilling undue alarm, which could have a "suggestive" influence, ask the patient to report changes in her emotional state that may already worry her, such as poor concentration, irritability, or obsessional thoughts, especially about harming the baby.
2. Urge both the mother and the father, if possible, to reduce psychosocial stressors by thorough planning before the birth. If no extended family is available to help, remind the patient of the normal exhaustion and tension that occur with a new birth. Classes for new parents not only teach parenting skills but also help couples communicate directly so that the father can be of additional emotional support.
3. Consider using care extenders in your office or referring the patient to a women's health cooperative or support group for young mothers to discuss pragmatic psychosocial supports. Parenting classes are educationally and emotionally supportive to both parents; they not only instruct the prospective parents about the needs of the baby and teach caretaking skills but also prepare the couple for emotional transitions. Research confirms what generations of families, using common sense, have known: Support from relatives and friends, a stable home situation in which to raise the baby (i.e., safe place), and staying active and involved offer the greatest likelihood of avoiding postpartum depression. Clearly, biologic vulnerability is not eradicated, but social supports are in place to facilitate adaptation and to ameliorate stress surrounding the birth.
4. Monitor the patient's emotional well-being during pregnancy and thereafter.

Allow the patient time to express her fears and worries about social concerns (e.g., financial problems) and, when warranted, involve ancillary supports (e.g., home health nurse, social worker) to help her sort out these issues. In one study of highly anxious postpartum women, professional intervention from a social worker was more effective than nonprofessional intervention or no intervention at all in lowering anxiety (Barnett and Parker, 1985).

5. The "Guidelines for Patients" sections from Chapter 1 (Anxiety) or Chapter 2 (Depression) may be given to the patient, depending on the nature of her distress and your judgment that more information at this point will be an enhancement, not another burden.

6. When multiple risk factors for postpartum illness are present, be particularly vigilant about patient follow-up. These psychosocial factors include the following:
   a. History of postpartum onset of major depression.
   b. Family history of depression.
   c. Recent adverse life event.

7. Initiate trials of antidepressant medication (e.g., SSRIs) or refer the patient to a psychiatrist. Psychotherapy is also useful in addressing psychosocial needs and evaluating any difficulty mother and baby may be having during the early attachment period. Estrogen replacement is of benefit in some women with postpartum depression and may be empirically given in selected cases (Gregoire and Kumar, 1996; Vliet, 1995).

What Can Safely Be Advised Concerning Prenatal and Postnatal Exposure to Psychotropic Drugs?

Women with psychiatric conditions have a high rate of relapse during pregnancy. They are understandably concerned about the risk to the fetus if they have been taking psychotropic drugs and the baby is exposed. When a woman taking psychotropic medication becomes pregnant, the primary care clinician should consult the psychiatrist about the prevalence of toxic effects of the specific medication and the need for follow-up.

Usually, the primary care clinician can safely advise the patient that growing evidence supports the notion that most antipsychotics and antidepressants can and should be continued during pregnancy and through labor and delivery (Altshuler et al., 1996; Cohen et al., 1994). Discontinuation should be avoided because it places the patient at greater risk for postpartum psychosis or depression. Conservative practice indicates avoidance of lithium carbonate, especially during the first trimester, although most authorities now believe that the association between lithium usage and the development of Epstein's abnormality has been overblown (Cohen et al., 1994). Central nervous system depressants (e.g., benzodiazepines) should be avoided, particularly during labor and delivery (Altshuler et al., 1996).

Some anecdotal reports have noted a withdrawal syndrome and prematurity in infants whose mothers took SSRIs during pregnancy (Chambers et al., 1996). These reports have had some methodologic flaws, however, and psychiatric opinion now converges on treatment continuing during pregnancy and through-out the postpartum period (Altshuler et al., 1996; Cohen et al., 1997). No long-term behavioral or cognitive problems have been observed in the majority of infants whose mothers took SSRIs or tricyclics during pregnancy and in the postpartum period. Nulman and colleagues (Nulman and Koren, 1996; Nulman et al., 1997) have pointed out a clinical caveat: perinatal risks arise when pregnant women who have clinical anxiety, depression, or other disorders remain untreated. Significant psychiatric illness in a mother adversely affects the devel-opment of cognition, language, and behavior in her infant and young child. Therefore, current evidence points to the need to treat depression during pregnancy and after the birth of the baby.

If a woman needs an antidepressant but wishes to breastfeed, it may be best to prescribe either tricyclic antidepressants or SSRIs. Both classes appear to have no untoward effects, although tricyclics have a more established record of safety (Mammen et al., 1997; Wisner et al., 1996; Yoshida et al., 1998). To date there have not been thorough behavioral assessments and longitudinal development follow-up studies of breast-fed babies of mothers who have taken antidepressants. Treatment therefore must be individualized, with careful obser-vation of the mother and baby during pregnancy and nursing. If adverse effects appear to develop, consider checking the level of antidepressant in the infant (Spigset et al., 1996; Wisner et al., 1996).

On the whole, there appear to be no detectable adverse consequences to infants whose mothers must take antidepressants. ECT and psychotherapy re-main viable options for the pregnant patient who is depressed, but there is growing evidence that mothers with depression or anxiety who take antidepres-sants (e.g., fluoxetine, sertraline) can breastfeed, resulting in health and psycho-logical benefits for both mother and child.

MENOPAUSE

Psychological Approach to Menopause

Women now live one third of their lives after cessation of reproductive capacity. In addition to adjusting to the hormonal changes ushered in by the female climacteric, women must make psychological adaptations at midlife to continue to live as fully and vibrantly as possible. Society is beginning to progress beyond the antiquated societal and psychoanalytic ideas from the earlier part of this century. When women were valued primarily for their capacity to bear and raise children, and when lifespans were shorter, the end of the reproductive years was assumed to herald depression, if not demise. In essence, both men and women believed that after menopause a woman's life was basically over. As psychoanalysts and other mental health professionals have taken adult develop-ment into account, these notions are being placed in perspective. Most women indeed mourn the loss of their reproductive capacity, but the majority make the transition to an active and fulfilling life.

Psychodynamic psychiatry and psychoanalysis now emphasize that growth and development are possible for each man and woman over the entire life cycle. Moreover, as men and women live longer, they are teaching professionals how much can be gleaned in one's later years. New models of successful aging are discussed in the popular and professional press, and negative stereotypes are being discounted. But myths die hard. It will probably take another generation before society fully embraces the view that the postmenopausal years can be a time women look forward to rather than dread. Instead of viewing menopause "in terms of loss rather than change" (Laughlin, 1997, p. 3), both men and women will gradually "be helped to envision what life can be for them at this new stage of development and beyond—to expect anew" (Laughlin, 1997, p. 2).

Is the Association of Depression with Menopause a Myth?

Much has been written about the psychological changes that accompany menopause. Women with a history of major depression before their perimenopausal years are at increased risk for depression during the transition to menopause, as are women who experience a long perimenopausal phase. But the climacteric does not place the majority of women at greater risk for a first episode of depression. Nor is there any evidence to support the notion that "the empty nest syndrome" (Nicol-Smith, 1996; Semel, 1986; Tallmer, 1986) causes anguish and bona fide depression in the majority of middle-aged women.

Cross-sectional studies show that most women experience much happiness, greater marital harmony, and more enjoyment in life after all their children have left home. Having met their obligations to others, they are now able to enjoy new opportunities and new freedoms. Sexual functioning can continue unabated, and sometimes may be enhanced, when the woman and her partner no longer fear pregnancy (Bennett, 1997; Gallant and Derry, 1995). Despite these sanguine findings, some epidemiologic studies show an increased incidence of dysphoria and minor psychological symptoms in menopausal women (Sherwin, 1993). These women, who are only mildly depressed or not depressed at all, appear to experience improvement in mood when treated with conventional doses of estrogen replacement therapy. However, estrogen is ineffective in the treatment of a major mood disturbance (see Chapter 2).

Estrogen increases the amount of serotonin at the synapses, thereby enhancing mood. The apparent mechanisms of action are as follows: (1) decrease in monoamine oxidase activity, with maintenance of higher serotonin levels; (2) displacement of tryptophan from binding sites, increasing free tryptophan in the brain, which is then metabolized to serotonin; and (3) increase in density of titrated imipramine-binding sites on platelets. Estrogen also causes some beneficial sexual side effects that may enhance responsiveness for many women. Exogenous estrogens increase vaginal lubrication, alleviating atrophic vaginitis and associated dyspareunia. Some physicians recommend the addition of testosterone for women who have diminished sexual desire and sexual arousal after menopause, even though this use has not been thoroughly studied in controlled trials. The recommended dosage is 1.25 to 5.0 mg daily (Johnson, 1998). Although testosterone is the hormone involved in sexual responsiveness, for most women personal relationships and life circumstances remain the predominant determinants of sexuality.

Primary care clinicians are increasingly aware of the benefits of hormone replacement therapy (HRT) in postmenopausal women. Those who receive HRT generally experience increased longevity and enhanced quality of life. Incontrovertible evidence now exists that HRT reduces the risk of heart disease, prevents bone loss (osteoporosis), alleviates physical symptoms such as hot flushes and night sweats, and reverses atrophy of the urogenital tissues, which can lead to atrophic vaginitis and urge incontinence. Although benefits and risks (e.g., breast cancer, uterine cancer) must always be weighed in each individual case, growing evidence supports the notion that estrogen supplementation in postmenopausal women benefits cognitive functioning and can reduce mild dysphoria (Johnson, 1998; Kravitz, 1998; Sherwin, 1994).

The primary care clinician should be aware that the suggestion of HRT can cause anger and resentment in some patients. An ongoing controversy spurred by the women's movement continues to rage regarding whether menopause is a normal phase of life or a treatable condition. Moreover, some feminist leaders have further politicized the debate, arguing that the pharmaceutical industry is simply making money off middle-aged women with chemicals that do not help them (see Doress-Worters and Siegal 1994; Friedan, 1993). A clinician who suggests HRT to an ardent feminist who has heard only these views is likely to engender a healthy debate, if not wrath. It is helpful to know the facts and to encourage the patient to review all her options (Gallant and Derry, 1995; Reid, 1998).

What Clinical Advice Might I Give the Patient?

The following approach to the menopausal patient is based on the evolving literature on menopause, as well as on my own clinical practice. After explaining in a general way estrogen's wide range of actions through receptors in the brains of men or women, I draw a diagram to sketch how estrogen supplementation helps develop new synaptic connections and interneuron dendritic processes. Estrogens have indirect effects on nerve cells but generally play a protective role on the cell formation. Estrogens have the ability to neutralize the effects of glucocorticoids released during stress; indeed, estrogen cycling during the reproductive years may render women more vulnerable "to the neurotoxic processes engendered by stress hormones" (Seeman, 1997, p. 1645) leading to greater susceptibility to depression (Chapter 2), anxiety (Chapter 1), and posttraumatic stress disorder (Chapter 6).

I explain that there is an evolving body of evidence to suggest that estrogen may prevent or arrest the development of Alzheimer's disease in women. I also underscore its global effect of improving cognition (Johnson, 1998; Sherwin, 1988, 1993). For example, in two demographically similar groups of healthy women about 65 years of age, 43 women who had not used estrogen since menopause (approximately 15 years) had significantly lower scores on both immediate and delayed paragraph recall than 28 women who had received estrogen during that time (Kampen and Sherwin, 1994). I explain that evidence continues to expand on HRT's health benefits—cognitive functioning in particular—and to show that it enhances the ability of women to learn new material and maintain verbal memory. It is important to know of any absolute or relative contraindications (i.e., breast, uterine, or ovarian cancer) and to perform a full physical examination and Papanicolaou (PAP) smear before beginning treatment.

Clinical Example 11–1

Even when these data are presented and no reasons are found to avoid HRT, not all patients will agree to this course of treatment. One patient, a very savvy nurse anesthetist, decided against HRT after reviewing materials I suggested and doing her own literature search. She had no positive history of breast, ovarian, or uterine cancer in her family of origin but remained unimpressed by the scientific data she studied (see "Resources for Patients"). From her perspective, the most helpful intervention was the psychotherapy process she voluntarily undertook with me to look at issues related to aging.

For this patient, ongoing discussion of multiple losses, including her disappointment at never marrying or having children of her own, led to a working-through process of even deeper efficacy. As the only daughter in her family, it was expected that she would "look after mom" during her mother's waning years. Although my patient lived a great distance from her mother, she felt responsible for all the caretaking. What was particularly embittering was her mother's assumption of a "help-rejecting, complainer stance." Nothing my patient did either pleased or ameliorated her mother's characterologic haranguing about her unhappy marriage (her husband had died 15 years earlier), and the disappointments of her other children (all of whom were successful professionals), or her refusal to use her considerable financial resources to remodel the dilapidated family home (she refused to buy an air conditioner even though she lived in a sweltering southern town).

My patient had to come to grips with the fact that, try as she might, she could not change or "cure" her mother. In part, her choice of a career as a nurse had been unconsciously predicated on her wish to finally have a salutary, therapeutic effect on someone. Naturally, it did not escape my attention that, in a salient role reversal, the patient rejected my suggestion for HRT—just as her mother, week after week and day after day, had rejected offers of assistance. The mother remained isolated, without community support, and continued to deteriorate physically, despite the daughter's frequent calls and visits. She appeared to bedevil even the most well-meaning physician: She refused to take advantage of any suggested treatment (e.g., antidepressants) and would not follow up on annual visits or blood work unless her daughter literally put her in the car and took her to the doctor.

This clinical example illustrates a number of the psychological features of midlife that should be considered when evaluating a perimenopausal or menopausal patient:

1. It is unlikely that long-term, characterologic patterns will be reversed. Even with the most sophisticated and compassionate of medical care, some women will resist—and even resent—assistance from friends, family, and each member of their health care team.
2. Although it is important to offer feedback and suggestions, such as the use of adjunctive HRT and/or psychotropic medication, remember that any number of psychological factors may contribute to the patient's noncompliance and reluctance to accept your advice.
3. Recognize that as the population ages (one third of U.S. women are now older than 50 years of age, and the life expectancy for women by 2000 is 84 years), increasing numbers of women in midlife will find themselves in the role of caring for aging parents. In addition to their menopausal health concerns, clinicians must look beneath the surface to the psychological issues that

impinge on these women and prevent them from making choices that would appear to be in their interest.

4. Family concerns, whether related to one's adolescent or adult children, one's mate or partner, or one's parents, can have a negative impact on healthy adaptations to menopause and midlife.

5. As clinicians grow older themselves, they must recognize a tendency that is a common pitfall in treatment: expecting patients to manage decisions as they themselves have done or are suggesting. Reluctance to change or to look at all options is not just a patient issue! Clinicians may become overly ambitious in trying to help patients change when instead they should be backing off and looking at their own "furor therapeuticus." An aphorism used by Kelli Holloway, MD, of the Karl Menninger School of Psychiatry, trenchantly makes this point: "You can lead a horse to water, but if you start carrying the horse across, it is likely that both of you are going to drown."

Patient Guidelines for Coping with Menopause

1. Challenge yourself to adapt to the menopausal years as creatively and as productively as possible. Try to focus less on what is lost and more on what can still be gained. See menopause as a time of change when your challenge is to make choices and define goals appropriate to the second half of life.

2. Recognize that most women now live one third of their lives after menopause. Usually, the physical symptoms of menopause (e.g., hot flushes, insomnia) are temporary, and hormone replacement therapy (HRT) can often reverse them if this course of action is your choice. However, most women still need to make adjustments in their self-image and body image as they age.

3. Everyone's body changes as they age, so we must work with our changing body image over and over again (Freedman, 1986, 1997). Psychologist Rita Freedman, an expert in body image and eating disorders, admits that she, too, had to grapple with this issue in her 50s. "I sometimes feel as vulnerable as the teenage bulimics who come to my office for help," she said. "The challenge for me parallels problems for them. How to shed an old, familiar body image while growing into a new one" (Freedman, 1997, p. 10).

4. Recognize the normal transitions in midlife and at menopause, such as seeing children leave home and becoming a mother-in-law or grandparent. In cultures where menopause is heralded by ritual or ceremony, women have fewer physical and mood symptoms. Find some ways to "celebrate" this transition in a positive way.

5. Try to face role expectations and stereotypes in order to attain and assert your own individual identity. Remember that at midlife women continue to provide most of the informal caregiving for spouse, parents, parents-in-law, and sometimes even adult children. This other-directed focus takes enormous energy! To stay emotionally and physically healthy, you must find ways to nurture yourself.

6. Learn as much as you can about physical changes that occur with menopause and about possible treatments available to you. Discuss with your physician whether HRT is right for you. You may also want to consider some of the natural menopausal remedies written about in the popular press. Be sure to tell your physician if you decide on a natural or herbal treatment, and by all

means avoid taking prescribed and herbal remedies together unless you discuss them with your physician first. Severe side effects can result from potent chemical interactions. Although HRT cannot reverse the aging process, it has been shown to be of positive benefit for a number of physical conditions (e.g., osteoporosis, coronary heart disease). Estrogen also enhances mood and cognition in many women.

7. Remember that most women at midlife do indeed feel good about themselves. They seem to have the ability to deal with multiple transitions and losses. Professional guidance or support groups can help you through the changes that inevitably occur at this point (e.g., loss of close friends, divorce or widowhood, retirement).

Additional Guidelines for Primary Care Clinicians

1. As with all other age groups, provide the patient with as much information as possible. Many patients expect to "tough out" menopausal symptoms. Be sure to assess for the vasomotor, cognitive, mood, and sexual effects of the loss of estrogen, and to recommend HRT when indicated.
2. Assess mood symptoms. Remember that women who have had an episode of major depression are more likely to have another at menopause. They should be treated aggressively with psychopharmacologic and psychotherapeutic modalities. However, mild depression is also frequently seen at menopause. Consider estrogen replacement therapy and adjunctive supportive psychotherapy in these women.
3. A cluster of transitional issues can affect a woman at midlife. Not only are there real changes going on in her body, but her roles in the family and in the workplace are shifting. Research on midlife continues to throw light on life issues, but an appreciation on your part of these transitions will aid you in creating a partnership with the patient. Some midlife transitions of older women include the following:
   a. Becoming a mother-in-law.
   b. Grandparenting.
   c. Empty nest syndrome (although this is not a problem for most women, it is for some).
   d. Cluttered nest (an adult child who returns home).
   e. Caregiving to parents or spouse with debilitating illness.
   f. Widowhood.
   g. Divorce.
   h. Remarriage.
   i. Retirement.
   j. Death of an adult child.
   k. Changes in body image.
   l. Chronic illness and disability.
3. Ask routinely about use of complementary or alternative medicines. A growing number of women are turning to natural remedies (e.g., dong quai, ginseng, red clover) that are thought to be mildly estrogenic. They may not tell you about these medications unless asked directly. Keep informed about the

growing scientific information in this area and communicate nonjudgmentally about their use. Remind patients of the benefits of exercise and a healthy diet and the importance of fun and pleasure to relieve stress.

4. Remind your patients that psychological growth can occur throughout the entire life cycle. The postmenopausal years should not be seen as a time when there is a dwindling of the spirit but rather as a time for renewal and psychological growth. Point the patient in the direction of seeking out these new opportunities. In assisting the menopausal woman in her transition from reproductive life onward, you have a unique opportunity to intervene in the management of the patient's long-term physical health.

5. Have realistic expectations for yourself as a clinician. Although it is crucial to be aware of some of the psychological issues and life transitions of the menopausal patient, she will probably also need other resources (e.g., support groups, psychotherapy) to work through these issues. The primary care clinician must be sensitive to various cultural, social, and personal determinants of health during menopause but also should encourage referral to mental health clinicians when appropriate. Aging women must confront issues surrounding their changing body image, role as a caretaker, eventual death, and so on. Psychotherapy is another avenue to aid the process of transitions that "provide women with opportunities to mature emotionally, even in the prime or twilight of their lives" (Semel, 1986, p. 268).

SUMMARY

Menstruation, pregnancy, childbirth, and menopause are normal stages in the lives of women. A considerable number of women experience psychological difficulties associated with their reproductive functioning. The spectrum of mood and behavioral changes associated with menstruation, pregnancy, and menopause most likely result from a complex interplay among psychosocial and hormonal factors. Clinicians who openly communicate with women about these "high-risk" times for emotional illness play a crucial role in prevention and are in the best position to gather information when a difficulty arises.

Evidence exists that disorders associated with reproductive functioning occur in all socioeconomic groups worldwide. The months surrounding birth are times when women face the greatest lifetime risk for development of a bona fide mental illness (e.g., postpartum depression, anxiety, psychosis). Psychosocial supports help ameliorate psychological dysfunction. In addition, pharmacologic treatment has been found highly effective in the treatment of PMS, postpartum depression, anxiety, and psychosis as well as the cognitive and emotional aspects of menopause. Women of childbearing age can usually take psychotropic medications safely when they are needed. Consultation with a psychiatrist is frequently helpful to weigh particular risks and benefits for an individual patient, particularly if she wants to conceive or becomes pregnant. Women who become mildly depressed at the onset of menopause may benefit from HRT, but those who experience major depressive disorder should be treated with antidepressants.

The primary care clinician must be aware that mood and anxiety symptoms associated with reproductive functioning occur on a spectrum ranging from mild to severe. There is considerable evidence indicating that estrogen has a complex influence on mood. Some psychological symptoms are alleviated by HRT, but further research is needed to understand the impact of genetics, culture, psychosocial stresses, and environmental support in the subgroup of women who are vulnerable to hormonal changes across the female life cycle.

Most patients who experience psychiatric symptoms do quite well with contemporary therapies (e.g., SSRIs for PMS, HRT for a mild perimenopausal depression, antidepressants or ECT for severe postpartum depression). Moreover, the use of psychotropic medication during pregnancy is appropriate in many clinical situations because the risk to the fetus is quite low. The majority of women can take antidepressants after the birth of the baby and safely breastfeed. In each situation, however, individualized treatment is required, and the risk-benefit ratio must be weighed. Nevertheless, given the pervasive effects on quality of life for the patient, her children, and others in her immediate family, it behooves primary care clinicians to pay particular attention to psychiatric symptoms associated with menstruation, pregnancy, and menopause.

Resources for Patients

General References

Northrup C: *Women's Bodies, Women's Wisdom: Creating Physical and Emotional Health and Healing*, rev. ed. New York, Bantam Books, 1998. (Original edition published in 1994.)

This encyclopedic volume has been heralded by physicians and lay persons because of its holistic approach to emotional and physical disorders. The author, an obstetrician-gynecologist, reviews pertinent aspects of the biology of the menstrual cycle, fertility, pregnancy, menopause, and nutrition. Her goal is to help women embrace their power by understanding how their bodies function. Dr. Northrup firmly believes that "medical science, when combined with wisdom of our hearts and our minds, is powerful medicine indeed" (p. xxii).

Some readers are bound to disagree with the author's belief in energy fields, chakras, and herbal and vitamin treatments; they will nonetheless be reassured by her expertise in conventional treatments, medical science, and appreciation for mind-body interactions (e.g., steps for healing include listening to the body and reclaiming the intellect). Numerous patient examples are included, as well as suggestions women can use to think through their problems, get a fuller grasp of the mistaken ideas that may be impinging on them, and begin to take decisive steps for healing. For example, in order to empower the patient with a reproductive or psychological problem, Northrup insists that the patient must sort through her belief systems and understand the purpose that any illness may serve. Quite psychodynamic in the breadth of her approach, she describes the part that childhood plays in the development of problems in addition to any negative cultural messages that have been internalized and persist in adulthood. She guides her readers in deciding to make changes and become healthy. As a mother, physician, and patient, the author has experienced labor, delivery, and physical illness "from both sides of the bed." This compassionate first-hand voice augments her authority about the myriad of ways women can decide to take command of their lives and restore well-being. She reminds her broad audience of readers (not only lay people but also physicians) of Albert Schweitzer's maxim: "It's a trade secret, but I'll tell you anyway. All healing is self-healing" (p. 673).

Semler TC: *All About Eve: The Complete Guide to Women's Health and Well-Being.* New York, HarperCollins, 1995.

This comprehensive paperback is a marvelously accessible resource to the major areas of women's health concerns. The praise it has received from physicians, educators, and politicians such as former Congresswoman Pat Schroeder and Senator Carol Moseley-Braun are deserved. Its readable summaries, interesting patient examples, fact-filled lists of available therapeutic options, and evaluations of how these treatments work—including the pros, cons, and costs—are excellent. This book has particularly comprehensive chapters on gynecologic concerns (e.g., menstrual and menopausal issues, sexual health, childbirth, fitness and nutrition). A thoughtful section for infertile patients reviews the latest available technologies and options for infertility treatment. The emotional issues that affect such patients (e.g., grief, stress, guilt, how to handle difficult social events surrounding or including children) are also emphasized.

Vliet EL: *Screaming to be Heard: Hormonal Connections Women Suspect and Doctors Ignore.* New York, M Evans & Co., 1995.

This widely read, popular guide to contemporary hormone therapies deserves a place in every woman's and every clinician's library. Written by a psychiatrist and expert psychopharmacologist, the book provides a brilliant, scientifically based, but easy to understand perspective on hormone therapies and traditional medical and complementary (holistic) treatment techniques.

Dr. Vliet postulates that estrogen and progesterone effects are culprits in migraines, fibromyalgia, and bladder problems. But she also takes up less controversial subjects, such as the need for HRT (including testosterone) to potentiate sexual vitality, decrease osteoporosis and heart disease, and alleviate mood and cognitive problems as women grow older. She includes numerous examples of patients who have experienced dramatic positive effects from hormone therapy. These case descriptions demonstrate the amelioration of typical menopausal syndromes (e.g., hot flushes, night sweats, joint pains), as well as the alleviation of insomnia, depression, low productivity, and poor self-esteem in menopausal women. This book is highly recommended for its balanced view of the decision-making process every woman must go through before she undertakes any treatment for PMS or menopause. Because many women are reading this book, it is suggested that the primary care clinician not ignore it. Like so many texts written by women about the biology of HRT, it includes sections on the psychological and spiritual needs incumbent in the process of healing.

Abortion

Stotland NL: *Abortion Facts and Feelings: A Handbook for Women and the People Who Care About Them.* Washington, DC, American Psychiatric Press, 1998.

Dr. Nada Stotland is a distinguished psychiatrist who has studied the impact of abortion and miscarriage on her patients over the course of her career. She clearly understands what a heart-wrenching experience abortion can be for any woman, her significant other, and her family. In this book, Stotland attempts to help the patient, parents, men, and friends sort out all the decisions that must be made before terminating a "problem pregnancy." In addition to sections addressing feelings about abortion, national and state laws, abortion procedures, and alternatives (e.g., adoption), as well as religion, ethics, and values, she includes an excellent chapter about the emotional reactions the patient is likely to face after the procedure (e.g., regrets, anniversary reactions, how to move on). Dr. Stotland's chapter, "For the Professional Counselor," is also useful to primary care clinicians who have patients who have had or plan to have an abortion. She is particularly expert at listing the information that clinicians and counselors need to know in order to help patients with their decisions. Although Stotland believes the final decision is ultimately the patient's alone to make, professionals must also take stock of their own values, beliefs, and unconscious assumptions to maintain their objectivity. What is so useful about this book is the step-by-step thought process it initiates for the patient, her loved ones, and those who care for her. This text is also highly recommended for women who have had an abortion and want to have an opportunity to thoughtfully process their reactions.

Postpartum Depression

Sebastian L: *Overcoming Postpartum Depression and Anxiety*. Omaha, NE, Addicus Books, 1998.

> *This is the first authoritative and highly accessible guide for the patient who experiences a mood change or anxiety after giving birth. Ms. Sebastian, an Advanced Registered Nurse Practitioner, has broad experience treating patients with postpartum mood disorders, particularly with cognitive-behavioral therapy. In this book, she helps patients sort out the differences between postpartum blues and bona fide depression. She forthrightly discusses how to navigate the mental health system and the roles of therapy and medication when treatment is needed. She also includes helpful advice for fathers and family members that is often forgotten when the primary caretaker is temporarily unable to function. Sebastian frames her book with the actual questions that patients ask clinicians and themselves: "Why does depression occur?" "Will it affect my baby?" "What can I tell other people?" "Will it happen again?" Virtually no aspect of postpartum anxiety or depressive disorders goes unaddressed. The author's reassuring and hopeful tone will leave new mothers believing that a postpartum mood disorder is a problem they can master.*

Menopause

Cherry SH, Runowicz CD: *The Menopause Book*. New York, Simon and Schuster, 1994.

Cone FK: *Making Sense of Menopause*. New York, Simon and Schuster, 1993.

Dennerstein L, Shelley J (eds.): *A Woman's Guide to Menopause and Hormone Replacement Therapy*. Washington, DC, American Psychiatric Press, 1998.

Horrigan BJ (ed.): *Red Moon Passage: The Power and Wisdom of Menopause*. New York, Three Rivers Press, 1996.

Sheehy G: *Menopause: The Silent Passage*. New York, Pocket Books, 1995. (Original work published in 1991.)

> *One fruit of the feminist movement of the 1960s has been the gestation of numerous books about and interest in menopause as once-novice adherents of women's rights now enter midlife. Ms. Sheehy's book is perhaps the best known and most easily acquired. It achieved its success as a* New York Times *bestseller for good reason—many women who were experiencing the symptoms of perimenopause and menopause felt they were "going crazy" rather than passing through an expectable and predictable physiologic change. Sheehy sees menopause as a "gateway to second adulthood" and comprehensively explains the risks and benefits of HRT. She believes it is crucial for women to know about their bodies in order to face down the myths of an earlier generation, when entering menopause typically meant that the end of one's life was just around the corner.*
>
> *Each of the other recommended books has a unique perspective to offer patients. Without exception, they suggest alternatives to traditional medical treatments in addition to outlining the physiologic, emotional, and sexual benefits of HRT. Drs. Cherry and Runowicz present a straightforward monograph that includes suggestions for exercise, nutrition, and general health care (especially breast care). Ms. Cone approached the subject by interviewing more than 150 lay women and medical experts to compile an informative and reassuring book about the symptoms, psychological effects, and treatments of menopause. Her book includes vivid quotations on sex, the reactions of men, and the role of alternative therapies.*
>
> *Drs. Dennerstein and Shelley have edited a most balanced, up-to-date guide for women. Included are the controversies sparked by the latest information about menopause, especially the medical and sociologic reasons some women decide not to take hormone supplements. A final section features recommendations from the World Health Organization; this information places menopause in its cultural and biologic context and outlines trends in therapy concerning women's menopausal health care in different countries. Of all of the books recommended for the patient, this is the most scientifically*

referenced volume and will be of particular use to the woman who wants sound advice based on outcome studies and validated research.

Finally, Ms. Horrigan's book approaches menopause as a spiritual and psychological journey. Eight extraordinary women from different backgrounds and traditions share how they were personally transformed by making a decision that "the change of life" would be a constructive time for restoration, rejuvenation, and personal growth. One can't help but be inspired by the creative possibilities and transformations exhibited by these women who experienced menopause as a time of illumination, not illness, when "wonderful and expected things can and will happen" (p. 69).

Resources for Primary Care Clinicians

Brown WA (ed.): Premenstrual syndrome. *Psychiatric Annals* 1996;26(9).

This special edition of Psychiatric Annals *is a practical summary about what is and is not known to date about PMS. Primary care clinicians will be less interested in the articles about specific diagnosis and assessment tools than in the pharmacologic and nonpharmacologic treatments. As Dr. Walter A. Brown opines in the introduction, there has truly been a "quiet breakthrough" in our understanding of PMS since the mid-1980s. Although premenstrual dysphoria was once thought to be psychosomatic, up to 90% of women have complete or almost complete relief from symptoms when SSRIs are prescribed. Approximately 5% of all women have disabling PMS. Therefore, the primary care clinician is advised to stay vigilant about the rapidly evolving clinical understanding of this heretofore disregarded syndrome.*

Stewart DE, Stotland NL: *Psychological Aspects of Women's Health Care: The Interface Between Psychiatry and Obstetrics and Gynecology.* Washington, DC, American Psychiatric Press, 1993.

For the primary care clinician who desires an additional reference about virtually every topic on the interface between women's psychology and gynecology, this is a thorough and important resource. Chapters summarize state-of-the-art diagnosis, pathophysiology, and treatment (topics such as perinatal loss, normal and complicated pregnancies, postpartum disorders, chronic gynecologic pain, infertility and abortion, female sexual disorders, and when to seek additional psychiatric consultation). Most clinicians will not read this text cover to cover but rather will turn to it when faced with a specific concern in practice. Special sections devoted to fetal anomalies, minorities, the male perspective, and ethics will raise the consciousness of most physicians in these important, but often neglected, areas. The diversity of cultures and human experiences in one's practice inevitably has implications for treatment and prevention of illness. This book covers the waterfront.

References

Altshuler LI, Cohen L, Szuba MP: Pharmacologic management of psychiatric illness during pregnancy: dilemmas and guidelines. *Am J Psychiatry* 1996;153:592–606.

Apfel RJ, Handel MH: *Madness and Motherhood: Sexuality, Reproduction, and Long Term Mental Illness.* Washington, DC, American Psychiatric Press, 1993.

Areias ME, Kumar R, Barros H, et al.: Correlates of postnatal depression in mothers and fathers. *Br J Psychiatry* 1996;169:36–41.

Astin JA: Why patients use alternative medicine: results of a national study. *JAMA* 1998;279:1548–1553.

Barnett B, Parker G: Professional and non-professional intervention for highly anxious primiparous mothers. *Br J Psychiatry* 1985;146:287–293.

Bennett R: Some issues on transitions in midlife and older women: stress, coping, and social supports. *Renfrew Perspective* 1997;3:15–16.

Bilge B: The secret garden. *The Sciences* 1998; Jan/Feb:38–43.

Block M, Schmidt PJ, Rubinow DR: Premenstrual syndrome: evidence for symptom stability across cycles. *Am J Psychiatry* 1997;154:1741–1746.

Brockington IF: Disorders specific to the puerperium. *Int J Mental Health* 1992;21:41–52.

Brown WA (ed.): Premenstrual syndrome [special issue]. *Psychiatric Annals* 1996a;26(9).

Brown WA: What are the best drug treatments for premenstrual syndrome? *Harvard Mental Health Letter* 1996b; Nov. 8.

Brown WA: PMA: a quiet breakthrough. *Psychiatric Annals* 1997;26:569–570.

Chambers CD, Johnson KA, Dick LM, et al.: Birth outcomes in pregnant women taking fluoxetine. *N Engl J Med* 1996;338:1010–1015.

Cherry SH, Runowicz CD: *The Menopause Book.* New York, Simon and Schuster, 1994.

Cicchetti D, Rogosch FA, Toth SL: Ontogenesis, depressotypic organization, and the depressive spectrum. In: Luther SS, Burack JA, Cicchetti D, et al. (eds.): *Developmental Psychopathology: Perspectives on Adjustment, Risk, and Disorder,* pp. 273–313. New York, Cambridge University Press, 1997.

Cicchetti D, Toth SL: The development of depression in children and adolescents. *American Psychologist* 1998; 53:2:221–241.

Cohen LS, Friedman JM, Jefferson JW, et al.: A reevaluation of risk of in utero exposure to lithium. *JAMA* 1994;271:146–150.

Cohen LS, Heller VI, Bailey J, et al.: Birth outcomes following prenatal exposure to fluoxetine. Poster presentation at the American Psychiatric Association Annual Meeting, San Diego, CA, May 7–22, 1997.

Cone FK: *Making Sense of Menopause.* New York, Simon and Schuster, 1993.

Cosmar MP: Book review of *Eve's Herbs: A History of Contraception and Abortion in the West. JAMA* 1998;279:81–82.

Coverdale JH, McCullough LB, Chervenak FA, et al.: Clinical implications of respect for autonomy in the psychiatric treatment of pregnant patients with depression. *Psychiatr Serv* 1997;48:209–212.

Dennerstein L, Shelley J (eds.): *A Woman's Guide to Menopause and Hormone Replacement Therapy.* Washington, DC, American Psychiatric Press, 1998.

Doress-Worters PB, Siegal DL: *The New Ourselves, Growing Older: Women Aging with Power,* rev. ed. New York, Touchstone, 1994.

Eigen M: Miscarriages. In: Finell JS (ed.): *Mind-Body Problems: Psychotherapy with Psychosomatic Disorders,* pp. 333–351. Northvale, NJ, Jason Aronson, 1997.

Erickson E, Holberg MA, Andusch B, et al.: The serotonin reuptake inhibitor paroxetine is superior to the noradrenaline reuptake inhibitor maprotiline in the treatment of premenstrual syndrome. *Neuropsychopharmacology* 1997;16:345–356.

Freedman R: *Beauty Bound.* Lexington, MA, Lexington Books, 1986.

Freedman R: On reaching a certain age. *Renfrew Perspective* 1997;3:10–12.

Freeman E: Sertraline versus desipramine in PMS treatment. Report of symposia at the annual meeting of the American Psychiatric Association, Toronto, Canada, May 30–June 4, 1998.

Freeman EW, Rickels K, Sondheimer SJ, et al.: A double-blind trial of oral progesterone, alprazolam, and placebo in treatment of severe premenstrual syndrome. *JAMA* 1995;247:51–57.

Freeman EW, Rickels K, Sondheimer SJ, et al.: Sertraline versus desipramine in the treatment of premenstrual syndrome: an open-label trial. *J Clin Psychiatry* 1996;57:7–11.

Friedan B: *The Fountain of Age.* New York, Simon and Schuster, 1993.

Gallant SJ, Derry PS: Menarche, menstruation, and menopause: psychosocial research and future directions. In: Stanton AL, Gallant SJ (eds.): *The Psychology of Women's Health: Progress and Challenges in Research and Application,* pp. 199–259. Washington, DC, American Psychological Association, 1995.

Gold JH: Premenstrual dysphoric disorder: what's that? *JAMA* 1997;278:1024–1025.

Gold J: Historical perspective of premenstrual syndrome. In: Gold JH, Severino SK (eds): *Premenstrual Dysphorias: Myths and Realities,* pp. 171–183. Washington, DC, American Psychiatric Press, 1994.

Gregoire AJP, Kumar R, Everitt B, et al.: Transdermal oestrogen for treatment of severe postnatal depression. *Lancet* 1996;347:930–933.

Harrison WM, Endicott J, Nee J: Treatment of premenstrual dysphoria with alprazolam: a controlled study. *Arch Gen Psychiatry* 1990;47:270–275.

Horrigan BJ (ed.): *Red Moon Passage: The Power and Wisdom of Menopause.* New York, Three Rivers Press, 1996.

Janssen HKEM, Cuisinier MCJ, Hoogduin KAL, et al.: Controlled prospective study on the mental health of women following pregnancy loss. *Am J Psychiatry* 1996;153: 226–230.

Johnson SR: Menopause and hormone replacement therapy. *Med Clin North Am* 1998;82:297–320.

Kampen DL, Sherwin BB: Estrogen use and verbal memory in healthy postmenopausal women. *Obstet Gynecol* 1994;83:979–983.

Kendell RE, Chalmers JC, Platz C: Epidemiology of puerperal psychosis. *Br J Psychiatry* 1987;150:662–673.

Klebanov PK, Ruble DN: Toward an understanding of women's experience of menstrual cycle symptoms. In: Adesso VJ, Reddy DM, Fleming R (eds.): *Psychological Perspectives on Women's Health*, pp. 183–221. Washington, DC, Taylor & Francis, 1994.

Klein-Stern S: An algorithm for the treatment of premenstrual dysphoric disorder. Report of symposia at the annual meeting of the American Psychiatric Association, Toronto, Canada, May 30–June 4, 1998.

Klock SC, Chang G, Hiley A, et al.: Psychological distress among women with recurrent spontaneous abortion. *Psychosomatics* 1997;38:503–507.

Koeske RD: Premenstrual emotionality: is biology destiny? In: Walsh MR (ed.): *The Psychology of Women: Ongoing Debates*, pp. 137–146. New Haven, CT, Yale University Press, 1987.

Kravitz HM: Dysphoric moods in women: menopause or myth? Paper presented at the annual meeting of the American Psychiatric Association, Toronto, Canada, May 30–June 4, 1998.

Laughlin LR: Women at and after menopause: the need for new expectations. *Renfrew Perspective* 1997;3:2–4.

Lenhart SA, Bernstein AE: *The Psychodynamic Treatment of Women*. Washington, DC, American Psychiatric Press, 1993.

Mammen OK, Perel JM, Rudolph G, et al.: Sertraline and nonsertraline levels in three breast-fed infants. *J Clin Psychology* 1997;58:100–103.

McNeil TF, Kaij L, Malquist-Larsson A: Women and nonorganic psychosis: mental disturbance during pregnancy. *Acta Psychiatr Scand* 1989;70:127–139.

Mortola JF, Girton L, Fischer U: Successful treatment of severe premenstrual syndrome by combined use of GnRH agonist and estrogen/progestin. *J Clin Endocrinol Metab* 1991;72:252A–252F.

Munjiza M, Ljubomirovic N: Pharmacotherapy of premenstrual syndrome. Paper given at 10th Congress of the European College of Neuropsychopharmacology, Vienna, Austria, Sept 13–17, 1997.

Nicol-Smith L: Causality, menopause, and depression: a critical review of the literature. *BMJ* 1996;313:1229–1232.

Northrup C: *Women's Bodies, Women's Wisdom: Creating Physical and Emotional Health and Healing*, rev. ed. New York, Bantam Books, 1998. (Original edition published in 1994.)

Nulman I, Koren G: The safety of fluoxetine during pregnancy and lactation. *Teratology* 1996;53:304–308.

Nulman I, Rovet J, Stewart DE, et al.: Neurodevelopment of children exposed in utero to antidepressant drugs. *N Engl J Med* 1997;336:258–262.

Parry BL: Reproductive factors affecting the course of affective illness in women. *Psychiatr Clin North Am* 1989;12:207–220.

Pearlstein T: Nonpharmacologic treatment of premenstrual syndrome. *Psychiatric Annals* 1996;26:590–594.

Pines D: *A Woman's Unconscious Use of Her Body*. New Haven, Yale, 1994.

Reid RL: Decision making at menopause. Report of symposia at the annual meeting of the American Psychiatric Association, Toronto, Canada, May 30–June 4, 1998.

Rickels K, Freeman EW, Sondheimer S, et al.: Fluoxetine in the treatment of premenstrual syndrome. *Current Therapeutic Research* 1990;48:161–166.

Riddle JM: *Eve's Herbs: A History of Contraception and Abortion in the West*. Cambridge, MA, Howard University Press, 1997.

Righetti-Veltema M, Conne-Perreard E, Bousquet A, et al.: Risk factors and predictive signs of postpartum depression. *J Affect Disord* 1998;49:167–180.

Rivera-Tovar A, Rhodes R, Pearlstein TB, et al.: Treatment efficacy. In: Gold JH, Severino SK: *Premenstrual Dysphorias: Myths and Realities*, pp. 99–148. Washington, DC, American Psychiatric Press, 1994.

Robinson GE, Stewart DE: Postpartum disorders. In: Stewart DE, Stotland NL: *Psychological Aspects of Women's Health Care: The Interface Between Psychiatry and Obstetrics and Gynecology*, pp. 115–138. Washington, DC, American Psychiatric Press, 1993.

Rubinow DR, Schmidt PJ: The treatment of premenstrual syndrome: forward into the past [editorial]. *N Engl J Med* 1995;332:1574–1575.

Ruble DN: Premenstrual symptoms: a reinterpretation. *Science* 1977;197:291–292.

Sebastian L: *Overcoming Postpartum Depression and Anxiety*. Omaha, NE, Addicus Books, 1998.

Seeman MV: Psychopathology in women and men: focus on female hormones. *Am J Psychiatry* 1997;154:1641–1647.

Semel VG: The aging woman: confrontations with helplessness. In: Bernay T, Cantor DW (eds.): *The Psychology of Today's Woman: New Psychoanalytic Visions*, pp. 253–272. Hillsdale, NJ, Analytic Press, 1986.

Semler TC: *All About Eve: The Complete Guide to Women's Health and Well-Being*. New York, HarperCollins, 1995.

Severino SK: Late luteal phase dysphoric disorder: a scientific puzzle. *Med Hypotheses* 1993;41:229–234.

Severino SK, Bucci W, Creelman ML: Cyclical changes in emotional information processing in sleep and dreams. *J Am Acad Psychoanal* 1989;17:555–577.

Severino SK, Gold JH: Summation. In: Gold JH, Severino SK (eds.): *Premenstrual Dysphorias: Myths and Realities*, pp. 231–248. Washington, DC, American Psychiatric Press, 1994.

Sharp D: The prevention of postnatal depression. In: Kendrick T, Tylee A, Freeling P (eds.): *The Prevention of Mental Illness in Primary Care*, pp. 57–73. Cambridge, MA, Cambridge University Press, 1996.

Sheehy G: *Menopause: The Silent Passage*. New York, Pocket Books, 1995. (Original work published in 1991.)

Sherwin BB: Affective changes with estrogen and androgen replacement therapy in surgically menopausal women. *J Affect Disord* 1988;14:177–187.

Sherwin BB: Menopause: myths and realities. In: Stewart DE, Stotland NL (eds.): *Psychological Aspects of Women's Health Care: The Interface Between Psychiatry and Obstetrics and Gynecology*, pp. 227–248. Washington, DC, American Psychiatric Press, 1993.

Sherwin BB: Estrogenic effects on memory in women. *Ann N Y Acad Sci* 1994;743:213–231.

Sichel DA, Cohen, LS, Dimmock JA, et al.: Postpartum obsessive compulsive disorder: a case series. *J Clin Psychiatry* 1993a;54:156–159.

Sichel DA, Cohen LS, Rosenbaum JF, et al.: Postpartum onset of obsessive-compulsive disorder. *Psychosomatics* 1993b;34:277–279.

Smith S, Rinehart JS, Juddock VE, et al.: Treatment of premenstrual syndrome with alprazolam: results of a double-blind, placebo-controlled randomized crossover clinical trial. *Obstet Gynecol* 1987;70:37–43.

Spigset O, Carleborg L, Norstrom A, et al.: Paroxetine levels in breast milk [letter to the editor]. *J Clin Psychiatry* 1996;57:39.

Steiner M, Steinberg S, Stewart D, et al.: Fluoxetine in the treatment of premenstrual dysphoria. *N Engl J Med* 1995;332:1529–1534.

Steiner M, Wilkins A: Diagnosis and assessment of premenstrual dysphoria. *Psychiatric Annals* 1997;26:571–575.

Stewart DE, Stotland NL: *Psychological Aspects Of Women's Health Care: The Interface Between Psychiatry and Obstetrics and Gynecology*. Washington, DC, American Psychiatric Press, 1993.

Stone AB, Pearlstein TB, Brown WA: Fluoxetine in the treatment of late luteal phase dysphoric disorder. *J Clin Psychiatry* 1991;52:290–293.

Stotland NL: *Abortion Facts and Feelings: A Handbook for Women and the People Who Care About Them*. Washington, DC, American Psychiatric Press, 1998a.

Stotland NL: Abortion: Social context, psychodynamic implications. *Am J Psychiatry* 1998b;155:964–967.

Stotland NL, Harwood B: Social, political, legal considerations. In: Gold JH, Severino SK (eds.): *Premenstrual Dysphorias: Myths and Realities*, pp. 185–200. Washington, DC, American Psychiatric Press, 1994.

Tallmer M: Empty-nest syndrome: possibility or despair. In: Bernay T, Cantor DW (eds.): *The Psychology of Today's Woman*, pp. 231–252. Hillsdale, NJ, Analytic Press, 1986.

Vliet EL: *Screaming to be Heard: Hormonal Connections Women Suspect and Doctors Ignore*. New York, M Evans & Co, 1995.

Wisner KL, Perel JM, Findling RC: Antidepressant treatment during breast-feeding. *Am J Psychiatry* 1996;153:1132–1137.

Wood SH, Mortola JF, Chan YF, et al.: Treatment of premenstrual syndrome with fluoxetine: a double-blind, placebo-controlled, crossover study. *Obstet Gynecol* 1992;80:339–344.

Yonkers KA: Treatment of premenstrual dysphoric disorder. *Current Review of Mood Anxiety Disorders* 1997;1:215–237.

Yonkers KA, Brown WA: Pharmacologic treatments for premenstrual dysphoric disorder. *Psychiatric Annals* 1996;26:586–589.

Yonkers KA, Halbreich U, Freeman E, et al.: Symptomatic improvement of premenstrual dysphoric disorder with sertraline treatment: a randomized controlled trial. *JAMA* 1997;278:983–988.

Yoshida K, Smith B, Craggs M, et al.: Fluoxetine in breast milk and developmental outcome of breast-fed infants. *Br J Psychiatry* 1998;172:175–178.

Chapter 12

Psychosis

In 1996, psychiatrist Roberta J. Apfel wrote for an audience of obstetrician-gynecologists about the sudden but unrecognized onset of psychosis in her father after hip replacement surgery (Apfel, 1996). Hoping to increase recognition of a potentially treatable illness that can affect any person at any age (i.e., acute psychosis), she shared how her father's physician was highly attuned to the physical status of his patient but had totally missed the mental status changes that were evident to even the casual observer. Apfel's young children were quite aware that grandpa was "out of his mind" when he revealed visual hallucinations of being in the countryside rather than in a hospital. Naturally, Apfel was alarmed. Was his sudden deterioration the result of medication; had it been brought on by surgery; or was it evidence of some underlying, and threatening, disease process?

Apfel summarizes how severe mental illness can frequently be missed because physicians fail to take note of the obvious. They miss something "essential about the patient" that does not fit with their customary expectations. An emotional malady may not be the manifest reason that the patient seeks care, nor does it match our characteristic, more defined role in physical care. Making the diagnosis of psychosis—a break with reality frequently accompanied by delusions, hallucinations, incoherent speech, or bizarre actions—begins with "brief, matter-of-fact interchanges that can reveal something unusual. . . . Tuning in to the commonsense impression of the patient, then checking this impression with someone else who knows the patient, is the best way to recognize psychosis" (Apfel, 1996, p. 171).

These diagnostic caveats are indispensable cues for the primary care clinician working in an era of managed care. No longer are psychotic patients hospitalized for long periods in state or private facilities. Differential diagnosis of an acute psychotic illness may be undertaken by the primary care clinician, not necessarily by the specialist. Moreover, with the advent of effective pharmacologic and psychosocial interventions, many children and adults with psychotic illness are able to live within the community. Primary care clinicians are increasingly consulted to provide long-term care for these patients and their family members. Because these women face the habitual task of managing a menacing illness, they need both medical and psychological support to reinforce their sense that they are worthwhile human beings.

But providing care for the psychotic patient is often more easily talked about than done, more straightforward in medical texts than in actual clinical practice. Why is this the case? Family members wish to deny that there is a problem and often do not seek help until there is no alternative. Clinicians must make empathic leaps to grapple with the bewildering plight of family members burdened by the demands of a loved one with psychotic illness. The patient's world seems bizarre, even alien. Communication is challenging at best. Unless one has been faced with a similar situation in one's own family, it is easy to want not to face these seemingly inscrutable problems. After all, physicians share society's "moral repugnance" because "subliminally we may hear the leper's mourning cry, 'unclean, unclean,' when we behold the mentally ill" (Backlar, 1994, p. 14).

Inevitably, both the patient and her family feel disenfranchised and alone, hoping to find a haven for solace and safety but rarely encountering one. They come yearning for ideas to aid

> a grown-up child whose dependency binds and entwines the caretaker parent. Usually, the sympathetic parents may be aware that their adult child cannot properly care for herself or himself. They understand, only too well, that the disease has altered and inhibited their relative's ability to cope with the everyday business of life . . . helplessly, they may twist and turn through labyrinthine social services, watching their ill family member deteriorate. Confused, even disoriented, oftentimes the families feel they have lost their way in what they had believed to be the familiar territory of their everyday lives.
>
> (Backlar, 1994, pp. 14–15)

Fortunately, the identification of new therapeutic agents and greater understanding of the pathophysiology of psychosis offer better prospects for patients than ever before. Indeed, primary care clinicians usually consult psychiatrists because of the expanding repertoire of drugs from which to choose when treating psychosis. However, to determine correct diagnosis; to facilitate compliance with medication; and to offer comfort, reassurance, and information to families, it is incumbent on those on the front lines to stay involved in their patients' follow-up care. This chapter offers some brief guidelines to help primary care clinicians deal with psychotic patients and their family members. As more patients are treated in the community and along a continuum of care, the number of psychotic patients in one's practice is likely to grow. Emphasis is placed on how to help women who have a spouse, child, parent, or sibling with psychosis and how to address the special challenges of the psychotic patient during her childbearing years.

IMPORTANCE OF EARLY RECOGNITION

The ease of access and the nonstigmatizing nature of primary care make it the logical point of entry for services for many psychotic persons (Burns, 1996). Family and friends find that they can turn to their primary care clinician with concerns they have about the patient. A mother may confide her worries about the social withdrawal or oddness of her child; such a pattern of behavior may be the initial clue to the insidious onset of schizophrenia. Patients with a well-established psychotic illness may approach the primary care clinician with non-specific emotional complaints, somatization, anxiety, and so forth. Any of these conditions can herald the first telltale symptoms of relapse (Neuman et al., 1995; Strathdee and Kendrick, 1996).

A prodromal phase of several years usually precedes the active phase of psychosis. This stage frequently is characterized by social withdrawal, impaired role functioning, peculiar behavior, or neglect of personal hygiene and grooming (Table 12–1). An "active phase" is defined when psychotic symptoms (e.g.,

---

Table 12–1. **Recognizing Early (Prodromal) Symptoms of Psychosis**

Deterioration in role functioning
Heightened social withdrawal
Sleep disturbance
Irritability
Depression or anxiety
Paranoia, magical thinking, or suspiciousness
Bizarre physical complaints that do not remit by reassurance
Bizarre behavior, thinking, or speech patterns (e.g., a relative, friend, or member
   of your office staff may be the first to observe the patient acting peculiar)
Disturbed communications

---

delusions, hallucinations, incoherence, catatonic behavior) become prominent (Lieberman, 1997). Although many patients recover from this initial episode, the majority experience one or more subsequent recurrences, from which they do not return to their prior level of premorbid functioning (Burns, 1996).

Initiating treatment for patients who experience their first episode of schizophrenia is critical to improving their quality of life. Antipsychotic drugs ameliorate the putative toxic effects of psychosis and thereby have a beneficial effect on the course of illness and on patient outcome. The sooner that treatment begins, the better the long-term prognosis (Kuipers, 1996).

MAKING THE DIAGNOSIS

The psychotic patient's first contact with the health care team typically begins at the emergency room door. This acute situation may be manifested by symptoms such as hallucinations, delusions, disorganized thinking, or violent behavior. Treatment must be tailored to address the positive, negative, and cognitive symptoms that are central features of schizophrenia (Table 12–2). Distractability, poor memory, slow reaction time, and attentional dysfunction are some of the functional consequences of the neurocognitive deficits; intervention with newer

---

Table 12–2. **Psychotic Symptoms**

Positive symptoms	Neurocognitive symptoms
Hallucinations	Memory deficits
Delusions, often bizarre or persecutory	Generalized cognitive dysfunction
Disorganized speech	Deficits in verbal IQ and arithmetic
Disorganized behavior/catatonia	Slowed reaction time
Inappropriate affect	Impaired "executive tasks" involving
Negative symptoms	planning and problem solving
Blunted emotions	Neurological "soft signs": diminished
Poor motivation	motor speed, coordination, and
Social withdrawal/isolation	sequencing, reflecting involvement
Poor grooming and hygiene	in frontal/subcortical circuitry
Poverty of speech	
Apathy/lack of energy or initiative	

(atypical) neuroleptics in the early stages may promote improved functional and cognitive abilities (Carpenter, 1997; Flashman et al., 1996; Green, 1996; Harvey and Keefe, 1997; Serper and Chou, 1997). The positive and negative symptoms appear to act independently of one another and to respond to different psychopharmacologic approaches (Carpenter, 1997; Munich, 1997; Tollefson, 1997).

The primary care clinician's role centers on helping to stabilize the patient who decompensates or who has a relapse or an exacerbation of illness. Ensuring safety, containing dangerous behavior, and using antipsychotic medications to minimize disruption in the patient's life are priorities after a thorough medical evaluation. Long-term psychotherapeutic and pharmacologic management is usually best left in the hands of a specialist.

The clinician must first determine whether the current episode of psychosis is primarily psychiatric or organic (Table 12–3). A detailed physical and neurologic

---

Table 12–3. **Organic Causes of Psychosis**

Metabolic disorders
  Cardiac, hepatic, renal, respiratory
    failure
  Fluid electrolyte imbalance
  Hyper/hypoglycemia
  Porphyria
  Wilson's disease
Nutritional deficiencies
  Starvation
  B_1, B_6, B_{12} deficiency
Endocrine disorders
  Hyper/hypothyroidism
  Hyper/hypoparathyroidism
  Cushing's disease
  Addison's disease
  Panhypopituitarism
Central nervous system disorders
  Cerebrovascular disease
  Delirium/dementia
  Head trauma
  Tumors
  Central nervous system infection
  Huntington's chorea
  Multiple sclerosis
  Seizure disorder/postictal states
  Normal-pressure hydrocephalus
Infectious diseases
  Syphilis
  Human immunodeficiency virus infection
  Lyme disease (neuroborreliosis)
  Cytomegalovirus
  Herpes simplex
  Urinary tract or respiratory infection
    (especially in the elderly population)

Drugs of abuse
  Alcohol
  Barbiturates
  Amphetamines
  PCP
  Cocaine
Other causes
  Anesthesia
  Antidepressants (tricyclics,
    monoamine oxidase inhibitors,
    tetracyclics)
  Antihypertensive agents
  Amantadine
  Aminophylline
  Beta-blockers
  Bromides
  Bromocriptine
  Cephalosporins
  Cimetidine
  Digitalis
  Disulfiram
  Ergotamine
  Ibuprofen
  Insulin
  Indomethacin
  Lidocaine
  L-Dopa
  Methotrexate
  Naproxen
  Oral hypoglycemic agents
  Procainamide
  Rifampin
  Tetracycline
  Vancomycin

examination, along with a complete blood count, liver and thyroid function tests, renal function tests, and urine toxicology, is essential (Kuipers, 1996; Stein et al., 1996). Most of the time, differential diagnosis is not easy because symptoms of psychosis are not specific to any particular psychiatric disorder. Schizophrenia, bipolar disorder, and major depression may all present with the same symptoms; it is therefore essential to obtain an extensive family history. Differential diagnosis can often be made only after long-term follow-up and specialty consultation.

WHAT TO DO FIRST

Safety is the primary issue in determining whether to hospitalize an acutely psychotic patient. Given the recent trend for decreasing lengths of stay, alternatives such as partial hospitalization, halfway houses, and day treatment centers are being developed as cost-effective alternatives to hospitalization. Primary care clinicians who treat acutely psychotic patients therefore must become aware of local community programs. Structured living situations in particular make it easier to avert suicide (Table 12–4).

Table 12–4. **Roles of the Primary Care Clinician in Management of Psychotic Patients**

---

1. Provide early recognition. Psychosis is underestimated and frequently goes unrecognized.
2. Rule out organic causes.
3. Assess whether the patient is dangerous to self or others; establish a safe environment.
4. Offer psychosocial support and pharmacotherapy, especially when a specialist is not readily available.
5. Provide continuum of care, particularly overseeing the patient's medical needs.
6. Offer hope, support, and reassurance; talk about the benefits of medication and psychotherapy to patient and family.
7. Counter the stigma and isolation of family members by discussing mental illness openly; empathize with the burden *each* family member feels, not just the desperate patient.
8. Encourage family members in their own self-care; emphasize the need for periods of rest or respite care.
9. Help both patient and family to develop a relapse prevention plan and to learn the early warning signs of relapse. Many patients have a specific recurrent symptom that heralds relapse (e.g., social withdrawal, days without sleep).
10. Work as an integral part of the health care team in managing the patient's long-term illness; collaborate with a psychiatrist, particularly to institute any new antipsychotic medication and to manage side effects.
11. Underscore the need for both patient and family to become advocates for themselves, learning all they can about illness and joining groups such as the National Alliance for the Mentally Ill (NAMI).
12. In addition to making sure patient and family members benefit from new psychoeducational tools, encourage them to take advantage of individual or group psychotherapy; everyone needs a place to address their fears and losses and to learn new ways to cope.

Hospitalization is sometimes essential to ensure medication compliance and to institute life-affirming psychosocial activities. Shortened length of stays are of particular concern for patients who do not immediately respond to treatment; they have a higher risk of being readmitted soon after discharge than do those who respond more quickly to initial therapy. In addition, they are reluctant to engage in the different facets of treatment and tend to have a higher chance of deteriorating (Buckley et al., 1996; Wyatt, 1995).

WHAT NOT TO DO

With the patient, be firm and tactful. A paranoid patient may be hostile and suspicious. Addressing anxiety with the empathic response, "It must be very troubling for you to have so many worries," or "I know you believe what you are saying, and I would like to talk to you about it" work better than attempting "to pluck out irrational delusions with tweezers of logic" (Mayerson, 1976, p. 166).

A withdrawn or floridly psychotic schizophrenic person can be approached by someone who is concrete and specific. Greet the patient by name, explain examinations simply, and keep the visit brief. Making challenging remarks and confronting the delusional system rarely lead to a good alliance.

WORKING WITH FAMILY MEMBERS

Listen carefully to the family's specific concerns. Remember that it may take months, even years, for families to work through their denial of the problem. (Denial is an expectable defense and not a sign of failure on the part of the clinician.) Encourage family members to learn all they can about the illness. Groups such as the National Alliance for the Mentally Ill (NAMI) are enormously helpful in providing information and emotional support. By recommending such groups and openly discussing the effects of illness, you make coping infinitely easier for families. They will be comforted by your attempts to make the unspeakable speakable. Education is essential to helping patients and families learn to live with psychosis and thereby prevent relapse.

WHY DOES MY PATIENT GET SAD AS SHE GETS BETTER?

Patients also need help in dealing with a reduction in psychotic symptoms. Those who respond well to antipsychotic medication are sometimes faced with a new and ironic challenge: learning to deal not only with the loss of familiar symptoms but also with the insight that they are facing a potentially severe, often lifelong, illness. The sadness that accompanies isolation yields to resignation when the patient must deal with many losses and the resurfacing of anger. Although it is not an easy task, reiterating that improvement brings about a change in the patient's sense of identity can be enormously supportive.

Here lies *a major contrast between caring for the physically ill and caring for the mentally ill.* When you restore physical health, you give something *back* to the patient. But when you treat an emotional problem, you take something away—something often perceived as precious and salutary, even though it is a symptom causing pain or rendering havoc. After all, the psychotic patient's perception is that her symptoms constitute her personal identity—her sense of self. For example, one patient remarked that even though she was getting better, she missed the vibrancy of her terrifying world. Normalcy required her to no longer experience the trees as swaying and glistening as she "saw and heard" them poignantly call out for her to caress them ritualistically. Small wonder that, to adjust to her new sense of reality, this patient mourned the loss of an essential part of her being.

GENDER DIFFERENCES

Recent studies of schizophrenia have demonstrated that men and women exhibit important differences in age of onset, premorbid characteristics, course of disease, response to treatment, and antipsychotic drug side effects. Hormonal and neurochemical factors during puberty may be at the root of these differences.

Female sex hormones cause the brain to mature earlier, making it more resistant to possible trauma during birth. Birth trauma may play an important etiologic role in the later development of schizophrenia in those who are genetically vulnerable.

The onset of schizophrenia occurs approximately 4 to 6 years earlier in men than in women. The disorder usually erupts during the critical developmental stage of late adolescence, which may explain the superior outcome seen in women with schizophrenia during the first 10 years of their illness. When onset occurs in the teenage years, it produces a cascade of effects. These include an interruption of cognitive and affective development, a disruption in interpersonal relationships, and insufficient growth and integration of premorbid strengths. All these effects result in substantial impact on the individual and portend a turbulent course of illness, particularly when treatment is not initiated.

Schizophrenia in women is characterized by more mood symptoms than those faced by men. Clinicians tend to diagnose the illness in women late, but by the age of 45 years the prevalence of the disorder in both sexes is essentially identical. New-onset schizophrenia (after age 50) almost always occurs in women and is probably the result of the hormonal changes ushered in by menopause (Perry et al., 1995; Seeman, 1995).

The course of the disorder also varies between the sexes. Women fare better in the initial years but deteriorate postmenopausally, requiring more medication, more hospitalizations, and more social service interventions. Compared to women, male patients tend to be more aggressive and to commit suicide at a higher rate; these traits are possibly related to male hormones (Szymanski, 1996; Szymanski et al., 1995). It has been hypothesized that the antidopaminergic effects of estrogen provide women with some protection during periods of vulnerability to schizophrenia (Cowell et al., 1996). The rate of age-related deterioration of brain dopamine receptors is slower in women than in men. This discrepancy may explain why women need to continue antipsychotic medication for as many as 10 years longer than men (Seeman, 1995).

Circulating hormones affect many body systems; all together, these influence antipsychotic drug response. For example, slower gastric emptying time in women results in a gradual onset of action of oral medication. Likewise, because women have a slower absorption rate than men, there are fewer instances of acute dystonia with the initiation of antipsychotic medication. This relative absence of acute effects is one factor implicated in the greater medication compliance of women. Furthermore, because antipsychotic agents are highly lipophilic, these drugs are stored longer in women because of their greater proportion of body fat. Women are thus protected longer from relapse when the drugs are discontinued or when their compliance is poor (Seeman, 1995; Szymanski, 1996).

Because of the putative antipsychotic action of estrogen, premenopausal women generally require lower doses of antipsychotic medication than do men of comparable age. A decline in estrogen levels has been linked to a worsening of psychosis. For example, exacerbation of schizophrenia is seen in premenstrual women (a time of lower estrogen). In addition, women appear to have fewer episodes of relapse during pregnancy, a time of high estrogen levels (Cohen et al., 1989).

Women have faster cerebral blood flow than men, which means that more of the medication reaches the actual target site. Both antipsychotic medications and estrogen are antidopaminergic. At menopause, when estrogen levels fall, estrogen withdrawal elicits withdrawal dyskinesia. This reaction is analogous to tardive dyskinesia, which emerges when antipsychotic doses are reduced. This phenomenon helps explain the greater prevalence of later-occurring, drug-related dyskinesias in older women. Although current practice guidelines are the same for both sexes, it may be that drug doses should vary in women according to their menstrual cycle and as they traverse the climacteric period (Seeman, 1995; Szymanski, 1996; Szymanski et al., 1995).

USE OF ANTIPSYCHOTIC AGENTS

Regardless of the particular antipsychotic agent, the time required to bring an episode into remission can be lengthy. Getting patients to comply with a treatment regimen is a major source of concern. Medications are often changed because of side effects and the need to increase compliance. Women are prone to certain side effects and symptoms as a result of taking antipsychotic medications (Table 12–5). To maintain a good treatment alliance, be sure to ask about these and other, non-gender-specific effects. Address any problems that are interfering with taking the drug. Patients must get used to taking medication

---

Table 12–5. **Physical Symptoms Secondary to Antipsychotic Medications**

Breast engorgement, pain, cysts, galactorrhea
Dyspareunia, decreased lubrication, and decreased sexual desire
Urinary frequency/hesitancy
Anorgasmia
Vaginitis
Amenorrhea, oligomenorrhea, menorrhagia
Early menopause
Increased incidence of tardive dyskinesia with age
Increased incidence of dystonia and akathisia

and must be reassured that the best medication specifically for them will be found (Casey, 1997; Spohn and Strauss, 1989).

CONSIDERATIONS FOR TREATMENT OF ACUTE PSYCHOSIS

The primary care clinician should refer to texts and contemporary treatment algorithms when a psychotic patient must be treated long term. These materials present the most common short-term and long term side effects, offer advice about when to modify or change an antipsychotic, and review innovative approaches (see Frances et al., 1996; Zarate et al., 1995). The following suggestions are made for the primary care clinician who must bring acute psychotic symptoms under rapid control and may not have the support of a psychiatrist to help manage immediate behavioral problems.

The initial aim of treatment should be sedation and behavioral control; the clinician's goal is to ensure the safety of the patient, her family, and others in her immediate environment, particularly clinic staff. Currently, most authorities suggest using a combination of a neuroleptic and a benzodiazepine. Benzodiazepines can be quite calming for agitated patients, and they tend to lessen the need for a larger amount of antipsychotic medication (Munich, 1997). The side effects that lead many patients to stop taking medication or that otherwise cause initial discomfort are therefore minimized.

One common combination is haloperidol (Haldol), 2 to 5 mg intramuscular, and lorazepam (Ativan), 1 to 2 mg intramuscular. Haloperidol may also be given intravenously. Another option is perphenazine, 5 to 10 mg intramuscularly every 4 to 6 hours, particularly in patients at risk for acute dystonic reactions. In general, only one or two injections are necessary before switching to oral medication. Usually, the benzodiazepine can be tapered quickly, with a shift to antipsychotic medication in divided doses throughout the day.

Still another option is to prescribe the elixir preparations thioridazine (Mellaril), 50 to 100 mg by mouth, or chlorpromazine (Thorazine), 50 to 200 mg by mouth. The latter medication is particularly useful when a sedating effect is desired (Schwartz and Hughes, 1996).

With the advent of new atypical neuroleptics, one option is to use risperidone (Risperdal) in combination with a benzodiazepine. Risperidone tends to have fewer extrapyramidal side effects than other antipsychotics, and the benzodiazepine works to sedate the patient quickly. Although this combination tends to be less sedating overall and requires a patient who is willing to take oral medication, it appears to work well in a variety of clinical settings. The average dose of risperidone is 6 to 8 mg per day, divided into several daily doses. In emergencies, risperidone should be initiated at 1 mg twice a day, then increased to 2 mg twice a day.

Some authorities suggest that risperidone may be particularly helpful for aggressive or hostile patients. Concomitantly, it is important to remember that benzodiazepines, although they can be very useful, tend to cause disinhibition in some patients. The acutely psychotic patient must therefore be monitored closely.

Avoid using two different antipsychotic medications in the same patient; this practice greatly exacerbates the potential for toxicity and side effects. If the patient does not respond to initial emergency measures, specialty consultation should be sought immediately. Other medications, particularly divalproex sodium or electroconvulsive therapy, should be considered in treating a refractory psychotic episode.

PATIENT AND FAMILY GUIDELINES FOR COPING WITH PSYCHOSIS

1. Learn all you can about the illness. Understanding all you can about your own or your loved one's illness will help you to develop realistic expectations and to cope with undeniable problems. Patients and family members who manage best tend to develop an accepting attitude and realistic expectations for both themselves and the ill person and therefore can handle inevitable crises with resolve and fortitude.

2. Find new ways of managing symptoms. Develop new coping skills. Many patients with psychotic illness are prone to feeling misunderstood and criticized. Learn to deal with situations that arise without criticizing yourself or your loved one. A high level of warmth, a sense of humor, and the ability to stay calm during times of difficulty have all been associated with a better chance of recovery. Becoming involved in meaningful activities and having a daily structure are also important. Despite some persistent disabilities or problems, most patients are independent and can perform their adult roles. Be sure to read about the "success stories" of other consumers who have overcome their illnesses. They provide inspiration that having a successful family and work life are reasonable and attainable goals for many (see Resources for Patients and Family Members).

3. Become familiar with the early signs of relapse. Each patient has her own unique warning signs that indicate relapse. Some worry all the time, others have difficulty sleeping, and others become socially withdrawn or have a recurrence of bizarre thoughts or sensations. Seek additional support from your health care team at this time; often a full-blown episode can be avoided. Most of all, do not lose your sense of perspective. Remember that relapses are a part of your illness and not a sign of failure. Comply with treatment. Try to accept new recommendations from your physician. Research has determined that those patients who do best tend to stick with treatment. They comply with the medication that works for them. If they develop side effects from medication, they tell their health care team instead of keeping it secret or stopping the medication on their own.

4. As much as possible, avoid the use of alcohol or illicit drugs. These can rapidly worsen your condition because of their effects on the brain.

5. Take threats of suicide or any warning signs of suicide very seriously. Seek help immediately.

6. If you are a caregiver, be sure to take care of yourself. Avoid isolation. Make sure that you have times of respite or vacations. You can do no good for either yourself or your loved one if you become beleaguered or burned out. Turning to support groups in your community can be quite valuable, as can reading about how others have dealt with the illness. These "friends at a

distance" can be real reservoirs of hope and can provide concrete tools for you to use in coping with the many vicissitudes and challenges of the illness in your loved one.

7. Above all else, maintain a sense of hopefulness about long-term gains. Psychosis is more treatable than ever. Stigma still exists, and some people will attempt to make you feel badly about having a mental illness or a family member with a mental illness. But there is much good literature showing that these disorders are biologically based. Psychosocial therapies can be most helpful, and newer medications also are making magnificent inroads on symptoms. Most patients do improve significantly with treatment. Face down the old myth that parents, especially mothers, cause mental illness. Reducing symptoms and improving overall outcome is the goal of the new pharmacotherapy.

ADDITIONAL GUIDELINES FOR PRIMARY CARE CLINICIANS

1. Emphasize the importance of drug treatment for the patient and family (Borison, 1995; Ereshefsky, 1995). It makes sense for the primary care clinician to become familiar with one or two conventional antipsychotic medications in order to intervene with an acutely agitated patient. A working knowledge of other types of antipsychotics can also be important if you have several families in your practice who have been affected by schizophrenia or another form of psychosis.

2. Seek consultation from a specialist who is familiar with the repertoire of antipsychotic drugs. The number of available and useful medications is rapidly expanding. Newer antipsychotic agents provide additional choices. They have unique side effect profiles that differ from those of conventional drugs and also from each other (Casey, 1997; Rotrosen and Adler, 1995). Tapering a patient with chronic illness and poor prognosis from a traditional antipsychotic (e.g., haloperidol) to an atypical antipsychotic agent (e.g., olanzapine; quetiapine) may provide better control and fewer side effects, and can engender hope. The use of these new antipsychotic agents must be individualized (Jibson and Tandon, 1996).

3. Be alert for the possibility of suicide. *As many as 1 in 10 schizophrenic patients eventually commits suicide.* Encourage the patient and family members whenever possible to have a plan in place should suicidal thinking develop. Take any threats very seriously. Should the patient have a suicidal crisis, underscore that suicidal thinking is a symptom of an acute phase of the illness that will probably pass in time as the treatment takes hold. Tell the patient that her life is important to you and that her death would be a tremendous loss, not a relief (Frances et al., 1996).

4. Be sure to ask about sexual functioning. The majority of patients of both sexes who take antipsychotic medications experience significant sexual dysfunction. Some patients even discontinue medication because it tends to interfere with sexual desire and orgasm. Sexual side effects can sometimes be reversed by choosing atypical antipsychotics or by reducing the dose of conventional antipsychotics. The effects of antipsychotic medication on sex-

ual functioning appear to be mediated by complex interactions involving the sympathetic, parasympathetic, dopaminergic, noradrenergic, and serotonergic systems. Inform patients that treatment is available for dealing with sexual issues.

5. Recommend psychosocial interventions. Daily structure and individual therapy can be particularly helpful. As noted, psychotic patients are faced with anxiety and depression when they come face to face with their illness, their losses, and questions about their future. Employment issues and family relationships must not be neglected. Families and patients should also be encouraged to take advantage of psychoeducational groups and classes available at most community mental health centers (Penn and Mueser, 1996). Psychosis is a terrifying experience. Psychotherapy provides an opportunity for the patient to form a healthy relationship within which she can communicate her central problems and develop the capacity "to think realistically . . . as time goes by" (Karon and Teixeira, 1995, p. 101). Empirical evidence demonstrates that psychotherapy has a dramatic effect for many patients, reducing thought disorder, lowering rehospitalization rates, improving overall adjustment to life, and even decreasing the amount of medication necessary to control symptoms in some cases (Karon and Teixeira, 1995).

6. Emphasize the importance of reducing stress to cope with illness. Patients and family members must learn to take care of themselves and do the things they enjoy. Family members must learn to care for their relatives without feeling total and complete responsibility for the illness. Supporting the family by suggesting psychotherapy has the advantage of helping family members establish realistic boundaries between themselves and the ill person. It also promotes good self-care, which has the parallel effect of helping the patient.

7. Be a source of hopefulness. When treated effectively, most patients soon recover from an acute episode of psychosis. The physician has an opportunity to make a powerful therapeutic intervention by discussing how more and more patients are being helped by new medications and psychosocial treatment. Although most patients do have at least some residual symptoms that affect their lives, they are still capable of having meaningful careers and raising families.

8. Address adequacy of delivery of care. In geographically isolated areas where trained clinicians are scarce, the risks increase for medication noncompliance, comorbidity, and relapse. Innovative programs such as interactive computer networks, telephone peer support, and care extenders can sometimes fill the gaps in the daily care of such patients. Clinicians should also encourage patients and families to make use of existing social support systems, such as school, church, or community support groups (Penn and Mueser, 1996; Strathdee and Kendrick, 1996).

GUIDELINES FOR TREATING PREGNANT AND POSTPARTUM PATIENTS

1. The risks and benefits of antipsychotic agents in the pregnant patient must be weighed in each individual case. Many clinicians are reluctant to prescribe

antipsychotics because of concerns about the fetus. However, women with chronic psychotic illness are at high risk for relapse if antipsychotic medication is withdrawn during pregnancy.

2. Most authorities believe that continuing antipsychotic treatment usually outweighs the risk to the fetus. A patient with a long history of psychosis who has been well maintained on antipsychotic medication and decompensates when it is discontinued should continue taking medication before, during, and after pregnancy (Cohen et al., 1989).

3. The postpartum period is a particularly high-risk one for women with a past history of psychotic illness or mood disorder. Encourage the use of psychosocial supports in addition to psychotropic medication at this time (see Chapters 2, 3, and 11).

4. Antipsychotic drug therapy without alteration can be maintained through labor and delivery. Incidents of neonatal complications, including jaundice, are infrequent. A more likely problem is a recurrence of psychosis if the drug is tapered off before delivery.

5. No special monitoring is required for the pregnant patient with psychosis. In general, however, increasing the dose of antipsychotic medication should be avoided whenever possible. To date, there is less experience with clozapine and risperidone than with older medications such as haloperidol during pregnancy.

6. Remember that the puerperium is a time of highest risk for the onset of mental illness. Women who have never been psychotic may become so (Apfel, 1996). The diagnosis of psychosis can be missed if the primary care clinician is attuned only to the physical needs of the mother and baby. Be alert to any changes in mood, inability to care for the baby, paranoia, or unkempt appearance. By all means, offer the patient as many psychosocial supports as possible at this high-risk time.

7. Discussions about contraception are an essential part of comprehensive treatment. The primary care clinician should discuss birth control methods with the patient to help her see this option as a possibility. Remind the patient that she has the right to make choices; in the past, a patriarchal approach on the part of physicians heightened patients' fears and increased their reluctance to use birth control (e.g., fear of sterilization) (Apfel, 1996, p. 173). Although some women with mental illness are not reliable about taking daily hormonal contraceptive pills, they may agree to other methods.

SUMMARY

The primary care clinician plays a central role in recognizing and caring for patients with psychosis. Early detection, addressing shame caused by illness, focusing on the stressors faced by family members, providing medical treatment, and staying involved over the long haul are some of the unique opportunities of working with this challenging patient group.

Although women with psychotic illness tend to have later onset and a more benign course of illness than do men, their treatment also raises complications, particularly during pregnancy and in the postpartum period. Female patients who have a parent, sibling, partner, or child with a psychotic illness frequently turn to the primary care clinician for advice. This possibility necessitates a general awareness of available community supports, ways to enhance coping strategies, and techniques for helping women feel empowered to deal with their illness (e.g., reading books, joining NAMI).

Because new psychotropic medications and methods of psychosocial support are rapidly evolving, working with a specialist is recommended whenever possible. Practical guidelines, such as learning how to use one or two antipsychotic agents, are outlined in this chapter to aid the primary care clinician in intervening early and successfully. The importance of assessing safety and suicidality while helping the patient more willingly accept treatment is briefly reviewed.

Care of patients with psychotic illnesses and their family members can be rewarding for both you and your staff. Your sense of hope, forbearance, and knowledge of available and potential treatment modalities is salutary balm for those human beings whose lives have been shaken and marginalized through no fault of their own.

Resources for Patients and Family Members

In previous chapters, a clearer distinction could be made between literature intended for a lay and for a professional audience. Clinicians who have in their practice one or more families touched by psychosis, particularly schizophrenia, will be moved and better informed by the humanitarian perspective and impressive knowledge base provided in any of these books. Although references particularly applicable to family members have been singled out, the professional's careful reading of any one of the following texts will expand skill and understanding in helping the psychotic patient and her family members.

Mueser KT, Gingerich S: *Coping with Schizophrenia: A Guide for Families.* Oakland, CA, New Harbinger, 1994.

This readable, detailed, practical workbook describes the symptoms, treatments, and course of schizophrenia. Especially useful are sections geared toward helping family members cope with the day-to-day manifestations of the illness (e.g., improving personal hygiene) and periods of relapse. Lists of strategies aid the patient and family member in managing unavoidable stressors and persistent symptoms. Special sections address comorbid depression, anxiety, and drug and alcohol abuse. Of particular note are suggestions on how to prevent and respond to crises, improve skills for communication, and help the patient with social, interpersonal, and vocational needs.

Secunda V: *When Madness Comes Home: Help and Hope for the Children, Siblings, and Partners of the Mentally Ill.* New York, Hyperion, 1997.

The sister of this award-winning author has had a long struggle with severe mental illness. The author's firsthand experience was a motivating factor in writing this book to bring comfort and understanding to "the walking wounded"—family members of the mentally ill. This unique vantage point helps her address the questions, burdens, and challenges faced daily by family members. Secunda blends the expert opinion of mental health professionals with the unique, authoritative voice of family members themselves. Although her book is laced with practical tips, its greatest strength lies in the hopeful perspective that life can be rich, worthwhile, and positively transformed despite inevitable loss and suffering. Secunda stresses that family members must take care of their own needs, which ultimately aids the designated patient. She demonstrates how those who may be initially "shattered" by having a mentally ill family member can ultimately find meaning and enhance personal growth. In this way, they "make their devastating experience count for something" as they "transfer their sorrows into causes for hope" (p. 296).

Torrey EF: *Surviving Schizophrenia: A Manual for Families, Consumers, and Providers,* 3rd ed. New York, Harper, 1995.

This update of a classic manual summarizes the most important changes in schizophre- nia research and how they have influenced contemporary treatment and rehabilitation. Torrey's discussion is comprehensive and erudite, addressing the major theories about what causes schizophrenia, its prognosis, and its course. Although sharply critical of some psychosocial perspectives and of society's serious neglect of the mentally ill, Torrey remains committed to understanding the patient's plight—and his grasp of it is unparalleled. He answers the most frequently asked questions by consumers and their families and provides advice about how to become an empowered advocate. Also outlined are the salient ingredients of any individualized treatment plan (e.g., medica- tion, job skills training, acquisition of interpersonal skills).

Resources for Clinicians

Backlar P: *The Family Face of Schizophrenia: Practical Counsel from America's Leading Experts.* New York, Putnam, 1994.

The seven chapters of this book are personal accounts of patients and their families who faced the special problems inherent in having a severe mental illness. Topics include the challenges of daily life with a person with schizophrenia, strengths and weaknesses of the mental health system, suicide prevention, violence, and commitment and other legal issues. Special sections address the unique struggles of single parents and adult children. Each absorbing story is complemented by commentary from a mental health professional whose expertise lies in the specific problem area being addressed. Although the book offers no easy answers, it does provide insight and realistic counsel about how the illness can be managed—with considerable success—over the long term.

Frances A, Docherty JP, Kahn DA: *Treatment of schizophrenia: The expert consensus guideline series. J Clin Psychiatry* 1996;57(Suppl 12B):7–58.

These guidelines are written primarily with the psychiatrist in mind but may be useful for primary care clinicians or care extenders when specialty referral is unavailable. Executive summaries highlight essential somatic, psychosocial, and pharmacologic modalities. Algorithms outlining drug choices during acute psychotic episodes and for continuation and maintenance treatments are state of the art. Special sections ad- dressing the nuances of medical evaluation, medication side effects, and titration of dosages of conventional and new antipsychotics are valuable for clinicians who have a number of patients with schizophrenia in their practice. The fundamental "Guide for Patients and Families" can be copied and distributed in a variety of practice settings.

Hatfield AG, Lefley HP: *Surviving Mental Illness: Stress, Coping, and Adaptation.* New York, Guilford Press, 1993.

If your goal is to empathize with the patient's experience of psychosis and her attempt to cope with underlying impaired judgment, reasoning, and cognitive processes, this book will prove an exceptional guide. The authors include insights from three consum- ers (i.e., former patients) who have been seriously mentally ill but nevertheless found ways to manage their illness, develop a stable identity, find purpose in life, and avoid relapse. Particularly powerful are sections that describe how the patients themselves experienced their health care; suggestions are made about how to make the system, including general medicine, more customer friendly and receptive to the mentally ill. Clinicians who provide knowledge about the illness and its treatment help the patient to cope with stigma by discussing adaptive strategies. They model a belief in the potential for recovery and resiliency—essential agents of growth and change for this afflicted population.

Munich RL: *Contemporary treatment of schizophrenia. Bull Menninger Clin* 1997;61:189–221.

In just a few pages, Dr. Munich reviews recent advances in neuroscience that have led to greater understanding and sophisticated treatment for schizophrenia. Practical treatment methods are briefly reviewed, including treatment of the acute, subacute, and convalescent phases of illness; drug therapies for the nonresponder; an overview of supportive psychotherapy; group modalities; family treatment; psychoeducation; rehabilitation efforts; and treatment settings (e.g., hospital, residential treatment, alternatives to hospitalization). The primary care clinician who wants to learn more about the neurobiology, psychopharmacology, and psychotherapy of psychosis in a compact but thorough fashion could find no better guide.

References

Apfel RJ: Recognizing psychosis. *Primary Care Update for OB-GYNS* 1996;3:171–175.

Backlar P: *The Family Face of Schizophrenia: Practical Counsel from America's Leading Experts.* New York, Putnam, 1994.

Borison RL: Introduction: new antipsychotic treatments of schizophrenia. *Psychiatr Ann* 1995;25:283–284.

Buckley PE, Buchanan RW, Schulz SC, et al.: Catching Up on Schizophrenia: The Fifth International Congress on Schizophrenia Research, Warm Springs, VA, April 8–12, 1995. *Arch Gen Psychiatry* 1996;53:456–462.

Burns T: Early detection of psychosis in primary care: initial treatment and crisis management. In: Kendrick T, Tylee A, Freeling P (eds.): *The Prevention of Mental Illness in Primary Care,* pp. 246–263. Cambridge, England, Cambridge University Press, 1996.

Carpenter WT: Understanding the concepts of negative symptoms. *J Clin Psychiatry* 1997;15:12–15.

Casey DE: The relationship of pharmacology to side effects. *J Clin Psychiatry* 1997;58(Suppl 10):55–62.

Cohen LS, Alshuler L, Heller VL, et al.: Psychotropic drug use in pregnancy. *Psychosomatics* 1989;30:25–33.

Cowell PE, Kostianovsky DJ, Gur RC, et al.: Sex differences in neuroanatomical and clinical correlations in schizophrenia. *Am J Psychiatry* 1996;153:799–805.

Ereshefsky L: Treatment strategies for schizophrenia. *Psychiatr Ann* 1995;25:285–296.

Flashman LA, Flaum M, Gupta S, et al.: Soft signs and neuropsychological performance in schizophrenia. *Am J Psychiatry* 1996;153:526–532.

Frances A, Docherty JP, Kahn DA: Treatment of schizophrenia: the expert consensus guideline series. *J Clin Psychiatry* 1996;57(Suppl 12B): 7–58.

Green MF: What are the functional consequences of neurocognitive deficits in schizophrenia? *Am J Psychiatry* 1996;153:321–330.

Harvey PD, Keefe RS: Cognitive impairment in schizophrenia and implications of atypical neuroleptic treatment. *CNS Spectrums: Int J Neuropsychiatr Med* 1997;2:41–55.

Hatfield AG, Lefley HP: *Surviving Mental Illness: Stress, Coping, and Adaptation.* New York, Guilford Press, 1993.

Jibson MD, Tandon R: A summary of research findings on the new antipsychotic drugs. *Psychiatry Forum* 1996;16:i–viii.

Karon BP, Teixeira MA: Psychoanalytic therapy of schizophrenia. In: Barber JP, Crits-Christoph P (eds.): *Dynamic Therapies for Psychiatric Disorders (Axis I),* pp. 84–130. New York, Basic Books, 1995.

Kuipers E: The prevention of social disability in schizophrenia. In: Kendrick T, Tylee A, Freeling P (eds.): *The Prevention of Mental Illness in Primary Care,* pp. 327–345. Cambridge, England, Cambridge University Press, 1996.

Lieberman JA: Factors that influence the outcome of first-episode schizophrenia. *J Clin Psychiatry* 1997;15:2–4.

Mayerson EW: *Putting the Ill at Ease.* Hagerstown, MD, Harper & Row, 1976.

Mueser KT, Gingerich S: *Coping with Schizophrenia: A Guide for Families.* Oakland, CA, New Harbinger, 1994.

Munich RL: Contemporary treatment of schizophrenia. *Bull Menninger Clin* 1997;61:189–221.

Neuman CS, Grimes K, Walker EF, et al.: Developmental pathways to schizophrenia: behavioral subtypes. *J Abnorm Psychol* 1995;104:558–566.

Penn DL, Mueser KT: Research update on the psychosocial treatment of schizophrenia. *Am J Psychiatry* 1996;153:607–617.

Perry W, Moore D, Braff D: Gender differences on thought disturbance measures among schizophrenic patients. *Am J Psychiatry* 1995;152(9):1298–1301.

Rotrosen J, Adler L: The importance of side effects in the development of new antipsychotic drugs. *Psychiatr Ann* 1995;25:306–310.

Schwartz NE, Hughes D: Assessment and treatment of acute psychosis in psychiatric emergency service. *Essential Psychopharm* 1996;1:152–166.

Secunda V: *When Madness Comes Home: Help and Hope for the Children, Siblings, and Partners of the Mentally Ill.* New York, Hyperion, 1997.

Seeman MV: Gender differences in treatment response in schizophrenia. In: Seeman MV (ed.): *Gender and Psychopathology*, pp. 227–251. Washington, DC, American Psychiatric Press, 1995.

Serper MR, Chou JCY: Novel neuroleptics improve attentional functioning in schizophrenic patients: ziprasidone and aripiprazole. *CNS Spectrums: Int J Neuropsychiatr Med* 1997;2:56–64.

Spohn HE, Strauss ME: Relation of neuroleptic and anticholinergic medication to cognitive functions in schizophrenia *J Abnorm Psychol* 1989;98:367–380.

Stein S, Solvason HB, Biggart E, et al.: A 25-year-old woman with hallucinations, hypersexuality, nightmares, and a rash. *Am J Psychiatry* 1996;153:545–551.

Strathdee G, Kendrick T: The regular review of patients with schizophrenia in primary care. In: Kendrick T, Tylee A, Freeling P (eds.): *The Prevention of Mental Illness in Primary Care* 1996, pp. 311–326. Cambridge, England, Cambridge University Press.

Szymanski S: Sex differences in schizophrenia. In: Jensvold MF, Halbreich U, Hamilton JA (eds.): *Psychopharmacology and Women: Sex, Gender, and Hormones*, pp. 287–297. Washington, DC, American Psychiatric Press, 1996.

Szymanski S, Lieberman JA, Alvir JM, et al.: Gender differences in onset of illness, treatment response, course, and biologic indexes in first-episode schizophrenic patients. *Am J Psychiatry* 1995;152:698–703.

Tollefson GD: Olanzapine: a new antipsychotic agent. *J Clin Psychiatry* 1997;15:19–24.

Torrey EF: *Surviving Schizophrenia: A Manual for Families, Consumers, and Providers*, 3rd ed. New York, Harper, 1995.

Wyatt RJ: Early intervention for schizophrenia: Can the cause of the illness be altered? *Biol Psychiatry* 1995;8:1–3.

Zarate CA Jr, Daniel DG, Kinon BJ, et al.: Algorithms for the treatment of schizophrenia. *Psychopharmacol Bull* 1995;31:461–467.

Chapter 13

Sexuality and Intimacy

Clinicians practice in a world in which sexual myths are exploding. Information about sexuality and intimacy literally floods the marketplace, and patients are asserting their rights to gratify physical and emotional needs as never before. New scientific information, the diagnosis and treatment of sexual disorders, and the widely accepted practice of individual, sex, and marital or couple's therapy have altered attitudes of both women and men. Many individuals now speak up about their sexual desires and problems and are not afraid to question the experts. What was once the exclusive purview of priests and poets is now also relegated to clinicians and therapists.

Although most would agree that a solid knowledge base about sexuality is essential for state-of-the-art practice, clinicians also are in awe of the transcendent mystery that lures two hearts in love. As much as has been learned in the past four decades about human sexual responsiveness, clinicians as well as others join in the chorus of the late Frank Sinatra's ode to the impalpable qualities and "chemical forces" of romantic, physical attraction in the Springer and Leigh hit, "How Little It Matters How Little We Know": "How little we understand what touches off the tingle; that sudden explosion when two tingles intermingle."

The problem is, of course, that after a while "tingling" hearts—and couples—begin to tangle. Eventually, even the most passionate of partnerships can hit a snag, and this is when clinicians are usually called on. In the early stages of "being in love," most men and women are content with those indelible, eternal moments "with your lips on mine, how ignorant bliss is," but when problems are encountered, they want to know what has happened and how they might correct it.

This chapter is about how primary care clinicians can help patients take a closer look at their sexual and relationship problems and point them in a constructive direction when referral to a mental health professional may be warranted. Emphasis is placed on the wide array of sexual and relationship difficulties that the primary care clinician is likely to see but that often are not addressed in medical texts, such as the toll of divorce, the special needs of the disabled patient, the needs of the lesbian patient, and some steps to take if the female patient experiences diminished sexual drive. Given the time constraints in a busy primary care practice, the intent is not to be all-inclusive but to help to conceptualize a contemporary understanding of women's relationship needs, delineating how the clinician can gather essential information and offer practical suggestions or exercises to ameliorate the most common problems.

THE IMPORTANCE OF STAYING
OPEN-MINDED AND OPEN-HEARTED
WHEN TAKING A SEXUAL HISTORY

Many women now seek guidance and support when a vexing relationship predicament confronts them. The primary care clinician is often the first person sought out to discuss the quandary, particularly if the patient's confidence and trust have already been earned over the course of a stormy illness or through the daily vicissitudes of caring for the family. An open-hearted, open-minded attitude on your part cultivates the patient's trust. She is then more likely to turn to you when any concerns about embarrassing or shameful issues arise. Rarely is this a matter of longevity or experience in practice alone. For example, after completing her primary care residency in a large metropolitan area, one young clinician was pleased but somewhat startled to find her practice burgeoning after only a few months. Patient satisfaction surveys indicated that her clientele found her easy to talk with and prudent in her workups and treatment recommenda-tions; but in addition, she never failed to ask her patients about their level of stress in the workplace or in their home lives. Not only did her patients appreciate what they correctly interpreted as her concern for their overall well-being, but this savvy and psychologically minded young physician used her interviewing skills as an entrée into taking a sexual and relationship history when it appeared warranted.

Opportunities abound for women to increase their "sexual literacy" (Kaplan, 1974, 1979; Schnarch, 1997; Westheimer, 1983). Despite the amount of sexually explicit material available, a woman with a real concern about her sexual func-tioning or her relationship still finds it difficult to reach a comprehensive understanding of her dilemma and to have some practical answers. Despite major changes in the understanding of human sexuality and relationship needs, clinicians and patients do not discuss these issues as often or as directly as would be ideal. Clearly, one limiting factor is time. Because of constraints on the routine office visit, sexual problems can easily go unaddressed. They are bypassed in order to focus on "real" complaints. In addition, clinicians have their own anxieties and inhibitions regarding sexuality, which make it difficult for them to be as open about that topic as they are about other physical or emotional concerns.

As society evolves toward greater awareness and knowledge about sexuality, clinicians are faced with having to learn more about the wide variations of sexual responsiveness and the pluralistic needs of individuals and relationships. Good interpersonal skills will probably always be needed to help draw out the hidden questions and concerns that patients may harbor regarding their intimate lives. As managed care clinicians are expected to do more with less, it will be all too easy to bypass taking even a basic sexual history. But difficulties in the sexual and relationship arenas invariably influence both physical and emotional well-being. Helping patients in this most sensitive but personal of areas is the first step in tackling any dysfunction and thereby preventing it from becoming intractable (Segraves and Segraves, 1993; Seiderman, 1995) (Table 13–1). Once again, your active, open approach plays a pivotal role in ensuring the patient's entitlement to a full interpersonal life, thereby promoting her growth in the sexual and intimacy spheres.

There is little doubt that women's sexual behavior is changing. Women of all ages are more willing to experiment with various types of sexual self-pleasuring, erotic fantasies, and even nonmonogamous relationships. Women are sexually experienced at far younger ages than were their mothers or their grandmothers. Women are also more aware of their own bodies and have available more informational tools to learn about them. Women are more apt to complain of

Table 13–1. **Most Common Sexual Disorders in Women**

Diagnosis	Definition
Sexual dysfunctions	
Hypoactive sexual disorder	Persistent lack of desire for sexual activity
Sexual aversion disorder	Aversion to and avoidance of genital sexual activity due to anxiety, fear, or disgust
Sexual arousal disorder	Persistent inability to attain or maintain physiologic sexual arousal
Orgasmic disorder	Delay or inability in experiencing orgasm despite sexual excitement
Dyspareunia	Pain associated with intercourse
Vaginismus	Involuntary vaginal muscle spasms accompanied by pain, often preventing complete intercourse
Sexual disorder due to medical condition	Clinically significant sexual dysfunction due to a medical condition (e.g., rheumatoid arthritis, coronary artery disease, multiple sclerosis, alcoholic neuropathy, thyroid deficiency)
Substance-induced sexual dysfunction	Clinically significant sexual dysfunction due to substance or medication (e.g., SSRIs, some antihypertensives, alcohol, barbiturates)
Paraphilias	
Exhibitionism; sexual masochism or sexual sadism; voyeurism; fetishism	Recurrent fantasies or behaviors that cause suffering to one's self or partner, leading to significant distress and impairment at work or in relationship
Gender identity disorder	Desire to be a member of the opposite sex; discomfort with anatomic gender
Addictive sexual disorders	Compulsive or excessive sexual behavior manifested by loss of control, preoccupation with the behavior, and continuation despite adverse consequences

loss of zest, dyspareunia, vaginismus, or other overt sexual dysfunction; sexual addiction and paraphilias concomitantly appear on the increase (Irons and Schneider, 1997) (see Table 13–1). These divergent behaviors indicate that, among other things, society has not yet achieved a state of equilibrium with respect to women's sexual liberation. Despite the advances in knowledge about human sexuality and societal attitudes over the past few decades, women "still have to contend psychologically with the heritage of an earlier science of evasion, which denies female sexuality, and with a lingering confusion about female sexual parts" (Sevely, 1987, p. 178).

LOVE IS NEVER ENOUGH: INTIMACY'S ROLE IN WOMEN'S RELATIONSHIPS

Women desire intimacy and reciprocity in their adult relationships. Contemporary psychoanalysts believe that the importance of connection derives from the first primary bond that women establish with their mothers (Chodorow, 1978). To a certain extent, men must move away from mother to achieve autonomy and to secure a sense of their maleness. If they do not, they are routinely and pejoratively given the sobriquet "mama's boy," which signifies a persistent and infantilizing tie to the mother. For women, the relationship to mother is rarely totally relinquished. It is transformed in adulthood into the woman's close relationships with women friends, her children, and even her mate. Women who are unable to naturally loosen the tie to mother may never feel at ease or free to pursue their own desires. They are frequently conflicted about establishing independence and engaging in mature sexual roles. In contrast, the desire for mutuality, depth, and intimacy is rooted in an early secure attachment, usually with the mother or primary caregiver.

Any presenting sexual complaint may shroud a conflictual relationship issue within the primary relationship; it also demonstrates how all of the woman's intimate connections—including those to husband, children, and friends—have been ignored or treated as irrelevant in medicine. When these issues are addressed, new possibilities for intimate connections grow, and the woman's happiness and well-being are enhanced. Many times, brief individual or couple's counseling can point the patient in a direction that renews and strengthens her relationship with her partner.

Heterosexual women seek happiness, security, and sexual fulfillment in a committed partnership with a man. Mutuality between the sexes is difficult to achieve in part because of the differential socialization of males and females (Baber and Allen, 1992). Primary care clinicians are usually quite sensitive to the dilemmas of their male and female patients who are striving to carve out a meaningful, mature partnership but nevertheless find themselves at odds. So many day-to-day concerns can stand in the way. Sexual, relationship, and social needs of the woman and man may seem worlds apart. Little is taught in school about negotiating differences, let alone about resolving conflict. This lack of attention to the development of relationship skills, which can help men and women meet and transcend their goal of a mutually satisfying, committed partnership, is not unique to either gender. Yet, as Baber and Allen (1992) note, "Women and men are expected to live together, communicate clearly their needs and concerns, and negotiate economic, sexual, reproductive, parental, and social demands in their day-to-day lives together" (p. 25). Given the rigidity of traditional gender roles and standards, it is difficult for both sexes to transcend stereotypes to establish autonomy and mutuality within their relationship.

These multiple demands are crucial to keep in mind, because a marital or sexual problem (see Table 13–1) that comes to your attention may obscure the real problem. Your collaboration with skilled mental health professionals in your community and your awareness of groups, classes, and other available resources are first steps toward providing the patient with the help she needs. Both resources can help patients sort out what is going awry in their relationships and how to have their needs met.

For example, a patient presents to you with a feeling of ennui in her primary relationship and anorgasmia of more than a year's duration. You recommend some appropriate self-help books (see "Resources for Patients") or basic sex therapy techniques (see "A Practical Technique for Helping Women Achieve Sexual Satisfaction"). When the patient does not readily improve, you refer her to a skilled marital and sex therapist. Later you learn that her marriage was actually quite fulfilling and required only some relatively minor adjustments in communication and timing of sexual interludes to improve compatibility. Your patient's boredom arose because she wanted to return to school to finish her degree, but she worried that doing so would anger her husband and cause her adolescent children to suffer. In fact, members of her immediate family were quite supportive and encouraging when she finally confronted the issue head-on. Her marital life resumed a comfortable pace in regard to communication and sexual satisfaction. She still had to have the courage to tell her parents her decision; they had never supported her dream of finishing college.

In this example, the patient's presentation of hypoactive sexual desire, her lack of sexual interest and energy, and the "problem" in her primary relationship could easily have been misdiagnosed or missed completely. To get to the real issue—and institute appropriate treatment—clinicians must look beneath the surface. Doing so in this case led to a successful, brief psychotherapy process and avoided extensive diagnostic work-ups and more elaborate treatment protocols (e.g., medication, sex therapy). Underscoring the importance of social ties may be a crucial preventive health maneuver; isolation is linked to a number of physical maladies in both men and women (see Chapters 8 and 10).

Friendships

Friendships with women and men not only enlarge the patient's world but also mitigate against "feelings of worthlessness, confusion, and dysphoria" (Frank et al., 1998, p. 367), which erupt in nonaffirming or overtly abusive relationships. Urge the patient to seek out affirming, mutual friendships for the sake of her emotional and physical health. In essence, "women's psychological and physical well-being depends on the quality and extent of her social relations. . . [which] enhance women's self-esteem and self-concept" (pp. 366–367).

Sometimes new ties with women friends can help patients forge satisfying adult connections, thereby alleviating some marital tension. Women's friendships tend to be characterized by a web of interconnections in which interdependence (healthy dependence) with other women is the norm (Bernardez, 1985; Jordan, 1991). In relationships with men or other women, women seek mutual bonds that correct traditional imbalances and lead to feeling that they are "heard, seen, understood, and known" (Jordan, 1991, p. 96).

A Range of Possibilities

In contemporary culture, women meet their needs for intimacy in ways that would truly shock those of previous generations. Cohabitation outside of marriage, commuter marriages, and high rates of separation, divorce, and single motherhood—to name only a few nontraditional situations—are all part of the contemporary scene (see Murstein, 1978). Primary care clinicians must be aware of women's intimacy needs and the wide range of adult relationships that have evolved to meet them.

The current generation of young men is also changing the definition of what it means to be a man and to be married. More and more men are assuming the role of equal partner with respect to childcare and nurturing activities in the home. Most physicians will probably not be as surprised as this author was when a coworker observed that her teenage daughter's male friends genuinely appeared to have different goals and ideals with respect to women than did men of the preceding generation. The coworker observed, "These guys want something totally different from our generation. Men are really changing." Informed by feminism, many young men apparently want to build an equal partnership that allows both individuals to grow and change. They are less bound by traditional stereotypes. Any improvement in this sphere is likely to benefit women's mental health. Women's vulnerability to depression has been linked to their subordinate social status and the problems they have juggling the multiple needs of children, partner, aging parents, and the workplace.

Qualitative investigations of marriage suggest that the burden of caregiving and nurturing that has fallen on women leads to emotional difficulties over the long term. Although women long for intimacy and family life, it "also entraps them in an arrangement of subordination and provokes feelings and assessments by them that are at least partially and sometimes [totally] negative" (Dressel and Clark, 1990, p. 778). Psychosocial factors (e.g., sanctions against expressing anger, prohibitions that prevent personal growth, economic inequality, low-status work) increase women's vulnerability to a range of emotional problems, particularly depression (see Chapter 2). Clinicians must continually examine their own gender-biased assumptions to acquire increased flexibility and encourage their patients to explore choices "without dictating or unconsciously expecting conformity to sexual stereotypes" (Bernardez, 1985, p. 4). In order for marital relationships to attain a vitality that can meet the interpersonal needs of men and women, marriage itself must evolve, particularly in the quest for greater equality between partners.

A PRACTICAL TECHNIQUE FOR HELPING WOMEN ACHIEVE SEXUAL SATISFACTION

After the clinician has taken a brief sexual history and has placed any difficulty the patient has in the context of her life situation, a likely query will be "what to do next?" Particularly if you believe the patient's difficulties are not stemming from a pertinent relationship or an overarching societal conflict, you may want to consider using a brief, relatively easy, and safe exercise to help enhance the woman's sexual responsiveness. To date, the most effective brief treatment for helping women achieve sexual satisfaction and orgasm after lifelong sexual aversion is a step-by-step program derived from the work of cognitive-behavioral therapists (see Barbach, 1976, 1982; Heiman and LoPiccolo, 1988; LoPiccolo, 1994; LoPiccolo and LoPiccolo, 1978). Sometimes the patient derives benefit from psychodynamic elements included in the approach (see Kaplan, 1974, 1979), particularly if her difficulties center on a lack of sexual desire, inhibition, fear of romantic success or intimacy, and anxiety based on unconscious or relationship concerns.

Because a significant minority of women report having difficulty achieving orgasm at some point in their lives, medical assessment should always include questions about sexual desire, sexual symptoms, and the availability and sexual interest of the patient's partner. If you have determined that a sexual disorder exists and have ruled out organic causes, you might suggest an approach adapted from the work of Heiman et al. (1988) and Barbach (1982). These steps can be employed by heterosexual women or lesbians, but they do require a working knowledge of relaxation therapy and/or guided imagery (see Chapter 7 for relaxation suggestions). To be sure, these steps are just a beginning, although they are sometimes all that is necessary for a satisfactory result. If the patient is amenable to these suggestions, urge her to take advantage of available books that go into more detail (Barbach, 1982; Heiman et al., 1988).

- *Step one*: Identify various parts of your genitals. This aids in an attitudinal acceptance of female sexuality. Face any long-standing fearful situations that have developed over time (e.g., parental disapproval). Use relaxation imagery and breathing techniques to master a tendency to catastrophize sexual situations and to correct distorted thinking about sexuality.
- *Step two*: Explore your body and genitals by touching. Counter your tendency to negatively label your body and your sexuality as horrible, bad, or ugly. Use selected readings to accurately label with positive emotions the sexual parts of your body and your sexual response.
- *Step three*: Locate erogenous zones, including the clitoris, as the focus for sexual pleasure. If you have acquired irrational beliefs based on misinformation, learn new facts about sexuality by reading, watching videos, and so on.
- *Step four*: Deactivate any belief that masturbation or sexual responsiveness in women is wrong. Use suggested readings to learn techniques of masturbation that work for you (see Barbach, 1976, 1982).
- *Step five*: Develop sexual fantasies by reading popular literature or watching videos.
- *Step six*: If you have not yet reached orgasm, consider buying a vibrator.
- *Step seven*: If you have a willing partner, demonstrate the techniques you have learned that produce arousal and orgasm. Couples improve when coequal and reciprocal learning is encouraged. Because negative thoughts about sexuality are often strongly linked to fear, anxiety, guilt, or depression, you and your partner can list any situation or disruptive thoughts and beliefs that occur during lovemaking. You strengthen your relationship by seeing what your partner must face and by helping him or her. Develop counterarguments to any disruptive thoughts or beliefs about sexuality that spontaneously arise.
- *Step eight*: Become assertive. Your partner wants to know what is satisfying. Ask your partner to caress and touch your genitals to produce orgasm through direct stimulation.
- *Step nine*: Continue direct manual stimulation of your clitoris with or without vaginal penetration to facilitate orgasm.

In essence, the patient and her partner are gradually introduced to increasingly more challenging sexual situations. A gradual process associated with pleasure and arousal rather than anxiety is based on the theory that most sexual dysfunction and aversion results from anxiety in the sexual situation (Kaplan, 1976, 1979) that can be overcome with learning and improved communication.

WHAT IS THE ROLE OF THE PRIMARY CARE CLINICIAN WHEN A RELATIONSHIP ENDS?

Many intimate relationships endure until the death of one partner, but increasingly in our society relationships are more temporary, often ending in separation or divorce. Whatever your personal biases regarding this issue, you will be called on to recognize, and to some extent to intervene with, the multiple stressors that occur when a relationship ends.

The loss of a love relationship signals a major life transition and emotional suffering for at least one partner, and probably both, with inevitable health consequences. For women who have been dependent economically on a partner, the end of the relationship can be financially devastating. In addition, the emotional needs of these women are also usually neglected.

For example, one divorced woman observed how friends and relatives treated her as if she had brought the pain and grief on herself. Crass contradictory statements ("You're better off without him" and "He's such a nice guy, how could you let him get away?") left her feeling alone and bewildered about her situation. It behooves clinicians to have some appreciation for what such women may be going through and to be willing to listen and express sympathy for their unique situation. When working with a woman who separates or divorces, remember that she is navigating the bereavement process (see Chapter 9). She has not only lost a spouse but also is usually severed from important friendships and from her former spouse's family. Other friends may feel threatened by her new "single" status and view her as a threat to their own marriages. Sometimes this perception creates a rift in long-standing, important friendships—yet another loss to bear!

Holidays can be particularly difficult. They are both a painful reminder of loss and a time of isolation if the children leave to be with their father. Even gatherings of the woman's extended family can be distressing, because seeing other "complete" families interacting may intensify her sense of loss. If the children are with her, she worries about how they are faring without their father. One elderly patient drove this point home. She remarked that her early loss of a husband through divorce had been more difficult than the subsequent death of a husband to whom she had been married much longer. She said she could mourn the death and move on, but that contact with her ex-husband—also the father of her children—was a constant reminder of her loss. It can be supportive for you to simply be aware that the separating or divorcing woman is experiencing very real pain and grief, which in many ways is more complicated than that caused by losing a mate through death.

Much of the divorce literature treats women as a homogeneous group. In fact, however, women's divorce experiences differ greatly, depending on age, ethnicity, socioeconomic level, and whether they initiated the divorce. In Wallerstein and Blakeslee's (1989) classic study of the effects of divorce, women older than 40 years of age were less likely than younger women to make social and psychological shifts. More than half of these older women experienced a decreased standard of living, with 80% becoming financially insecure. Moreover, older women faced different social, psychological, and economic barriers than did the younger women, who had more opportunities to find new partners or to develop new careers. Our task as clinicians is to help patients make this transition by pointing them in the direction of support and by affirming their future despite this loss. A woman whose primary relationship has ended must deal with (1) an experience of loss; (2) a tendency to disavow or inhibit anger; (3) a tendency to redirect anger toward the self, leading to guilt and/or low self-worth; (4) a tendency to be immobilized and to deal passively with circumstances; and

(5) a difficulty in recognizing and embracing her own sense of power (Kaplan, 1991; Miller, 1991).

After divorce, most women continue to be the primary parent to their children, even in cases of shared custody. The children may actually fare better after the divorce, but women themselves struggle with conflicting demands of working, parenting, and conserving enough energy for self-care and personal interests (e.g., hobbies, time with friends). Here your active involvement can play a crucial role in the woman's emotional well-being and physical health. Urge the patient to facilitate the grief process by seeking out as much emotional support (e.g., friends, psychotherapy) as possible. Empathize with the feelings of pain, sadness, anger, frustration, fear about the future, and sense of personal failure that accompany the ending of most intimate partnerships.

Even if the woman feels as though she has made a good decision and life is going better, she may tend to leave her own needs unattended. Inadequate finances can be a huge problem that precludes decisions such as returning to school or looking for a different job. Social service agencies and women's health cooperatives may be able to offer help. In particular, encourage the patient to work through the grieving process by taking advantage of divorce workshops, women's support groups, or brief grief therapy processes. Alert the patient to any tendency to sacrifice her personal needs to the point of exhaustion or depression for the sake of her children or others (e.g., aging parents) for whom she has primary responsibility. Just knowing that you have some appreciation for the complexity of her situation and for the economic, emotional, and social dilemmas she faces can be enormously supportive.

INFERTILITY

At least 1 of 12 couples in the United States has some kind of problem with "impaired fecundity" (Downey, 1993; Morokoff and Calderone, 1994). Infertility is included in this chapter on sexuality and intimacy because it can be devastating to the woman, and it also has the potential for cascading negative effects on a couple's relationship. Primary care clinicians usually refer infertile patients (those unable to conceive after 12 months of intercourse without contraception) to an infertility specialist for a thorough workup and possible treatment. You will nevertheless be in a position to help evaluate and manage the emotional sequelae of women and men who cannot conceive. Your role also extends to determining which psychological factors are likely to increase a couple's chances for childbearing by increasing their awareness of emotional (i.e., stress-related) issues that may be a part of their problem. Once before considered a reason for infertility, stress is again being taken seriously as evidence reveals that treating it with behavioral modification brings positive results in a significant number of infertile couples (Domar, 1997; Domar et al., 1992, 1993).

Primary infertility appears to be on the rise (Morokoff and Calderone, 1994; Roberts et al., 1998). One potential factor is delayed childbearing. More women now focus on attaining their educational and career goals and so delay marriage and pregnancy. Other possible causes of increased primary infertility include smoking, strenuous exercise, and exposure to stress. Although exposure to environmental hazards (e.g., radiation, chronic loud noise, physical strain) has been hypothesized as a cause of infertility, there are few scientific data to support this notion (Morokoff and Calderone, 1994).

Sexual dysfunction may also play a role in some cases of infertility. If there is a lack of desire or an aversion to sex (see Table 13–1), sexual intercourse may occur too infrequently to make conception likely. New data support the notion that chances of conception are enhanced by regular sexual activity. Women who have regular sexual intercourse (at least once in every day of a nonmenstruating week) have more regular cycles than women who have sporadic sex, and women whose cycles approach 29 days have the highest likelihood of having fertile cycles. These women also have the highest incidence of fertile-type basal body rhythms. Compared with women who are celibate or who engage in sporadic sex, they also have higher estrogen levels and adequate-length luteal phases. These data suggest that frequent and regular sexual activity are more important to fertility than once thought. The primary care clinician must educate the patient about the importance of regular sexual activity and the role it plays in infertility.

Spontaneous sex becomes difficult after years of reproductive frustration. Sexual dysfunction may be the result of infertility as well as the cause of it. Should sexual activity take on a mechanical or demand quality in the relationship, as often becomes the case when the desired end is pregnancy, the couple may find themselves with decreased sexual desire, increased resentment and anger, and a communication crisis in their marriage. Caregivers who are aware of these potential problems and who focus on a couple's sexual health can provide early education and suggest appropriate intervention and treatment resources. Here, as in other aspects of human sexuality, the clinician must be comfortable speaking directly about the physical and emotional aspects of sex. Quality of life is restored when the clinician evaluates the patient and her partner to determine the presence of sexual dysfunction or a personal issue that may be interfering with reproduction (Morokoff and Calderone, 1994). In evaluating the infertile couple, the clinician must be especially sensitive and tactful. Women, in particular, have an intense yearning to achieve "fulfillment of the childhood wish to conceive and bear a child within their body. . . .[L]ack of control over the reproductive capacities of one's own body is an enormous crisis—a blow to the individual's narcissism, a diminution of pride in the mature bodily self-representation" (Pines, 1993, pp. 136–137). The physician must keep in mind that the crisis of infertility causes the patient shame and embarrassment, the potential loss of ever being able to conceive, and a pervasive sense that she has failed—that she is not "a whole woman." If the woman is never able to conceive, she must eventually mourn the loss of all her dreams and fantasies of having a baby; in essence, she must find a new and broader way of defining her identity as a woman (see Chapter 9 for a discussion of the nature of loss). Psychotherapy, and even psychoanalysis, can provide invaluable emotional support for the infertile woman and for the woman who becomes pregnant with one of the new fertility techniques. Both present "complicated issues" of coming to terms with "hard realities" so that the woman can "recover her self-esteem and find satisfaction elsewhere" (Pines, 1993, pp. 148–149).

As noted, there is growing evidence to suggest that, in some women, mild to severe emotional stress may lead to impaired fertility. Stress directly affects reproductive hormones, particularly by reducing testosterone levels and interfering with spermatogenesis in men. Corticotrophin-releasing factor, endogenous opiates, and glucocorticoids are involved in the pathophysiology of distress amenorrhea. This phenomenon has been observed in college students, recruits into the armed forces, women entering religious life, concentration camp internees, and prisoners under sentence of death (Tolis and Diamanti, 1995).

Although the effects of stress on the woman's reproductive functioning are quite complex, a range of counseling techniques has helped some women to cope with infertility and, in a significant percentage of cases, to become pregnant. Harvard psychologist Alice Domar teaches women techniques from progressive muscle relaxation to guided visual imagery in order to master "the stress associated with infertility." In tracking 174 of her infertile patients, she found that, within 6 months of completing her program, 44% had achieved conception. Previously, most of these patients had undergone a wide range of fertility treatments. Domar's goal had been to help the patients handle the emotional side effects of not "getting pregnant" (e.g., depression and anger). It was not her goal to help her patients have a baby. But she found that after women were able to reduce—and in some cases to master—stress, they began to get pregnant as a "happy side effect" that has earned her the laudable eponym, the "goddess of fertility," in some women's circles in the Boston area where she practices (Gill, 1998).

Although additional replication with larger and more diverse populations is needed, other mental health professionals are corroborating Domar's pioneering work on infertility and the mind-body interface. In one study using problem-focused group psychotherapy, participants reported enhanced positive feelings, greater effectiveness, and greater likelihood of having a child, compared with controls (McQueeney, 1997). The investigators suggested that thorough education of this kind provides information and promotes assertive communication. Women who have felt a loss of control in their lives because they cannot become pregnant learn that they can control certain decisions with greater effectiveness.

Clinicians and patients may wonder which particular mind-body techniques (e.g., relaxation, imaging) work for various infertility problems, for which patients, and under what conditions. Controlled trials of treatment protocols may provide a better understanding of this issue. In the meantime, the primary care clinician's responsibility is to make patients aware of the available research and to point them toward acquiring skills such as relaxation therapy and coping techniques. Successful conception is far from guaranteed. But even if couples are unsuccessful in their quest to have a baby, they will definitely be helped to deal with any emotional fallout. Although the most sophisticated medical treatments for infertility are relatively new, quite expensive, and available primarily in cities, most towns have classes or groups for learning mind-body techniques, such as breathing, guided imagery, stress management, and assertiveness training. Moreover, these sessions are usually time-limited and relatively inexpensive. For millions, infertility is a heart-wrenching problem; telling the patient about these modalities cannot hurt her, and they are likely to be of some help.

SPECIAL ISSUES OF WOMEN WITH PHYSICAL DISABILITIES

Women with physical disabilities (e.g., spinal cord injury, arthritis) have sexual needs and must receive adequate sexuality education and instruction as a part of their overall rehabilitation. Often women with disabilities have more difficulty finding partners and establishing relationships that lead to intimacy than do able-bodied women (Leyson, 1991; Rintala et al., 1997). Access to interpersonal and social interactions is usually limited, but the greatest threats related to disability are feelings of worthlessness and unattractiveness. Any illness affects one's body image and can interfere with sexual receptivity. The disabled woman must overcome these body image concerns in order to develop confidence that she can date, engage in sexual behavior, and establish a satisfying relationship regardless of ongoing physical limitations. Groups such as SIECUS (Sexual Information and Educational Counseling of the United States) advocate that disabled persons have as much access as able-bodied individuals to sexual health care and opportunities for socializing and sexual expression. SIECUS has also compiled an extensive bibliography (which is available from the organization on written request or through the Internet) that describes a number of available resources for patients, parents, significant others, and professionals.

When working with a disabled patient in primary care, by all means inquire about sexual adjustment and any physical problems that might hamper spontaneous sexual activity (Table 13–2). For example, a woman with severe arthritis may be unable to have sexual intercourse in the missionary position but may be quite comfortable in other sexual positions; moist heat, vaginal lubricants, and non-weight-bearing exercises may also help her prepare for intercourse (Ehrlich, 1973; Sipski and Alexander, 1997). Open an individualized discussion with the patient. In addition, recommending up-to-date manuals or texts is an extremely supportive counseling maneuver (see Haseltine et al., 1993; Kroll and Klein 1992; Leyson, 1991; Schover and Jensen, 1988). Despite the increasing availability of these materials, disabled women still report that professionals lack knowledge in the areas of sexuality and relationship needs (Richards et al., 1997). With some exceptions (Schover and Jensen, 1988; Sipski and Alexander, 1997; Welner, 1997), available materials are usually oriented toward disabled men. Primary care clinicians should be sure to include an opportunity to discuss birth control, desire and concern about becoming pregnant, and genetic factors. A working knowledge of position variations and comfort with urogenital and masturbatory techniques gives the patient permission to creatively adapt and be sexually gratified despite the disability. Referral to a physiatrist or rehabilitation expert (e.g., physical and occupational therapist) with special training in the sexual health of disabled patients can be reassuring.

Because disabled women are a disenfranchised, minority group, their psychosocial problems are often discounted. Take into consideration that, if the disability has been lifelong, the woman's parents may have been overprotective in some cases. Most of these single women worry about finding a partner who will love and cherish them despite their disability, but once they have experienced romance and sensate pleasuring, they find that they can accommodate their own needs and those of their partner. For example, in writing about the experience of women with complete spinal cord injury, Richards et al. (1997) included some poignant statements from their research subjects that express the meaningful sexual expression many are able to find. One woman reported that "it took me a long time to realize. . . there are other things. . . .[Y]ou don't have to have intercourse to have sexual feelings and get sexual arousal and be able to enjoy it" (p. 279). These women had to learn how to manage physical changes,

---

Table 13–2. **Counseling the Physically Disabled Patient About Sexuality**

1. Remember that physically disabled persons are still sexual beings. Take the initiative to discuss sexual functioning and concerns.
2. Empathize with any change in the patient's body affecting appearance or body image.
3. Be aware that dating and the limited number of available partners are special concerns for singles, adolescents, and young adults. Opportunities for socialization, support groups, and educational resources are often available at rehabilitation centers and women's health cooperatives.
4. Explore sexual options (e.g., change in sexual positions for arthritis patients, development of erogenous areas [neck, breast] that are not anaesthetic, and nondemand pleasure techniques after spinal cord injury).
5. Discuss the management of any medical apparatus that may interfere with a sexual relationship (e.g., catheters, ostomy bags). Encourage open communication with the partner. With time and patience, concerns about appliances can be managed.
6. Encourage participation in specific support groups (e.g., Ostomy Association, spinal cord networks) where other patients, who may have dealt with the problem themselves, are expert in openly addressing sexual and relationship issues. They may have good suggestions that professionals are not aware of because of lack of experience with the problem.
7. Encourage the patient to take advantage of counseling and sex education classes at local rehabilitation centers. Excellent films, pamphlets, books, and other materials are now available to aid persons with virtually any physical disability to achieve a more gratifying sexual life.
8. Remind the patient that the brain is still the most important and essential sexual organ. Despite physical disabilities, sexual fulfillment remains a gratifying aspect of one's life as long as the patient is willing to learn and to experiment. Encourage fantasy.
9. In those rare cases in which disability is very extensive and/or a partner is absolutely unavailable, emphasize the importance of fantasy. Suggest available reading materials or films. Permission to fantasize underscores your regard for the patient as a whole, sexual person despite physical limitations.
10. Include discussion about childbearing, contraception, and sexually transmitted diseases in your interview with the patient.

---

such as bowel and bladder functions, but after they did so, the matter became routine and did not interfere. As one woman explained, "I could self-stimulate and get sensation back, and it was kind of becoming a full person again; [the disability] kind of forces you to be inventive. . . and more experimental" (p. 278). Others found men who were able to champion their needs and affirm them as women: These women reported that they still felt desirable and sexy despite their injury, and they continued to have a positive sexual self-concept. Pivotal to most was the understanding and flexibility of a partner who loved them. As one woman remarked, "When he saw me naked, he caressed my legs and cried, and told me how sad he was that this had happened to me. . . .[H]e was absorbing me as a whole person, especially parts I was embarrassed about" (pp. 278–279).

In summary, women with physical difficulties can have fulfilling, satisfying sexual lives. Primary care clinicians can offer suggestions to help them solve problems related to sexuality and intimacy after disability. First and foremost, the clinician must feel comfortable enough to open the topic for discussion and then to point the patient toward the wealth of contemporary resources that are increasingly available; understandably, not everyone is comfortable working with the sexual needs of disabled people. Old stereotypes and anxieties are not easy for any of us to relinquish. In such situations, it is advisable to direct the patient to another professional who is less reticent. Knowing one's own biases and limitations in any area is one of the hallmarks of a mature caregiver.

SPECIAL ISSUES OF THE LESBIAN PATIENT

Lesbians are a diverse group of women who traditionally have not received good health care because they have feared rejection from the medical community. Like other marginalized groups, lesbians are becoming more self-accepting and self-actualizing, so they are seeking out comprehensive medical and psychotherapeutic care as never before (O'Hanlan, 1998; White, 1995). Frequently, these patients look for referral from within their own communities in finding a clinician who is open, empathetic, and knowledgeable about lesbian issues. Working with lesbians requires clinicians to "examine their attitudes about homosexuality, recognizing which views they hold which are not consistent with facts. Physicians have the unique opportunity to influence others to align their attitudes with objective information. By teaching adults and children about diversity of orientation, providers can reduce the pervasive yet unfounded disdain for homosexuals, facilitating maintenance of lesbian and gay individuals' self-respect" (O'Hanlan, 1998, p. 103).

Homosexuality is no longer considered a mental disorder in the third and fourth editions of the American Psychiatric Association's *Diagnostic and Statistical Manual of Mental Disorders* (American Psychiatric Association, 1987, 1994), and the majority of psychiatrists and psychoanalysts believe it to be a normal sexual variant. A number of retrospective historical studies are making apparent the range of homosexual relations over the generations and the potentiality of men and women in same-sex partnerships to lead productive, creative, and meaningful lives. Extensive research has confirmed that lesbians are comparable psychologically to heterosexual women in their level of maturity, psychological adjustment, goal orientation, and self-actualization (Hanley-Hackenbruck, 1993). Lesbians have more in common with heterosexual women than they do gay men, and they struggle with the same discrimination and prejudice in our society as other females.

The primary care clinician should be aware that a specific burden of gays and lesbians is internalization of the hostile and prejudicial attitude of society, which leads to guilt and self-hatred about being different (Stein, 1993). This impingement on the self is called "internalized homophobia." It takes its toll on a daily basis and is thought to be responsible for a significant portion of the emotional struggles that lesbians face.

Studies have shown that, despite living in a homophobic culture, most lesbians are highly productive members of society. More than half of lesbians participate in a monogamous, enduring relationship (Kirkpatrick and Morgan, 1980). As more lesbian couples choose to rear children (either as the product of a prior heterosexual marriage or as the result of alternative insemination), the research of Kirkpatrick et al. (1981) on lesbian mothers and their children is frequently cited. This long-term study found no significant differences in self-concept, intelligence, or moral judgment among children raised in lesbian families, compared with their peers raised in heterosexual families. Although a small percentage of children were taunted by peers, which naturally created discomfort, their parents' sexual orientation did not influence their own orientation or overall psychological adjustment. Children who are raised by mothers who are psychologically healthy themselves, who have the support of an affirming community, and whose fathers are involved and supportive fare better than children who do not have these advantages.

Many primary care clinicians are likely to have a number of lesbians in their practices without being aware of these patients' sexual orientation. For this reason, the unique medical and psychosocial needs of lesbians are frequently missed (Table 13–3). An open and nonjudgmental attitude can help the patient to "come out" to the clinician. Using inclusive language and working to avoid any covert biases during history taking are essential. For example, you might ask the patient (1) whom she includes in her immediate family, (2) whether she is in a relationship, and (3) whether she has been sexually active with men, women, or both (White, 1995).

The majority of lesbians have had relationships with men. Increasingly, sexual orientation is viewed by psychiatrists and psychoanalysts as something that is fluid across the life cycle and not as an "either/or" decision. It is therefore imperative for clinicians not only to know about the diversity of sexual orientation in clinical practice but also to be willing to accept the "ambiguity" and plurality of their patients' experiences (Hanley-Hackenbruck, 1993; O'Hanlan, 1998; Stein, 1993). More adolescents are "coming out" because of a relative increase in social acceptance. In addition, Kirkpatrick and Morgan (1980) suggested that because the primary object of love and attachment for women is usually the mother and heterosexual choice requires women to turn away from mother to father, women may be less fixed in their heterosexual object choice

---

Table 13–3. **Special Concerns of the Lesbian Patient**

1. Acquisition of lesbian identity. The "coming out" process is never a one-time event but instead occurs over the person's entire life, with every new person the woman decides to reveal her homosexuality to.
2. Recognition of an emerging sexuality and the resulting identity issues in adolescents and young adults.
3. Fluidity of sexual attraction. Most lesbians have had relationships with men. Some worry about persistent attraction and fantasies about the opposite sex, yet maintain a lesbian identity.
4. Child custody concerns.
5. Sexuality and sexual dysfunction.
6. Effects of violence, harassment, and discrimination.
7. Internalized homophobia, the tendency for woman to harbor shame and self-hatred, which has a negative impact on psychological and physical health.
8. Establishing intimate relationships, including nonsexual friendships.
9. Conflicts in relationships with parents, siblings, and friends, particularly regarding lesbian identity.

and more "flexible" or ambiguous in that choice than men. This theory will not surprise the primary care clinician or mental health professional who has probably, in the course of years of practice, met many women who acknowledged a sustained relationship or transient fantasy with someone of the same or opposite sex, despite an espoused definitive sexual preference. Women nonetheless worry about themselves and whether they are "normal." They may relate a history of preferential involvement with one or the other sex—only to change in young adulthood, midlife, or late life.

You may also encounter other, unusual relations that defy conventionality (see Magee and Miller, 1997; Murstein, 1978). Historically, one of the most famous was the marriage of Nigel Nicholson to Vita Sackville-West in 1913. The couple, although notoriously happy in their early years together and the parents of two gifted sons, found greater fulfillment in midlife in homosexual relationships. Although they remained married and the closest of friends, their deepest passions were saved for members of their own sex. This fascinating "portrait of a marriage" is recounted in a poignant memoir by their elder son (Nicholson, 1973). The concrete example of Sackville-West and Nicholson demonstrates the growing psychodynamic perception of the plasticity of human sexual response (especially in women) over the course of a lifetime:

> In women, homosexuality and heterosexuality do not appear to be at opposite ends of the continuum as Kinsey et al. (1953) suggested they were. Rather, the two trends might be seen as running a parallel course, capable of intermingling and of changing positions of ascendancy in consciousness and behavior under certain circumstances.
>
> (Kirkpatrick and Morgan, 1980, p. 360, quoted in Hanley-Hackenbruck 1993, p. 60)

Primary care clinicians must also be aware of the hate crimes against gays and lesbians. According to the U.S. Department of Justice, homosexuals are the most victimized group in the nation (White, 1995). Other mental health issues requiring routine screening in lesbians are (1) depression and suicide risk (Chapter 2), (2) substance abuse (Chapter 4), (3) domestic violence (Chapter 6), and (4) sexual functioning (see "A Practical Technique for Helping Women Achieve Sexual Satisfaction").

Finally, the decision to have a child is one for which the patient may elicit the clinician's help and support. If you feel unable to provide the services needed by a lesbian patient, then she should be referred to another provider who can (O'Hanlan, 1998; White, 1995).

SEXUAL SIDE EFFECTS OF PSYCHOTROPIC DRUGS

Most classes of psychotropic drugs commonly cause some side effects (Jensvold et al., 1996; Segraves, 1995). The primary care physician must be particularly aware of the problems associated with the selective serotonin reuptake inhibitors (SSRIs), because they are so frequently used in the treatment of depression. Other medications (monoamine oxidase inhibitors, lithium, antipsychotics) may also decrease libido, impair orgasm, or have reproductive side

Table 13–4. Partial List of Psychotropic Medications Causing Orgasmic Dysfunction and Decreased Libido in Women

Tricyclics	**Other antidepressants**
Desipramine	Trazodone (occasionally)
Clomipramine	**Mood stabilizers**
Imipramine	Lithium
Tetracyclics	Valproic acid
Amoxapine	**Antipsychotics**
Monoamine oxidase inhibitors	Chlorpromazine
Phenelzine	Fluphenazine
Tranylcypromine	Haloperidol
SSRIs	Molindone
Fluoxetine	Risperidone
Sertraline	Thioridazine
Paroxetine	**Benzodiazepines**
Fluvoxamine	Alprazolam
	Psychostimulants
	Amphetamines

effects. Bupropion (Wellbutrin), nefazodone (Serzone), and mirtazapine (Remeron) do not seem to inhibit sexual functioning and may on occasion enhance it (Boyarsky et al., 1998; Labbate and Pollach, 1994; Modell et al., 1997; Walker, 1993) (Tables 13–4 and 13–5).

Because sexual dysfunction accompanies depression, it can be difficult to determine the extent to which the antidepressant treatment is the cause of the patient's complaint. It now appears that SSRI-induced adverse sexual side effects are the rule rather than the exception (45% to 55% of patients when carefully questioned). In practice, these side effects are substantially underreported by patients and, in clinical research trials, underestimated (1% to 2% reported by the pharmaceutical industry in most early literature). In some cases, sexual side effects may not be reported because of disinterest in sex. Not all people have a desire to participate in sexual activity; as large population samples tell us, at least 1% of adults never have any sexual relationships (Lewontin, 1995; Michael et al., 1994). Certainly, these preferences need to be taken into account, but sometimes clinicians fail to ask about sexual problems or concerns.

With respect to daily medication management, no clinical or statistically significant difference is found among the various SSRIs, but a number of strategies have been recommended to minimize sexually related adverse events. These include (1) reducing the dose, (2) switching to another class of drugs

Table 13–5. Psychotropic Drugs that May Increase Sexual Functioning

Bupropion	Trazodone (clitoral enlargement)
Buspirone (BuSpar)	Clonazepam
Desipramine	Mirtazapine
Imipramine	Amphetamines

(e.g., from an SSRI to nefazodone or bupropion), and (3) adding another agent (e.g., yohimbine, bupropion, cyproheptadine) (Cohen, 1997; Jensvold et al., 1996; Modell et al., 1997; Segraves and Segraves, 1998). In a number of case reports, bupropion was found to be relatively devoid of adverse sexual side effects and, on some occasions, was decidedly "prosexual." For example, Grimes and Labbate (1996) described the case of a 35-year-old woman whose depression was abated by sertraline (Zoloft, 100 mg/day). She experienced diminished quality and frequency of orgasm within 2 weeks and did not receive benefit from a 2-week trial of cyproheptadine (Periactin, 4 mg/day). After 3 months of continued therapy with sertraline, bupropion (Wellbutrin, 75 mg/day orally) was added. Within 1 week, the patient's ability to achieve orgasm and her enjoyment of sex had returned to normal. Several weeks later, the patient experienced spontaneous orgasm. When the bupropion was stopped, her spontaneous orgasms were curtailed and her sexual functioning returned to what it had been previously on sertraline alone.

In summary, patients should be advised about the possibility of adverse sexual events when taking a psychopharmacologic agent (see Table 13–4). For example, patients taking fluoxetine or paroxetine report significantly decreased levels of libido, arousal, and intensity of orgasm. Moreover, there is a prolonged time between arousal and orgasm and a trend toward decreased duration of orgasm. In contrast, patients taking bupropion report significant increases from baseline in libido, arousal, duration of orgasm, and intensity of orgasm. Overall, 77% of bupropion-treated patients report one or more positive effects of sexual functioning. Bupropion may be a reasonable choice for those with a history of SSRI-induced sexual adverse side effects who present with significant sexual problems as part of their depression or who develop difficulties during an SSRI trial.

The SSRIs have sparked researchers to create other novel approaches to the sexual dysfunctions. These include granisetron (Kytril), an antiemetic used to treat chemotherapy-associated nausea, which blocks the serotonin (5-HT 3) receptor. The 5-HT 3 receptor has been shown to enhance sexual behavior in animal studies, and antidepressants that block this receptor, such as mirtazapine (Remeron), appear to cause fewer sexual side effects (Nelson et al., 1997). No drug has been proved, in a controlled clinical trial, to decrease sexual dysfunction caused by SSRIs. This finding derives from clinical work with patients, so the cohort is small and nonrandom (Table 13–6).

Less is known about women's vulnerability to sexual side effects. Not only has little research been done on women, compared with men, but clinicians exhibit a gender bias here, too: They tend to mistakenly believe that sexual functioning is less important to women than it is to men. In clinical practice, it must be

---

Table 13–6. **Medications Reported to Decrease Sexual Dysfunction Caused by SSRIs**

Cyproheptadine (Periactin)	D-Amphetamine
Yohimbine	Pemoline
Amantadine	Granisetron
Nefazodone	Mirtazapine
Bupropion	Sildenafil
Buspirone	

Table 13–7. **Clinical Management of Psychotropic-Induced Sexual Dysfunction**

---

1. Assess whether the patient is truly bothered by sexual side effects.
2. Wait for spontaneous remission.
3. Reduce to minimal effective dose.
4. Give partial drug holidays (e.g., lowering the dose of an antidepressant during holidays or over weekends to avoid withdrawal syndrome).
5. Switch to another medication.
6. Consider using pharmacologic treatment.
7. Consider addition of gingko biloba, the potent herbal leaf extract, 120–240 mg/ day.

---

remembered that any drug side effect that alters sexual functioning has a "domino effect" on the patient's partner (Jensvold et al., 1996); therefore "inattention to sexual side effects may lead to undue distress, misunderstandings, and/or treatment noncompliance" (Jensvold et al., 1996, p. 368). Larger studies and more placebo-controlled studies of the sexual side effects of psychotropic medications will increasingly inform the practice of physicians and the treatment of women. In the meantime, clinicians must manage psychotropic-induced sexual dysfunction empirically and on an individualized basis (Table 13–7). Referral to a psychiatrist is usually warranted to help distinguish medication effects from relationship difficulties that may be covertly impeding the sexual relationship.

GUIDELINES FOR PATIENTS

1. Attend to the development and maintenance of your intimate relationships, and recognize that they are likely to change over the course of your lifetime. The more confidence and experience you have, the more likely you are to make friendships and establish a marriage or long-term partnership that is in your best interest.
2. In addition to your primary relationship, seek out and cultivate other important, sustaining friendships. Women's connections to other women have always been essential for healthy psychological functioning. Strive to listen to your needs for intimacy and find ways to get those needs met.
3. Make a personal assessment of how you feel about sexuality, intimacy, and relationships. Are you getting what you want? If not, think through how you can begin the process of change. Have you been taught how to make knowledgeable decisions about relationships, or do you feel powerless to change? Develop new relationships so that you can make informed decisions about them. Cultivating a sustaining, mutual partnership based on love and caring may mean learning new skills. Read, attend groups with other women, and find role models who can help.
4. If relationship conflicts or sexual dysfunctions develop, seek professional support through psychotherapy. Remember that the concept of marriage requires us to shift from a "legal arrangement between a man and his wife" to a "committed partnership based on economic cooperation, sexual expression, and emotional intimacy" (Baber and Allen, 1992, p. 58).

5. Learn as much as you can about your own sexuality. Despite changes in contemporary society, most women need more information about their own bodies to make knowledgeable sexual decisions and to enhance their sexual enjoyment. Opportunities to learn from the support and experiences of others abound in various women's groups and women's health cooperatives.

6. If you have had difficulty with sexual expression, keep as your goal your right to a positive sexual experience. As it is in all other areas, knowledge in this sphere is power. The more you can learn about yourself as a sexual being, the more you will be able to make positive changes based on new information. In essence, you are trying to shift any outmoded sexual script you may have learned over the course of a lifetime to enlarge your worldview. Ultimately, you must take charge of your own sexuality and your own body.

7. Face outmoded myths, especially related to sexuality and pregnancy. For years, women abstained from intercourse during all or part of their pregnancies, even if they had not been medically advised to do so. In fact, sexual intercourse during all three trimesters is usually quite safe, but because of lack of knowledge, many couples have sacrificed their sexual enjoyment. Moreover, most new mothers can comfortably and safely resume sexual relationships by about 3 weeks post partum.

8. Remember that no one can help unless you speak up! If you notice a change in your sexual responsiveness (e.g., reduced desire, a problem with orgasm), speak to your clinician. Sometimes medication or a treatable medical problem is the culprit. Low sexual desire can also be an indication of a relationship problem that needs attention. Your clinician can help you sort out what step to take next.

9. Face the problem with courage and hope. A number of behavioral and psychotherapeutic techniques can help you make a positive shift. Most of the time these treatments are brief, affirming, and rewarding. You can usually see improvement after a few sessions.

ADDITIONAL GUIDELINES FOR PRIMARY CARE CLINICIANS

1. Take a sexual history. Even if your questions are brief, asking signals a willingness to listen and to discuss any concerns. Your openness especially aids those patients who harbor shame and anxiety.

2. Discuss treatment options openly. To point the patient in a constructive direction, assess whether the problem is lifelong or recently acquired and whether it occurs in all sexual situations or tends to be more situational. For example, if the patient confides that she has sexual fantasies about men but is not aroused by her partner, you can reasonably assume that her libido is intact but that her relationship is causing difficulty.

3. Recognize that a common sexual complaint of women is hypoactive sexual desire. After you have ruled out major depression, medication-related problems, and androgen deficiency associated with menopause, inquire about the patient's specific complaints. Some women have a very active fantasy life and masturbate regularly. Their sexual problem has a deeper root, namely, a relationship problem. Intervene with these patients by pointing them in the direction of a marital or an individual psychotherapy process.

4. Maintain a nonjudgmental, open attitude and speak directly with the patient. Offer as many resources as possible to facilitate open communication and to give the message that you take her problem seriously. This tactic also enhances the patient's sense of power; she has a "right" to be sexually alive! You might further suggest the behavioral exercise outlined previously as a starting point. Reassure the patient that sexual concerns are among the most common of human afflictions but that these problems are usually highly responsive to education and other clinical interventions.

5. In patients who have lifelong hypoactive sexual desire or sexual aversion, be sure to consider a history of sexual trauma or abuse (Chapter 6). Sexual dysfunction is common in this group, in part because intimacy is perceived as unsafe. However, many patients can overcome the untoward sequelae of abusive or aversive sexual experiences with comprehensive psychotherapy. One of the benefits of a psychotherapeutic approach is the working through of the long-term sexual conflict and the affirmation of the patient's right to a satisfying sexual life.

6. Keep in mind the hefty toll on your patient when a relationship ends, causing possible consequences to physical health and emotional well-being. Divorce or the termination of a long-term committed heterosexual or lesbian relationship can rupture a woman's social support, economic stability, and sense of identity as a "partner." She will need your direction in negotiating a variety of concerns, including child custody, economic help, and her new status as a single person.

7. Do not hesitate to suggest that the patient obtain good legal advice or avail herself of social services. An astute social worker can help her acquire available benefits she may be unaware of but for which she may be eligible. Relationship transitions are rarely easy for anyone, and yet our society is beset by more of them than ever before. Be vigilant about the psychiatric problems of complicated bereavement, depression, and anxiety. Whenever possible, suggest pertinent reading, participation in divorce workshops, and the like. There is no substitute for your investment and your empathic attunement to the difficulties your patient faces in making this life transition.

8. Recognize that particular groups of women (infertile, disabled, and lesbian) have specific concerns about their health care and their relationships. You should develop a working knowledge and familiarity with these concerns. Openness on your part will help these patients to talk about any problems that are impeding their lives and influencing their overall health and well-being (see Tables 13–2 and 13–3).

SUMMARY

Despite progress in understanding the importance of women's sexual responsiveness and desire for intimacy, all too often these issues are overlooked or ignored by clinicians in a busy practice. Physicians have always found it anxiety-provoking to delve into the most personal areas, but this avoidance is also fueled by time constraints, lack of knowledge, and doubt that revealing a sexual issue can lead to change or growth. What should be one of life's most rewarding and gratifying experiences has traditionally been shrouded in shame, ignorance, and denial; inevitably, both women and men have paid a heavy price. When problems in sexual and relationship spheres go unaddressed, each family member's psychological and physical health is potentially compromised. However, clinicians now have new opportunities to help their patients and themselves increase relationship and sexual literacy, thereby enhancing quality of life and personal satisfaction.

The primary clinician's comfort and care in taking the sexual history help the patient to volunteer sensitive, often embarrassing thoughts and experiences. Usually all that is required to broach difficulties in the sexual sphere are some well-timed and specific questions. Asking the patient whether she is sexually active or whether she enjoys her sexuality is a good start. Wondering whether she has noticed any change in her or her partner's interest or frequency can open the topic for further discussion as a barometer of overall well-being. You can further inquire whether the problem is lifelong or recent and whether it occurs in specific or in all situations. If difficulties are uncovered, medical and pharmacologic causes of sexual dysfunction must first be ruled out. A mental health clinician may be consulted to further hone the specific dysfunction by taking a sexual, marital, and psychiatric history (particularly given the time constraints in primary care). Close collaboration between primary care clinicians and mental health professionals is as essential in this area of women's sexual health as in any other, lest the patient believe that you are making a referral because you find her problem unacceptable, odd, repugnant, or a sign of failure.

Primary care clinicians remain pivotal players in the collaborative team to improve the patient's sexual health and her intimate relationships. In the past, health care professionals ignored, trivialized, and often inadvertently injured patients when they failed to even broach these topics. Because sexuality has become a much more speakable issue in our culture, clinicians are now in a position to reverse anachronistic attitudes by dealing directly with these crucial life issues. Doing so also means looking at oneself and addressing any hidden biases and inhibitions regarding human sexuality. Increasing your knowledge base and capacity to be receptive to the patient's history enables you to explore any difficulties with sexual responsiveness more straightforwardly.

Any presenting sexual complaint may hide an important relationship issue. General health and well-being have been correlated with sexual desire, and although there will no doubt always be individuals for whom sex is an insignificant part of their life or primary relationship, a low frequency of sex usually signals a low overall satisfaction in the relationship. Those clinicians who show interest, support, and knowledge about sexuality and its role in helping the individual attain greater life satisfaction will inevitably have the gratitude of the patient.

All patients have unique needs, desires, and aspirations in the arenas of sexuality and relationships. The primary clinician must eschew stereotypes as an individualized treatment approach is formulated in concert with the patient's input.

In this chapter, special emphasis has been placed on the woman patient's needs for intimacy and mutuality in her adult relationships. These relationships include not only her primary sexual relationship but also her adult friendships with persons of both sexes. Special concerns of infertile couples, disabled women, lesbians, and patients taking psychotropic medications have also been reviewed. As with any other health care concern, treatment of a sexual issue must be individualized to help restore quality of life. Such an approach points the direction for the intimate connections that women yearn to cultivate to ensure personal satisfaction and well-being.

RESOURCES FOR PATIENTS

Primarily for Heterosexual Women

Wallerstein JS, Blakeslee S: *The Good Marriage: How and Why Love Lasts.* Boston, Houghton Mifflin, 1995.

Judith Wallerstein's landmark study on the effects of divorce sparked the psychodynamic psychotherapist's interest in what factors facilitate happy marriage. She wondered whether such marriages even exist or are but a figment of wishful fantasy. Through extensive interviews with 50 couples, she discovered eight tasks that couples must accomplish to mold and sustain a satisfying marriage. These tasks include separating from one's family of origin, building togetherness, coping with crises, finding a way to deal with conflict and differences, maintaining a vibrant sexual life, sharing laughter, and providing nurturance. Any woman or man desiring to shape a fulfilling and mature partnership can use this book as a wellspring to do so. The authors include stories of a number of couples interviewed for the study and actual dialogue from these sessions to "spice up" the research findings. Although the book is about the lives of successful heterosexual couples (there is no similar published study to date for long-term homosexual relationships), it is a thought-provoking and inspiring read for any adult contemplating commitment. Wallerstein concludes by viewing marriage as a potentially transformative and life-enhancing experience for both partners; in modern life, the good marriage is "our only refuge" because individuals answer our complex needs "for friendship, comfort, love, and reassurance" (pp. 336–337).

Wallerstein JS, Blakeslee S: *Second Chances: Men, Women, and Children a Decade after Divorce.* New York, Ticknor & Fields, 1989.

Many insightful books are now available for women who divorce. This work, based on the senior author's thorough research on the effects of divorce on the couple and their children, is well known for its ground-breaking findings and superb clinical recommendations. Based on extensive interviews with women, men, and children, the text offers suggestions about how individuals can navigate through the tumultuous after-effects of divorce. Particularly relevant are sections describing the acute and long-term effects of divorce on children and how parents can work to ameliorate any untoward and hurtful consequences on youngsters and teens while not undermining or minimizing their own needs as adults.

For Heterosexuals or Lesbians

Scharf M: *Intimate Partners: Patterns in Love and Marriage.* New York, Ballantine Books, 1987.

Scharf M: *Intimate Worlds: How Families Thrive and Why They Fail.* New York, Ballantine Books, 1995.

These widely available, best-selling paperbacks are likely to be read by women in your practice who want to increase their ability to nurture and sustain their intimate relationships. The author is a wonderful writer whose passion for helping others has led her to study and work with leading family therapists, psychiatrists, and other mental health professionals. In these thoroughly engaging and helpful books, she summarizes what she has mastered so that women and men can build the necessary and life-enhancing foundation for family life. (Essential as this task is to a fulfilling life, the basics are never taught in school!) In each book, Scharf applies psychodynamic and family systems theory to help her readers understand what contributes to common maladies. She gives plenty of sage advice about how to work out difficult problems. For example, in Intimate Worlds, *she offers practical tips and describes several tasks (e.g., have town meetings, directly share negative feelings, don't be afraid to share positive feelings, and find creative ways of dealing with parenting responsibilities and parenting conflicts) that every family can use to make meaningful life changes. For anyone who wants to improve marriage or family life, these books are highly recommended.*

Especially for Lesbians or Parents of Lesbians

Vida G (ed.): *The New Our Right to Love: A Lesbian Resource Book.* New York, Simon and Schuster, 1996.

This authoritative paperback takes up almost every issue or problem confronting lesbians and offers direction about how to get additional help or locate resources. Sections include relationships, sexuality, health, activism, religion and spirituality, education, law, and culture. Each topic is covered in some depth, although the patient will probably need to look up the book's suggested readings for additional coverage on a particular subject (e.g., there are several excellent books now available regarding lesbian sexuality, which are listed at the end of the chapter on sexuality and relationships). By suggesting this particular overview to patients, the primary care clinician demonstrates knowledge, acceptance, and a willingness to discuss all aspects of the lesbian patient's health and sexuality, thereby promoting openness and a solid health partnership in the clinician-patient relationship.

For Patients with Concerns about Sexuality

Barbach L: *For Yourself: The Fulfillment of Female Sexuality.* New York, Penguin, 1976.
Barbach L: *For Each Other: Sharing Sexual Intimacy.* New York, Penguin, 1982.

Both of Lonnie Barbach's best-sellers are likely to be well known to your patients. Each is a complete program for dealing with all aspects of oneself that promote—or prevent—a satisfying sexual relationship. The texts are full of technical pointers (Kegel exercises, vaginal sensitivity exercises, accepting pleasure from one's partner with the "yes exercise"), and excellent tips are also given about how to improve a sexual relationship by open communication, planning for sexual encounters, arriving at working solutions through compromise, and learning how to pleasure one's partner. These compact but information-filled books cover virtually every aspect of female sexual response and list ways a woman can gain more sexual satisfaction whatever her age, marital status, or past difficulties. Barbach is a highly skilled cognitive-behavioral therapist who derives many of her insights from her clinical practice. She is aware of the powerful psychodynamic issues that can also interfere with human sexual response, and she shows women how to resolve conflicts and face down feelings of jealousy, inadequacy, shame, and inner dictates precluding sex, because "each person's physical and emotional needs must be considered if sex is to be a joyous, unself-conscious experience" (1982, p. 279).

Schnarch D: *Passionate Marriage: Sex, Love, and Intimacy in Emotionally Committed Relationships.* New York, WW Norton, 1997.

Libraries and bookstores are cluttered with volumes espousing magic remedies for increased sexual potency and "do-it-yourself" sex therapy at home. This is not one of those "snake oil" panaceas, but it is one of the best books of its genre and comes highly recommended by sex therapists. As Schnarch describes the latest and best-validated techniques for improved sexual performance, he places primacy on the mature relationship as the bedrock of sexual fulfillment. Also unique is the author's masterful synthesis of family systems and psychological theories, which he employs to help readers understand pertinent aspects of development and achieve their sexual potential. Schnarch's use of humor and direct language may be off-putting to some shyer readers, but the majority of patients in a primary care practice will find his clinical examples and warm style both refreshing and instructive. There is also plenty of direct advice about how to loosen or even bypass gridlock in a relationship (e.g., stop taking your partner's reactions personally, confront yourself for the sake of your own integrity and personal development, stop trying to change your partner, keep your mouth shut about your partner's issues—particularly concerning things you are certain are true). Anyone desiring to increase the intimacy quotient can benefit from this book.

RESOURCES FOR PRIMARY CARE CLINICIANS

Magee M, Miller DC: *Lesbian Lives: Psychoanalytic Narratives Old and New.* Hillsdale, NJ, Analytic Press, 1997.
For a fuller appreciation of the diversity inherent in the lesbian experience and the most up-to-date psychodynamic, feminist, and social understanding of homosexuality, this book is an invaluable resource. You will learn that there is no such thing as "a homosexual"; rather, there are "many homosexualities," meaning that lesbians are as diverse in what they do and aspire to become as are heterosexuals. The authors vibrantly describe the "real world" lives of many different lesbian women, so clinicians inevitably garner much understanding about the richness, complexity, and psychological health of lesbian lives just by reading some of these cases. Although same-sex partnerships are depathologized in contemporary mental health practice, clearly both heterosexuals and homosexuals share the range of mental health problems. An appendix at the end of the book deals with pertinent social issues affecting lesbians, including child custody, adoption, and same-sex marriage. This book is also recommended for patients who are interested in how far psychoanalysis and psychiatry have evolved in their understanding of gender roles, sexual preferences, and lesbian relationships. This shift away from bias and prejudice will ultimately benefit the lives of all men and women.

Person ES: *Dreams of Love and Fateful Encounters: The Power of Romantic Passion.* New York, WW Norton, 1988.

Person ES: *By Force of Fantasy: How We Make Our Lives.* Basic Books, New York, 1995.
Neither of these books is typical medical fare. As applicable for the patient as for the clinician, they are full of insights on why we love and what happens when we fall in love. Both are laden with interesting vignettes, fascinating quotations from literature and poetry, and keen perceptions into the nature of each man's and woman's quest for fulfilling relationships. Although Person's books are recommended here to aid the primary care clinician in gleaning a deeper understanding of the vicissitudes of human passion that can benefit patient care, you may be surprised how much they will help you to live and to love more fully yourself. There are plenty of cogent insights to savor: "Passionate love cannot be sustained without the moments in which the lovers feel they have achieved merger, that they are one. Part of the ongoing intensity in love is the insistent hunger to re-experience such epiphanies" (p. 127). "When one is rejected in love, the sense of loss can afflict the very core of the self, fracturing that self, rendering one an emotional amputee" (p. 297). "Constitutional as well as experiential and conflictual factors determine whether one greets life with a fistful of commandments or a pocketful of dreams. Our fantasies may reinforce the former, or herald the latter" (p. 172). If your spirit requires a bit of replenishment from the day-to-day grind, or if your primary relationship could benefit from a fresh spark, turn to either of these resources. To paraphrase the late Dr. Karl Menninger's advice to psychiatric residents, readings such as these not only help us learn new information but also serve as part of the "psychotherapy of everyday life."

REFERENCES

American Psychiatric Association: *Diagnostic and Statistical Manual of Mental Disorders,* 3rd ed., rev. Washington, DC, American Psychiatric Association, 1987.

American Psychiatric Association: *Diagnostic and Statistical Manual of Mental Disorders,* 4th ed. Washington, DC, American Psychiatric Association, 1994.

Baber KM, Allen KR: *Women and Families: Feminist Reconstructions*. New York, Guilford Press, 1992.

Barbach L: *For Each Other: Sharing Sexual Intimacy*. New York, Penguin, 1982.

Barbach L: *For Yourself: The Fulfillment of Female Sexuality*. New York, Penguin, 1976.

Bernardez T: A psychosocial approach to psychotherapy: understanding society's bias against women. *Radcliffe Quarterly* 1985; June:3–4.

Boyarsky B, Hague W, Rouleau M, et al.: Sexual side effects of mirtazapine in depression. New research presentation, American Psychiatric Association Annual Meeting, Toronto, Canada, June 1, 1998.

Cohen AJ: Ginkgo biloba for drug-induced sexual dysfunction. Paper presentation, American Psychiatric Association Annual Meeting, San Diego, California, May 17–22, 1997.

Chodorow N: *The Reproduction of Mothering*. Berkeley, CA, University of California Press, 1978.

Domar AD: Stress and infertility in women. In: Leiblum SR (ed.): *Infertility: Psychological Issues and Counseling Strategies*, pp. 67–82. New York, John Wiley & Sons, 1997.

Domar AD, Zuttermeister PC, Freedman R: The psychological impact of infertility: a comparison with patients with other medical conditions. *J Psychosom Obstet Gynaecol* 1993;14(Suppl):45–52.

Domar AD, Zuttermeister PC, Seibel M, et al.: Psychological improvement in infertile women after behavioral treatment: a replication. *Fertil Steril* 1992;58:144–147.

Downey J: Infertility and the new reproduction technologies. In: Stewart DE, Stotland NL, et al. (eds.): *Psychological Aspects of Women's Health Care: The Interface Between Psychiatry and Obstetrics and Gynecology*, pp. 193–206. Washington, DC, American Psychiatric Press, 1993.

Dressel P, Clark A: A critical look at family care. *Journal of Marriage and the Family* 1990;52:767–782.

Ehrlich GE: *Total Management of the Arthritic Patient*. Philadelphia, JB Lippincott, 1973.

Frank JB, Weihs K, Minerva E: Women's mental health in primary care: depression, anxiety, somatization, eating disorders, and substance abuse. *Med Clin North Am* 1998;82:359–389.

Gill MS: Fertility goddess. *Vogue* 1998; May:120–173.

Grimes JB, Labbate LA: Spontaneous orgasm with the combined use of bupropion and sertraline [letter]. *Biol Psychiatry* 1996;40:1184–1185.

Hanley-Hackenbruck P: Working with lesbians in psychotherapy. In: Oldham JM, Riba MB, Tasman A (eds.): *Review of Psychiatry*, vol 12, pp. 59–83. Washington, DC, American Psychiatric Press, 1993.

Haseltine FP, Cole SS, Gray DB (eds.): *Reproductive Issues for Patients with Disabilities*. Baltimore, MD, Paul H Brookes, 1993.

Heiman JR, LoPiccolo L, LoPiccolo J, et al.: *Becoming Orgasmic: A Sexual and Personal Growth Program for Women*, rev. ed. New York, Prentice-Hall, 1988.

Irons RR, Schneider JP: Addictive sexual disorders. In: Miller NS (ed.): *Principles and Practice of Addictions in Psychiatry*, pp. 441–457. Philadelphia, WB Saunders, 1997.

Jensvold MF, Plaut VC, Rojansky N, et al.: Sexual side effects of psychotropic drugs in women and men. In: Jensvold MF, Halbreich U, Hamilton JA (eds.): *Psychopharmacology and Women: Sex, Gender and Hormones*, pp. 323–368. Washington, DC, American Psychiatric Press, 1996.

Jordan J: The meaning of mutuality. In: Jordan JV, Kaplan AG, Miller JB (eds.): *Women's Growth in Connection: Writings from the Stone Center*, pp. 81–96. New York, Guilford Press, 1991.

Kaplan AG: The "self-in-relation": implications for depression in women. In: Jordan JV, Kaplan AG, Miller JB (eds.): *Women's Growth in Connection: Writings from the Stone Center*, pp. 206–222. New York, Guilford Press, 1991.

Kaplan HS: *Disorders of Sexual Desire and Other New Concepts and Techniques in Sex Therapy*. New York, Brunner/Mazel, 1979.

Kaplan HS: *The New Sex Therapy: Active Treatment of Sexual Dysfunctions*. New York, Brunner/Mazel, 1974.

Kinsey AC, Pomeroy WB, Martin CE, et al.: *Sexual Behavior in the Human Female*. Philadelphia, WB Saunders, 1953.

Kirkpatrick M, Morgan C: Clinical aspects of female homosexuality. In: Marmor J (ed.): *Homosexuality Behavior: A Modern Reappraisal*, pp. 357–375. New York, Basic Books, 1980.

Kirkpatrick M, Smith C, Roy R: Lesbian mothers and their children: a comparative survey. *Am J Orthopsychiatry* 1981;51:545–551.

Kroll K, Klein EL: *Enabling Romance: A Guide to Love, Sex, and Relationships for the Disabled (and People Who Care About Them)*. New York, Harmony Crown, 1992.

Labbate LA, Pollack MH: Treatment of fluoxetine-induced sexual dysfunction with bupropion: a case report. *Ann Clin Psychiatry* 1994;6:13–15.

Lewontin RC: Sex, lies, and social science. *New York Review of Books* 1995;April 20, pp. 24–31.

Leyson JFJ (ed.): *Sexual Rehabilitation of the Spinal-Cord-Injured Patient.* Totowa, NJ, Hamana, 1991.

LoPiccolo J: Sexual dysfunction. In: Craighead LW, Craighead WE, Kazdin AE, et al. (eds.): *Cognitive and Behavioral Interventions: An Empirical Approach to Mental Health Problems,* pp. 183–196. Boston, Allyn & Bacon, 1994.

LoPiccolo J, LoPiccolo L: *Handbook of Sex Therapy.* New York, Plenum, 1978.

Magee M, Miller DC: *Lesbian Lives: Psychoanalytic Narratives Old and New.* Hillsdale, NJ, Analytic Press, 1997.

McQueeney DA, Stanton AL, Sigmon S: Efficacy of emotion-focused and problem-focused group therapies for women with fertility problems. *J Behav Med* 1997;20:313–331.

Michael RT, Gagnon JH, Laumann EO, et al.: *Sex in America: A Definitive Survey.* New York, Little, Brown, 1994.

Miller JB: Women and power. In: Jordan JV, Kaplan AG, Miller JB (eds.): *Women's Growth in Connection: Writings from the Stone Center,* pp. 197–205. New York, Guilford Press, 1991.

Modell JG, Katholi CR, Modell JD, et al.: Comparative sexual side effects of bupropion, fluoxetine, paroxetine, and sertraline. *Clin Pharmacol Ther* 1997;61:476–487.

Morokoff PJ, Calderone KL: Sexuality and infertility. In: Adesso VJ, Reddy DM, Fleming R (eds.): *Psychological Perspectives on Women's Health,* pp. 251–284. Philadelphia, Taylor & Francis, 1994.

Murstein BI (ed.): *Exploring Intimate Life Styles.* New York, Springer, 1978.

Nelson EB, Keck PE, McElroy SI: Resolution of fluoxetine-induced sexual dysfunction with 5-HT3 antagonist granisetron. *J Clin Psychiatry* 1997;58:496–497.

Nicholson N: *Portrait of a Marriage.* New York, Athenum, 1973.

O'Hanlan KA: Lesbian health: therapeutic perspectives. In: Wallis LA (ed.): *Textbook of Women's Health,* pp. 97–104. Philadelphia, Lippincott-Raven, 1998.

Person ES: *Dreams of Love and Fateful Encounters: The Power of Romantic Passion.* New York, WW Norton, 1988.

Person ES: *By Force of Fantasy: How We Make Our Lives.* Basic Books, New York, 1995.

Pines D: *A Woman's Unconscious Use of Her Body.* New Haven, CT, Yale University Press, 1993.

Richards E, Tepper M, Whipple B, et al.: Women with complete spinal cord injury: a phenomenological study of sexuality and relationship experiences. *Sexuality and Disability* 1997;15:271–283.

Rintala DH, Howland CA, Nosek MA, et al.: Dating issues for women with physical disabilities. *Sexuality and Disability* 1997;15:219–242

Roberts LW, Fromm LM, Bartlik BD: Sexuality of women through the life phases. In: Wallis LA (ed.): *Textbook of Women's Health,* pp. 763–780. Philadelphia, Lippincott-Raven, 1998.

Scharf M: *Intimate Partners: Patterns in Love and Marriage.* New York, Ballantine Books, 1987.

Scharf M: *Intimate Worlds: How Families Thrive and Why They Fail.* New York, Ballantine Books, 1995.

Schnarch D: *Passionate Marriage: Sex, Love, and Intimacy in Emotionally Committed Relationships.* New York, WW Norton, 1997.

Schover LR, Jensen SB: *Sexuality and Chronic Illness: A Comprehensive Approach.* New York, Guilford, 1988.

Segraves RT: Psychopharmacological influences on human sexual behavior. In: Oldham JM, Riba MB (eds.): *Review of Psychiatry,* vol 14, pp. 697–717. Washington, DC, American Psychiatric Press, 1995.

Segraves RT, Segraves KB: Female sexual disorders. In: Stewart DE, Stotland NL (eds.): *Psychological Aspects of Women's Health Care: The Interface Between Psychiatry and Obstetrics and Gynecology,* pp. 351–374. Washington, DC, American Psychiatric Press, 1993.

Segraves RT, Segraves KB: Sexual dysfunction: diagnosis and treatment. *Primary Psychiatry* 1998;5:71–76.

Seiderman SN, Rieder RO: Sexual behavior through the life cycle: an empirical approach. In: Oldham JM, Riba MB (eds.): *Review of Psychiatry,* vol 14, pp. 639–676. Washington, DC, American Psychiatric Press, 1995.

Sevely JL: *Eve's Secrets: A New Theory of Female Sexuality.* New York, Random House, 1987.

Sipski M, Alexander CA (ed.): *Sexual Function in People with Disability and Chronic Illness: A Health Professional's Guide.* Gaithersburg, MD, Aspen Publishers, 1997.

Stein TS: Overview of new developments in understanding homosexuality. In: Oldham JM, Riba MB, Tasman A (eds.): *Review of Psychiatry,* vol 12, pp. 9–40. Washington, DC, American Psychiatric Press, 1993.

Tolis G, Diamanti E: Distress amenorrhea. In: Chrousos GP, McCarty R, Pacak K, et al. (eds.): *Stress: Basic Mechanisms and Clinical Implications. Ann N Y Acad Sci* 1995;771:660–664.

Vida G (ed.): *The New Our Right to Love: A Lesbian Resource Book.* New York, Simon & Schuster, 1996.

Walker PW, Cole JO, Gardner EA, et al.: Improvement in fluoxetine-associated sexual dysfunction in patients switched to bupropion. *J Clin Psychiatry* 1993;54:459–465.

Wallerstein JS, Blakeslee S: *The Good Marriage.* Boston, Houghton-Mifflin, 1995.

Wallerstein JS, Blakeslee S: *Second Chances: Men, Women, and Children a Decade After Divorce.* New York, Ticknor & Fields, 1989.

Welner SL: Gynecologic care and sexuality for women with disabilities. *Sexuality and Disability* 1997;15:33–40.

Westheimer R: *Dr. Ruth's Guide to Good Sex.* New York, Gramercy, 1983.

White J: Medical care of lesbian patients. In: Carr PL, Freund KM, Somani S (eds.): *The Medical Care of Women*, pp. 787–793. Philadelphia, WB Saunders, 1995.

Chapter 14

The Older Patient

At her 80th birthday party, internationally acclaimed jazz pianist Marian McPartland provided an admirable perspective on growing older. She said, "I don't dwell on being over the hill, I just take it as another dimension in my life. I've got things to do and . . . I feel that working is the best thing anybody can be doing, especially when you are doing something you like, and you are able to give others work, and generally be helpful all around. I certainly don't want to just sit in the backyard and dig bulbs."

(Folly Theatre, 1998, p. 13)

Why can't more senior citizens embrace the perspective of McPartland? Why are the final years of life dreaded by so many people, including clinicians? Despite the continuous process of loss most people face as they grow older, the mature years can afford unique opportunities for growth and creativity (Pruyser, 1987). This kind of creativity is not necessarily about bringing forth special talents, although it certainly can be—as cases like that of Marian McPartland demonstrate (see Comfort, 1976).

For the majority of elderly patients, growing older does not have to be a time of inevitable decline of body and mental functions, nor a time of bitter disappointment or malcontent. For older people who maintain a modicum of physical and emotional health, growing old affords new opportunities as one realizes the successes and disappointments inherent in a life fully lived. As the late psychologist Paul Pruyser (1987) observed, older persons exhibit a greater sense of interiority than younger persons. This reflective capacity enables them to take on the important process of reviewing their lives as they adjust to new, and somewhat diminished, aspirations. The elderly are indeed survivors whose hardiness and resilience prepare them for the losses yet to come, including the loss of their own lives. But in the best of circumstances, their tenacity and reflectiveness permit what Pruyser called "attitudinal forms of creativity in ordinary people" (p. 429).

Psychoanalyst Carl Jung (1930/1978) described this kind of "artistry of life" another way. He contrasted the morning of one's life with the evening, pointing out that what was initially "great" or significant does not necessarily carry over into one's advancing years, when different challenges must be met. In his psychotherapeutic work with older people, Jung had occasion to look deeply "into the secret chambers of their souls" and found that those who viewed the second half of life as an opportunity were less likely to possess excessive self-absorption because they had already lavished their "light upon the world." Jung believed that these blessed elderly were creative, productive, and generative—true artists of life; he observed that "we must not forget that only a very few people are artists in life; that the art of life is the most distinguished and rarest of all arts" (Jung 1930/1978, p. 19).

319

As the older population continues to grow dramatically, the primary care clinician naturally asks: "What can I do to preserve the health and add to the quality of life, not just the longevity, of my elder patients?" As all clinicians unfortunately realize, too few of our elderly attain the "artist of life" perspective of a Marian McPartland. To some extent, this failure occurs because some very treatable problems remain unrecognized.

Another area of concern is dementia. Clinical trials for the treatment of Alzheimer's disease are just beginning. Alzheimer's disease is a women's mental health problem because it affects the oldest of the old in our society, who are predominantly women. More women than men have Alzheimer's disease; women also provide a disproportionate amount of care for loved ones with the disease (McCann et al., 1997). Older women in the United States outnumber older men by 6 million, and the difference increases with advancing age. Because women have a longer life expectancy than men and because older men are more likely to marry, a high proportion of older women live alone. They are at increased risk for disability and poverty, and the sequelae of loneliness and demoralization (e.g., depression). However, when the elderly can partake of meaningful activities, their physical and psychological health improves, as measured by quality of life indicators or a number of other research domains (Clark et al., 1997).

WHAT THE CLINICIAN CAN DO TO HELP THE OLDER PATIENT THRIVE

Remaining active as well as productive is a key component of successful aging. Older adults are presented with unique psychological stressors that can contribute to psychiatric disorders, such as depression, psychosis, substance abuse, anxiety, and eating disorders. When they discontinue important pursuits, they experience diminished satisfaction in life. When the physician encourages an active lifestyle, a good diet, an ongoing social support, and an exercise regimen, the patient is more apt to maintain a sense of personal autonomy, health, and independence.

For example, in the past, occupational therapy was generally used after a patient fell victim to a catastrophic illness or accident. In a preventive program with the goal of mitigating the health risks of older adults, an occupational therapy protocol was designed to help patients achieve a healthy and satisfying lifestyle and remain socially active (Clark et al., 1997). Patients were taught a number of important skills, including home and community safety, exercise and nutrition, joint protection and energy conservation, and the like. During activity sessions, they went to community outings, worked on craft projects, viewed films, played games, and attended dances. The highly individualized protocol also required participants to apply its content to their everyday experiences so as to better overcome barriers to successful daily living. When administered by professional occupational therapists, preventive programs for older adults were found to be highly effective across various health, function, and quality-of-life domains.

This chapter paints with a broad brush the canvas of problems the primary clinician is likely to face in working with older female patients. An all encompassing view is clearly beyond the scope of this book; it is worthy of an entire

---

Table 14–1. **Office Aids to Mental Wellness Intervention of the Elderly Patient**

Assess cognitive and mood function. Consider differential diagnosis of depression, dementia, and pseudodementia.

Pay special attention to medications, especially polypharmacy of over-the-counter and prescribed drugs; consider toxicity. Review indications of all drugs. Titrate psychotropic medications slowly.

Be alert to misuse of substances (e.g., undiagnosed alcoholism).

Assess sexual functioning. Encourage discussion of sexual concerns. Validate desire for sexual well-being. Discuss any physical illness of patient or partner that can interfere.

Be alert to covert eating disorder, especially in patients with poor nutritional status and/or preoccupation with physical appearance.

Identify self-neglect, domestic violence, elder mistreatment.

Attend to advance directives for medical treatment.

---

text by itself. But recognizing the scope of the most common problems, helping the patient or caregiver to obtain specialty consultation when needed, having an appreciation of the pharmacologic pitfalls in treating the elderly, and appreciating the psychological challenges of this period of life enables the primary care clinician to have a positive impact on the growing number of older women in his or her practice (Tables 14–1 and 14–2).

DEPRESSION

Depression is widespread in late life, affecting women at substantially higher rates than men. About 5% of primary care patients older than 65 years of age suffer from major depressive disorder. Clinically significant, subsyndromal depressions (i.e., those that do not meet all the criteria of the *Diagnostic and Statistical Manual of Mental Disorders*, 4th ed., 1994) are also common, adding to the public health burden. These treatable illnesses are still frequently missed by health care providers (Lebowitz et al., 1997; Rothschild, 1996). Among the depressed elderly, symptoms such as loss of appetite, sleeplessness, anergia, and

---

Table 14–2. **Office Aids to Helping Caregivers of the Elderly**

Give careful instructions, both verbal and written.

Show concern for caregiver's emotional and physical well-being. Remind caregiver of the possibility of burnout. Encourage days off, respite care, and so on.

Provide referral information and suggest pertinent reading to increase support network of caregivers (e.g., Alzheimer's Society).

Encourage caregiver to deal early on with legal issues (e.g., advance directives, living wills, durable power of attorney).

Remember that mistreatment and neglect of the elderly occur when caregivers are stressed, emotionally burdened, depressed, or "burned out." Help prevent this situation through early identification and support.

---

loss of interest or pleasure in usual activities are more common initial presentations than mood difficulties. The greater likelihood of these physical symptoms is a prime factor that leads to underdiagnosis and undertreatment of depression in this population.

Depressed patients are at a high risk for physical decline; prevention and treatment of depression may be one of the most cost-effective and practical interventions to reduce physical decline in later years (Penninx et al., 1998). Hypothetically, depression increases sympathetic tone, decreases vagal tone, and causes immunosuppression. Depression therefore may deepen susceptibility to and inhibit recovery from physical disease via psychological mechanisms. Patients who are depressed are less likely than healthy persons to seek medical attention and rehabilitation, or to follow prescribed treatments and practice healthful living habits (Penninx et al., 1998). In concrete terms, depressed persons do less "walking, gardening, and vigorous exercise" and complain more about "fatigue and pain," which may explain in part their physical decline (Penninx et al., 1998, p. 1725). Even though clinicians know how common depression is, when they hear about the problems of weight loss or insomnia, loss of taste, or low energy, they tend to think first of other diseases (e.g., diabetes, malignancy). Instead, depression should be high on the list of differential diagnoses in the elderly.

Research has revealed the heterogeneity of the clinical and biologic causes of late-life depression. In women, hormone-related causes have been suggested, and hormone replacement therapy has been associated with improved mood and quality of life for many. In others, depression appears to be a result of brain abnormalities, appearing on CT scans as ventriculomegaly or white-matter hyperintensity (Jeste, 1997). Vascular disease has also been implicated. Lesions in the basal ganglia and prefrontal areas of the brain result in the clinical profile of a depressed patient with psychomotor retardation, lack of insight, and impaired executive functioning (Roberts et al., 1997).

The primary care clinician must first rule out any medical illnesses or drug-induced side effects that may be causing depression (see Chapter 2). Grief reactions must also be taken into account. Older women suffer more losses than younger ones, often outliving their spouse and friends. But the thorniest presenting symptom to evaluate is difficulty with concentration. Half of all patients with Alzheimer's disease experience depression before organic brain syndrome becomes evident. These patients still benefit from having depression treated (Oxman, 1996).

For most physicians, selective serotonin reuptake inhibitors (SSRIs) have become the first-line antidepressant therapy for elderly patients because of their ease in prescribing, benign side-effect profile, and lack of toxicity when taken even in overdose (Newhouse, 1996). But inhibition of liver cytochrome P-450 oxidase enzymes has emerged as one of the potentially more problematic aspects of the SSRIs, especially in the elderly. Those elderly patients who take multiple medications may be more at risk for adverse interactions or effects if metabolism is altered by the inhibitions of these oxidases (Finkel, 1996; Flint and Rifat, 1998).

The long-established principle that medications should be initiated at lower doses and the doses increased more slowly in older persons than in younger has scientific merit. To avoid the anxiety or agitation that may be produced by an SSRI, physicians should begin at half of the routine or recommended clinical dose for adults (e.g., fluoxetine or paroxetine at 10 mg/day; sertraline at 25 mg/day). Because patients tend to tolerate SSRIs better than they do traditional tricyclic therapy, their greater cost may be justified by improved compliance, fewer doctor visits, and decreased hospitalization (Finkel, 1996).

Despite the notable advances in psychopharmacology, medication should not be viewed as the sole approach. Cognitive-behavioral and psychodynamic treatments are widely available and quite effective in promoting quality-of-life changes. The elderly patient must deal with many changes, stressors, and "phase-of-life" challenges (Arieti and Bemporad, 1978; Sunderland, 1996). These can be uniquely addressed in the presence of a benign and interested psychotherapist. The primary care clinician should encourage involvement in psychotherapy because it can prolong periods of good health and therefore is cost-effective.

Family members also feel the brunt of others' depression; their burden can be lifted by a referral to a psychoeducational workshop or a suggestion that they try self-help or professional psychotherapeutic support for themselves (Sherrill et al., 1997). Patients and families value hearing how others in similar circumstances have handled an illness; this information normalizes their experience and gives them an opportunity to openly address concerns. It is particularly important to help loved ones sort out deficits they attribute to aging from the toll that depression takes; when this issue is appropriately handled, family members tend to blame their loved ones less and to assist them more in maintaining ongoing treatment.

Patients benefit from the active learning process of cognitive-behavioral therapy to sort out relationship, life-stage, and health-related difficulties; they learn to overcome obstacles that get in the way of experiencing more pleasure. As in the treatment of younger adults, cognitive-behavioral therapy for older individuals challenges distortions and helps replace automatic, negative thoughts with more constructive ones. Some modifications are necessary (e.g., asking elderly patients to summarize material when there is any decline in memory or attention span), but in general the same opportunity to learn new skills and confront new stresses can be employed across the life cycle (Thompson, 1996).

Patients need time to elaborate their concerns in greater detail, particularly to disentangle real from perceived losses in life and to work through conflicts with a spouse, adult children, and friends. Many women must come to understand their propensity to brood over "lost opportunities." They may need to mourn the loss of ideal love or a youthful appearance, either of which could be a dominant and pervasive but unconscious goal. Psychodynamic psychotherapy enables the patient to "feel receptive again to the array of life's aims and loves" (Arieti and Bemporad, 1978, p. 286). Current behaviors and relationships are explored so that the patient may confront rigid expectations and personal myths; the goal is to achieve a more realistic but vital perspective for one's remaining years. In essence, the woman is urged to discover and cultivate strong and important relationships with friends and family members, and to pursue cultural interests. This perspective helps her accept age and transcend its many losses, including the eventual end of life itself. She is then freer to reap other rewards of a rich life.

In some cases of psychotic depression or depression unrelieved by trials of standard psychotropic medication and psychotherapy, electroconvulsive therapy (ECT) may prove lifesaving. Most psychiatrists believe that ECT is not used because of physicians' and patients' misconceptions about it. Those who have not themselves witnessed the easy application and beneficial effects of contemporary ECT have a distorted view based on inaccurate portrayals by movies and television. In reality, ECT is extremely safe and nonpainful when given using anesthesia in an operating room; it can rapidly alleviate depression, particularly in those with a life-threatening illness (e.g., not eating, severely suicidal). For the most part, any mild effects on memory (ECT-related confusion) are rapidly reversible, but this side effect may limit ECT's use in older patients who already have significant memory impairment. Clinical judgment becomes imperative in selecting those patients whose medical or psychiatric condition warrants the potential benefit weighed against side effect of short-term (and usually totally reversible) memory impairment (Flint and Rifat, 1998; Rothschild, 1996; Zisook, 1996).

WHY IS ALZHEIMER'S DISEASE A WOMEN'S MENTAL HEALTH PROBLEM?

Because women make up 72% of the U.S. population older than 85 years of age, they are the group most affected by this heterogeneous disease. One third to one half of this group have Alzheimer's disease (McCann et al., 1997). The risk of Alzheimer's disease increases dramatically with advancing age, and many more women than men survive to ages at which Alzheimer's disease is most common.

In the next 50 years, the number of people with Alzheimer's disease will more than double; most of those affected will be women, who generally have the most limited social and financial resources (McCann et al., 1997). As the population ages, this patient group will become older and more frail, with more functional impairments and chronic diseases.

One study estimates that more than 4 million people in the United States alone are affected with Alzheimer's disease, but because the distinction between normality and disease is not precise, estimates of prevalence vary widely (Khachaturian, 1997; Morrison-Bogorad et al., 1997; Small et al., 1997). However, it is generally agreed that there is underrecognition of the dementing diseases because clinicians do not routinely assess cognitive functioning and because mild cognitive impairments are viewed as a normal part of the aging process (Small et al., 1997). Alzheimer's disease is the most common form of dementia (70%), followed by diffuse Lewy body disease (15%–25%) and vascular dementias (5%–10%) (Cullum and Rosenberg, 1998). Comprehensive care requires a full evaluation to rule out treatable and reversible causes of memory loss or other conditions of dementia (Table 14–3).

The consensus statement on the diagnosis and treatment of Alzheimer's disease and related disorders recommends that family intervention is crucial to comprehensive care. Loved ones require education, counseling, and support (Khachaturian, 1997; Lake and Grossberg, 1996). Studies of caregivers of Alzheimer's patients have demonstrated an increased prevalence of depression and depressive symptoms and a greater use of antidepressants, tranquilizers, sleeping pills, and pain medications. Families should also be given concrete warnings about the hazards presented by the Alzheimer's patient who wanders, stays home

---

Table 14–3. Diagnostic Considerations for Memory Changes in the Elderly

Potentially treatable/reversible conditions

Medical
  Medication side effects (anxiolytics, sedatives, analgesics, antidepressants, alcohol, anticholinergics)
  Age-related polypharmacy and pharmacokinetics (decreased metabolism/ elimination)
Psychiatric
  Pseudodementia (i.e., depression associated with dementia)
  Depression
Metabolic/endocrine
  Hypothyroidism, Cushing's disease, kidney disease
Nutritional deficiencies
  Vitamin B_1, B_6, B_{12} deficiency
  Poor eating habits
  Weight loss secondary to psychiatric illness
Neurologic
  Infection
  Normal-pressure hydrocephalus
  Chronic subdural hematoma
  Tumor

Irreversible/progressive conditions

Neurologic
  Alzheimer's disease
  Lewy body disease
  Vascular dementia
  Frontotemporal dementia
  Prion disease

---

alone, or continues driving. Poor health, dementia, and visual impairment place both drivers and the public at risk; the primary care clinician is in a position not only to help patients maintain their independence but also to discourage older drivers who are impaired and to encourage others to voluntarily retake driving tests in order to prevent accidents (Forrest et al., 1997).

New treatments have been found to slow or to arrest the degenerative process; the use of cholinesterase inhibitors (i.e., tacrine HCl [Cognex] and donepezil [Aricept]) has been approved. Donepezil is becoming a first-line intervention because of the associated statistically significant improvement in cognitive functioning with no serious side effects or abnormal laboratory findings. (Tacrine causes notable gastrointestinal distress and reversibly elevates serum transaminase levels; it moderately improves cognitive functioning in patients with mild-to-moderate Alzheimer's disease.) Donepezil can be given once daily and does not require regular liver monitoring. The recommended starting dose of 5 mg/day may be increased to 10 mg/day after 1 month. However, the higher, more efficacious dose tends to cause cholinergic side effects (e.g., nausea, diarrhea, insomnia).

Various hormone therapies and vitamin supplements have been heralded as keys to longevity and even to a reversing of the aging process. Nonsteroidal antiinflammatory agents, selegiline, alpha-tocopherol, and *Ginkgo biloba* have each been the focus of placebo-controlled trials claiming their effectiveness (LeBars et al., 1997; McCann et al., 1997; Sano et al., 1997), but no single agent has been found to be uniformly effective. The clinician has a partially salutary message to give the patient and her family: "We have several agents we can try that have helped others, and new drugs are being developed every day. We hope we can slow the course of this disease, but as far as we know it is not reversible, even with medication."

In postmenopausal women, estrogen therapy has been posited as one of the major senescence decelerators (Olshansky et al., 1998; Yaffe et al., 1998). In addition to reducing the risk of heart disease, osteoporosis, and symptoms of menopause, estrogen has been shown in some studies to reduce by half the risk of Alzheimer's disease for women in the postmenopausal period and to significantly delay the age of disease onset, even after adjustment for other risk factors (McCann et al., 1997). Apparently, estradiol modulates neurotransmitter activity, particularly increasing central adrenergic tone through the monoamine oxidase and serotonin pathways. Estradiol also prolongs the survival of cholinergic neurons, acting independently or in synergy with other neurotropic factors to improve cognitive functioning by promoting cholinergic activity in the brain. But as yet estrogen cannot be recommended unequivocally. In a metaanalysis of 10 studies of postmenopausal estrogen use, conflicting results were found (Yaffe et al., 1998). More trials are needed to support the use of estrogen in women for the prevention or treatment of Alzheimer's disease or other dementias.

Primary care clinicians are likely to be called on to treat depression, agitation, or psychosis associated with dementia. Although nonpharmacologic strategies can reduce stimuli or modulate the environment of the agitated patient and can increase the social structure and activity level of the depressed patient, most patients require pharmacologic therapy (Alexopoulos, 1996; Alexopoulos et al., 1998; Duffey and Coffey, 1996). Clinical trials indicate comparable efficacy among antidepressant agents for patients with depression. Likewise, the antipsychotic drugs are comparably efficacious in treating a variety of behavioral and psychotic symptoms. Although newer antipsychotics (e.g., clozapine, risperidone, olanzapine) have not been well studied in elderly patients with dementia, mounting clinical evidence supports their use (Alexopoulos, 1996; Tariot, 1996). Two superb monographs review treatment selection according to algorithms of the significant behavioral disturbances common to patients with Alzheimer's disease (see Alexopoulos et al., 1998; Schneider and Small, 1996).

Supportive psychotherapy can also help the neurologically damaged patient (and her family) adapt to the reality of the illness and constructively deal with its deficits (Lewis et al., 1992; Lewis and Langer 1994; Lewis, in press). In addition to facilitating a process of mourning the loss of previous functioning, the psychotherapeutic relationship provides a haven that "is understandably experienced as a very special blessing to these patients" (Lewis et al., 1992, p. 327). Lewis cautions treaters that their own biases about the hopelessness of organic damage can creep into the doctor-patient relationship and poison a potentially useful dialogue that helps the patient deal constructively with limitations. Although patients and families should not be given "false hope," they must also be urged to see what they can still do to educate themselves about the nature of the illness and be aided in their capacity to cope with problematic behaviors and emotions (e.g., aggression). Psychotherapy helps patients and families of the organically damaged feel less alone and facilitates long-range planing and goal setting.

Successful patient management requires the primary care clinician to spend time establishing an excellent working alliance with the family and other caregivers. As mentioned, caregivers—who are most typically women—can easily succumb to burnout and are at a higher risk for the diagnosable conditions of depression and anxiety. Three fourths of dementia patients require admission to a residential, long-term care facility at some point. Their loved ones need time to complete the arrangements and to make the emotional adjustment. They can benefit from the supportive, compassionate care of a primary care clinician who urges them to make plans early.

Family members also worry about the genetic risk to themselves. You can remind them that having a first-degree relative with Alzheimer's disease increases their risk by only slightly more than 1% above that of the general population (Khachaturian, 1997; Post et al., 1997). Clearly, more research is needed to determine the types of health care services required by persons with Alzheimer's disease and to examine the health consequences of caregiving. As yet, the necessary community-based services, including adult day care, transportation, and home health care, are not covered. Yet our society will need to develop alternatives to institutionalization in light of the huge increase in the number of older, unmarried women who will develop Alzheimer's disease over the next 50 years. As McCann and associates aptly summarized, "Unless progress is made in preventing the disease or delaying its onset, the need for medical services and the cost of such services will be extraordinary. . . . Planning for these services must consider the changing patterns of family structure and economic support, especially with regard to women, the group most affected by the disease" (1997, p. 136).

SOME PRACTICAL STEPS IN TREATING THE BEHAVIORAL SYMPTOMS OF DEMENTIA

Behavioral management of dementia—a harrowing challenge both for the clinician and the patient's loved ones—is the leading reason for admission to a nursing home. Overt hostility, agitation, hallucinosis, and hyperactivity respond to neuroleptics, although there is currently no single best choice of medication. Diagnosis of the symptoms is often complicated by cognitive impairment, and antipsychotic medications can cause side effects, especially if they have high anticholinergic potency. Although newer antipsychotic agents (e.g., risperidone) look promising, there is no clear evidence that one agent offers unparalleled benefit.

Usually, a fairly low dose of medication brings the target symptoms of disruptive behavior under control (once-daily oral doses: haloperidol, 0.5–2 mg; loxapine 10.5–20 mg; risperidone 0.5–3 mg) (Harris, 1997; Jeste et al., 1996; Sunderland, 1996). The basic principle of starting with lower doses and increasing in small increments applies to the use of conventional and newer antipsychotic drugs in the elderly (Jeste et al., 1996). Polypharmacy should be avoided because of the risk of anticholinergic toxicity.

Alternatives to neuroleptics for behaviorally disturbed patients with dementia require more study. To date, possibilities include trazodone, buspirone, diphenhydramine, and oxazepam. Each has been found, in at least one study, to diminish agitation or other behavioral disturbances in the demented elderly. The primary care clinician who treats the behavioral symptoms in these patients is advised to refer to standard pharmacologic texts for the most current treatment and dosage recommendations in this rapidly evolving area of geriatric psychiatry. Specialty consultation with a mental health professional may also be warranted, especially because minor adjustments in the patient's daily routine or a more comprehensive environmental manipulation may be required for adequate symptom amelioration. For example, late-day agitation (sundowning) may be managed by reorienting the patient and by structuring activities as the sundowning occurs. Increased light and/or psychotropic medication (e.g., trazodone) may also be helpful.

Wandering can be dangerous and troublesome, requiring diversion and supervision or even the addition of sound or motion detectors to one's home (Cole, 1995). For patients who pace all night, a sedative (e.g., trazodone) may be necessary. Because the behavioral problems and life circumstances are unique for each patient, few generalizations can be made safely. An individualized treatment plan for behavioral management, which models a capacity to use assistance and to adapt to change, should be formulated in concert with the caregiver and a team of professional experts.

SUBSTANCE ABUSE

Because clinicians tend to associate addictive disorders with younger adults, alcohol and drug problems among the elderly have also received less attention by the medical community. At the Mayo Clinic, 10% of all annual alcoholism admissions occur in patients older than age 65 (Morse, 1988). Not surprisingly, the psychological issues of retirement, death of a loved one, health problems, and family conflicts were found in these patients' histories. The elderly are vulnerable to drug and alcohol abuse not only because of increased biologic sensitivity (e.g., alcohol and hypnotics accumulate because of reduced metabolism) but also because they turn to these substances as an outlet for the "common ailments of old age, such as loneliness, pain, insomnia, depression, and grief" (Morse, 1988, p. 260).

When taking a comprehensive medical history, clinicians must ask the older woman about how much alcohol she is drinking, also taking into account the addictive depressogenic effects of prescribed drugs (e.g., benzodiazepines) and the intoxicant effects of over-the-counter agents (e.g., antihistamines). Be sure to ask about the presence of a substance abuse history, because such patients are at much greater risk for abuse of psychoactive drugs. Women who have sustained a loss tend to "self-medicate" at home with alcohol, benzodiazepine, or pain medication. Among those elderly patients who do have a problem with abuse, a few will be relying on cold remedies, mouthwashes, and gargles that contain up to 25% alcohol. Misuse is typically denied by the alcoholic.

Prevention of substance abuse problems in the elderly begins with education about the increased biologic sensitivity to these drugs with aging and the psychosocial stressors that can potentiate their use. Although physicians may empathize with patients who drink because they feel depressed, they also need to let elderly patients know that depression itself can result from alcohol consumption. When alcohol abuse is curtailed, mood typically improves. Likewise, it is important to explain how alcohol can affect the metabolism of other drugs, such as by increasing the blood levels of benzodiazepines, amitriptylines, or barbiturates. If a patient complains that a medication is ineffective (e.g., a hypnotic drug prescribed for a brief period because of insomnia), she may actually have developed cross-tolerance with alcohol.

For the majority of patients, substance abuse treatment is effective. You should underscore the value of becoming completely abstinent, although a substantial number of patients are able only to "cut down" rather than "stop." In most cases, pharmacologic treatment and/or psychosocial therapy (e.g., individual therapy; Alcoholics Anonymous) is necessary to augment the education and treatment provided by the primary care clinician (see Chapter 4). Although the idea of "controlled" drinking or drug use should be discouraged, it is nevertheless wise to be hopeful and encouraging about the long-term results of comprehensive treatment. The majority of women who engage in treatment experience improved mood and improved cognitive functioning as the toxic effects of the addictive drugs lessen in their bodies.

ABUSE AND NEGLECT

Primary care clinicians must be aware of the potential for their elderly patients to be neglected and abused; there is mounting evidence that this societal malady is on the increase. Abuse can occur both by those who have a personal (i.e., caregiving) relationship with the woman and by those with a professional or business relationship; it is not limited to domestic violence (Hudson, 1997). Moreover, living alone, lack of social support, and limited finances put women at risk of neglecting themselves. Mistreated elders "stay hidden in the home or institution" and the signs are "too often denied, ignored, or blamed on aging or illness" (Hudson, 1997, p. 146). Elders can also become violent toward or mistreat their caregivers, leading in some instances to reprisals. A vicious cycle can be set in motion, impeding the health and mental well-being of both parties; intervention is essential. Primary care and mental health clinicians must confront their tendency to keep silent or remain unaware of this societal malady (Nadien, 1996).

Effective intervention begins when clinicians are informed about the potential of elder mistreatment. Factors associated with violence toward the elderly include an overwhelmed caregiver, the elderly person's dependence on a spouse or adult child, the poor health of the elderly person or the perpetrator, and rigid, unyielding caregiving expectations. Elder neglect and self-neglect are associated with (1) a refusal of the patient or her caregiver to accept assistance (e.g., because of denial, pride, mistrust), (2) a self-interest of the caregiver, (3) an overwhelmed caregiver who can no longer meet the elder's needs for time and/or financial support, and (4) a dysfunctional family system (e.g., due to estrangement, alcohol abuse) (Flitcraft, 1998). Routine assessment for abuse and neglect is advisable, with the clinician paying particular attention to injury, affect, hygiene, and nutritional status.

EATING DISORDERS

Eating disorders have been characterized classically as illnesses of adolescence and young adulthood, but truly late-onset eating disorders do occur (Beck et al., 1996; Zerbe, 1993/1995). Older women become preoccupied with age-related body changes in appearance, which inevitably raise narcissistic (i.e., self-esteem) concerns. Paramount are the losses one endures and how one adapts to inevitable change. Reduced appetite, diminished taste and smell, and a desire to exert control over the body (and the aging process) all factor into the cause of anorexic or bulimic tendencies in the aged.

Decreased food intake, poor appetite, and body preoccupation in the elderly patient should alert the clinician to consider the possibility of an eating disorder. For example, one patient in her 70s presented to a psychiatrist for headache, shortness of breath, malaise, back pain, and pedal soreness, for which no organic cause could be found. She had exhausted—both literally and figuratively—a sophisticated and committed medical community that was unable to pin down her problem, let alone alleviate her distress, despite numerous diagnostic work-ups and pharmacologic trials. In fact, she was battling a 20-year course of anorexia nervosa and brief episodes of purging that had developed after the death of her only child. Her husband had "solved" his grief by having an affair, but this bereaved woman had nowhere to turn. She had "buried" her feelings in her body. She developed numerous psychosomatic illnesses and ruminated about her body image and appearance. Eventually, she began an expressive psychother-apy process. Her physical preoccupations decreased, and she reestablished a relationship with her mate despite his affair. Although she remained thin and continued to exercise vigorously, she no longer teetered at the threshold of death from anorexia and metabolic disturbances brought on by purging and laxative abuse.

The primary care clinician may need to call on a specialist to differentiate a true eating disorder from clinical depression (Beck et al. 1996; Zerbe 1993/95) or dementia (Cullen et al., 1997). In both clinical depression and dementia, loss of appetite, weight loss, rejecting food, and turning on anyone who even men-tions eating may masquerade to even experienced clinicians as symptoms of anorexia nervosa. However, the patient with an eating disorder typically is hungry but does not eat because of worry about physical appearance. She is likely to overexercise, to abuse over-the-counter laxatives and diuretics, and to always be "on a diet," all the while manifesting concern about health (e.g., "Doctor, I take eight different vitamins and seven herbs every morning before I race walk"). In contrast, most depressed and/or demented patients take poor care of themselves, are not interested in food, and are anergic.

In your evaluation, be empathic about how society discriminates against older women by its emphasis on youth and beauty. The primary care clinician should be careful about dispensing advice about the need to lose weight, which may be "taken over-seriously, even compulsively, and result in anorexia nervosa" (Beck et al., 1996, p. 394). Those who have been sensitive to weight or appearance issues earlier in life may experience an exacerbation of body or eating preoccupa-tion if criticized by a spouse, friend, or physician. Should you be confronted with the differential diagnosis of depression or truly late-onset eating disorders, first rule out other medical conditions that also cause weight loss (e.g., diabetes).

Then consider specialty referral after initiating some basic treatment steps in these life-threatening conditions (see Chapters 2 and 5).

PSYCHOSIS IN LATE LIFE

Elderly patients can and do become psychotic. As the lifespan becomes longer, the number of older patients with psychoses is expected to increase. These conditions arise primarily from late-onset schizophrenia, general medical conditions, and mood disorders. Late-onset schizophrenia is 2 to 5 times more common in women than in men (see Chapter 12). Premorbidly, the patient may have a mild schizoid or paranoid personality pattern. Usually, there is a prodromal decline in functioning, followed by active auditory hallucinations and delusions. Cognitive (neuropsychologic) impairment is apparent, but deterioration is rarely observed. Schizophrenic patients do not have difficulty learning new information, but must struggle to retain it. In contrast, Alzheimer's patients have difficulty both with learning and with retention (Harris, 1997; Sunderland, 1996).

Pharmacokinetic and pharmacodynamic alterations in the elderly translate into the necessity of using lower doses of antipsychotic medications; these changes also place the patient at risk for serious adverse effects (e.g., neuroleptic-induced tardive dyskinesia). Most experts recommend a basic principle of "starting slow and going slow" when using any psychotropic medication in the elderly (Harris, 1997).

The new serotonin-dopamine antagonists (e.g., quetiapine, risperidone, olanzapine) have added to the therapeutic armamentarium for the management of elderly patients because of their lower incidence of side effects. Many other agents (e.g., haloperidol) can also be useful in reducing agitation and curtailing hallucinations. In addition, vitamin E (alpha-tocopherol) has proved effective in some patients with tardive dyskinesia. Most clinicians recommend social skills training for older patients with psychoses to increase their self-confidence and social interactions (Jeste et al., 1996).

PHARMACOLOGIC CONSIDERATIONS

The differences between men and women have only of late been applied to research in drug therapies. Although the elderly of both sexes are at increased risk for adverse drug effects, leading to increased morbidity and potential mortality, some other important generalities about gender difference can also be made. Among the very old, information is limited, so that gender-related drug effects in this group are not as yet fully understood.

The elderly are a heterogeneous group. Because they differ so much in such factors as activity level, general overall health or lack thereof, and dietary patterns, response to particular drugs is unpredictable. Pharmacokinetic changes affect medication absorption, distribution, metabolism, and elimination. For example, the greater loss of lean body mass after age 60 in women affects the distribution of water and lipid-soluble drugs. Older women who take psychoactive drugs for anxiety, depression, bipolar illness, or other conditions are therefore at greater risk for the development of side effects (Jeste et al., 1996; Noyes, 1997).

Lithium toxicity is more common, particularly when an older person becomes dehydrated with the flu or gastrointestinal upset. Although not all enzymatic pathways are affected by aging, hepatic metabolism can change with reduced blood flow. Psychotropic medications, such as the benzodiazepines, tricyclic antidepressants, and carbamazepines, are likely to accumulate because of reduced hepatic metabolism. Initiating low-dose pharmacotherapy and watching carefully for adverse drug reactions are recommended for the older woman patient (Finkel, 1996; Noyes, 1997).

Polypharmacy among the elderly is often underestimated, particularly among those who live alone. Be sure to ask about all over-the-counter medications and herbal remedies the patient is taking. These are often considered unimportant by patients but can increase the frequency of drug-to-drug interaction, thus exacerbating compliance problems. The more medicine an elderly person takes, or believes she must take, the greater the chance for clinical failure (Leventhal, 1994; Noyes, 1997).

Be sure to give the patient plenty of instructions about prescribed medications and urge her to use memory aids such as pillboxes or calendars. Physical impairment (e.g., loss of vision, loss of hearing, loss of dexterity secondary to arthritis), lack of knowledge, and memory problems are all factors that can negatively affect the older person's adherence to treatment recommendations. Take, for example, an elderly patient with a hearing problem who fails to respond to treatment. You may think she understands you because she nods affirmatively. In fact, she may not have heard your instructions and so was not compliant because she did not understand, not because she was reluctant to follow your advice or was having a memory lapse (see Mayerson, 1976).

Diagnosis of the patient's difficulty in following through with your advice begins in the office. If you write down your instructions, in addition to practicing the communication skills of face-to-face interaction with well-enunciated, distinct words, you are more likely to be successful in enlisting the patient's cooperation. You will also be more likely to pick up on any covert physical or memory impairments that impede the patient's self-care and quality of life.

Thirty-one percent of all prescription medications and more than 40% of all nonprescription drugs in the United States are consumed by people older than 65 years of age, although this group makes up only 14% of the population (Jeste, 1997; Noyes, 1997; Zubenko et al., 1997). Particularly in institutional settings, patients are at risk for drug-induced illnesses because of multiple drug use. Inadvertently, medications may be duplicated (e.g., generic and brand names used but not recognized by the patient or inexperienced staff members). Be particularly aware of the inadvertent overuse of sleep aids among the elderly. Because of age-related changes in metabolism, benzodiazepines such as flurazepam (Dalmane) can accumulate and cause adverse consequences, including falls and resultant hip fractures. For the agitated elderly patient in an institutional setting, a small dose of neuroleptic medication (risperidone, 0.5 mg orally, once a day; or haloperidol, 0.5 mg orally, once a day) may be all that is required to bring severe anxiety and/or psychotic thoughts under control and to assist nursing personnel in the overall care of the patient (Noyes, 1997; Sunderland, 1996; Tariot, 1996).

SEXUALITY

There are a growing number of popular accounts and spirited testimonials of older women who proclaim that sexuality remains a vitalizing, comforting, and important part of their lives (see Berman and Goldman, 1992; Comfort, 1976; Doress-Worters and Siegal, 1987/1994; Weaver, 1996). An active sex life improves the quality of life and contributes to enhanced self-confidence, self-image, and feelings of competency. But the desire to maintain physical intimacy into old age can be impeded by sexual problems and fewer available partners. The latter is particularly an issue for heterosexual women, who tend to outlive their male partners and are often reluctant to seek out other available men (Gatz et al., 1995; Leventhal, 1994). The most important factor for the primary care clinician to keep in mind is to ask about the patient's sexual life. When you inquire about the sexual needs and desires of the older patient, you confront the stereotype of the asexual older woman. This inquiry gives the patient permission to speak to you about issues she may otherwise feel are forbidden.

Because of the physiologic complaints associated with menopause (e.g., estrogen deficiency leading to thinner vaginal walls, decreased vaginal secretions, atrophy of Bartholin's glands), dyspareunia is the most common sexual complaint of older women. Although arousal and lubrication take longer to occur, orgasm itself is not significantly impaired. Many complaints and much embarrassment can be averted by counseling the female patient to use external lubricants, which are widely available in pharmacies and women's health cooperatives. Some women prefer petroleum jelly to water-soluble lubricants; encourage the patient to try several different brands until she finds the one that works best for her. This suggestion not only provides valuable technical information but also psychological affirmation of the woman's desire to remain sexually active and involved all her life.

For those patients whose physical mobility may be limited (e.g., because of arthritis), a range of interventions can be suggested, including buying a book or manual that describes less taxing sexual positions or seeking out a formal sex therapy process. Remind the older patient that a nonsteroidal analgesic or hot bath before sex may reduce any pain or soreness associated with the medical problems of late life. Shifting to a side-by-side position for intercourse may also be preferable to having one person on top.

Sometimes vaginal penetration is precluded by a medical condition or by a waning of interest on the part of the patient's partner. In these cases, try to affirm the importance of alternative modes of sexual expression, which range from massage to hand-holding to oral sex. You might also suggest a sex therapy process. Many older couples have been helped by books, videotapes, and recommendations from trained therapists (see Comfort, 1976). For the older woman who is alone, masturbation can be a satisfying alternative, particularly if she experiences permission and sensitive encouragement that her erotic desires are natural, lifelong, and a sign of good emotional health.

You should remind the patient of the common aphorism that the most important sexual organ is the brain. This somewhat facetious but accurate statement prepares her for the counseling points about the actual diminution in sexual responsiveness that occurs with aging. In regard to a woman's desire to feel "more normal," you might observe that diminished vaginal lubrication, decreased sexual interest, and increased difficulty attaining orgasm have been shown to be the norm for women over age 60 (Leiblum and Segraves, 1995). Moreover, most heterosexual women are concerned about their partner's ability to achieve, maintain, and enjoy an erection because they have observed the increase in the male's sexual response cycle. These shifts in responsiveness can be adapted to when partners free themselves to be creative and adventuresome. Lesbian couples also find that the climacteric period damps their sexual desire. Hormone replacement therapy, in addition to the aids described previously, can lessen their sexual complaints.

Primary care clinicians cannot expect to be familiar with all the nuances of contemporary sex therapy to be able to help every aging patient. What is more important is an accepting attitude that allows inquiry into sexual functioning to be taken seriously. It is important to have knowledge about the experts in your community. Referral for advice reassures your patients that you take their needs seriously and believe that sexual health is an important aspect of quality of life and ongoing satisfaction in a relationship (see Wallerstein and Blakeslee, 1995). Rule out any disease states that can interfere with sexual functioning (e.g., arthritis, chronic obstructive pulmonary disease, scarring after hysterectomy). But also pay special attention to emotional issues in the comprehensive medical evaluation. The majority of sexual problems in the elderly occur because of untreated and undiagnosed depression, loss of self-esteem, and marital discord (Barry, 1995; Leiblum and Segraves, 1995; Zisook, 1996). Assessment of the impact of any major life event on the woman is essential, because "sexual functioning is intimately interconnected to all aspects of physical and emotional health" (Leiblum and Segraves, 1995, p. 692).

Clinician and patient alike sometimes need the gentle reminder that, although sexuality changes over the course of a lifetime, it need never become a nonexistent or nonessential part of one's being. Growing older brings about unique stressors, but it also brings about new opportunities for learning about oneself and one's partner. As Leiblum and Segraves observed:

> Whereas sexual exchange over the years may have occurred in the confines of the bedroom behind locked doors, it now may be possible for couples to venture out of the bedroom and into other areas of the house. As one 68-year-old, newly sexually active widow explained, "The bedroom is boring!" . . . On the other hand, some long-partnered couples—homosexual or heterosexual—may have eliminated some positive components of their sexual script. For instance, during early courtship, much time is usually spent getting ready for a sexual encounter. Long baths or showers before sex, anointing the body with oils and perfumes, and putting on (or taking off) sexy undergarments may have been important components for the sexual encounter . . . with much sensual stroking and mutual arousal before intercourse. Over the course of a 30- or a 40-year-marriage, *a more "no-nonsense approach" to sex may have evolved, without the niceties, thoughtfulness, and just plain preparation of youth. Unfortunately, there is often a greater need for such ingredients as one grows older.*
>
> (1995, p. 692, emphasis added)

A LONG AND HAPPY LIFE—WHAT FACTORS PROMOTE IT?

Physician and patient alike are naturally curious about those factors that promote optimal aging. Histories of centenarians are instructive. They depict lives of hardy survivors able to withstand multiple losses and disappointments in life and yet emerge with a sense of wholeness and well-being. People who live a long life may have suffered a great deal, but in essence they still count their blessings and find that their cup continually runneth over with enjoyment for what life affords. They remain happy because they have a capacity to see the positive in virtually every situation. Grateful for the good times and believing that they will leave behind something that transcends themselves, they have a philosophy of life that embodies finding pleasure in the here and now and refusing to dwell on life's failures or setbacks (Prager, 1998).

Pruyser (1987) opined that maintaining a sense of humor in the face of life's disappointments and adversities is a form of creativity within the reach of ordinary, not just gifted, persons. This kind of life perspective eschews sarcasm and arrogance; jokes are not made at other people's expense. As the elderly person confronts her own mortality and waning energy, altruism and humor offer consolation and "the capacity to smile benignly at one's self, to accept one's inevitable foibles, and to accept realistically one's limitations in influencing the world without feeling lamed by such awareness" (Pruyser, 1987, p. 433).

A remarkable book by the African-American centenarians Sarah and Elizabeth Delaney (1993) points to other crucial factors contributing to longevity. As described by Gillum (1997), the personal remembrances of these women, who were ages 103 and 101 when their first book was published, illustrate seven likely contributing factors to a meaningful life that grew even fuller as they overcame obstacles and put their own hopeful philosophies about living into the practice of helping others (e.g., altruism). These factors of optimal aging include (1) middle-class financial circumstances and the acquisition of education; (2) avoidance of maternal morbidity and mortality and the tolls of domestic violence and stress (the sisters remained single all their lives); (3) avoidance of unnecessary medical treatment; (4) recognition of the value of good nutrition and exercise (i.e., for years the sisters took long daily walks, then turned to yoga when long walks were no longer possible; they also ate fruit and vegetables every day, drank boiled water, and took vitamin supplements); (5) lifelong companionship and family support; (6) optimistic outlook and the capacity to withstand disappointment (even in the face of family tragedies and discrimination that would have embittered others less resilient, they maintained a sense of hopefulness and a live-and-let-live attitude); and (7) strong religious faith and belief in the importance of individual life contributions. Raised by a clergyman in a socially activist parish, the Delaneys developed a lifelong sense of social activism and connection to others. At a time when most women, especially African-Americans, were not encouraged to follow a professional career, they pursued their respective careers in dentistry and teaching, "dedicated to helping others and asking little in return," until they retired (Gillum, 1997, p. 50).

The most important antidote to psychological aging appears to be staying involved throughout one's entire life. The older patient should be encouraged to follow the dictum that Erikson (1950) attributed to Freud: "To love and to work." The primary care clinician plays a pivotal role because maintaining a physically healthy body is the fulcrum of psychological well-being. But the clinician must embody the wisdom of staying physically active, maintaining a sense of humor, and dealing with issues of loss. Those who can mourn are equipped to carry on vibrantly and energetically with an ever-increasing awareness of the limits of time, accomplishments, and even life itself. Women especially must find ways to maintain a sense of self-esteem in the face of changes in appearance and body. Psychotherapy and even psychoanalysis may be useful in helping the older patient live more fully and meaningfully, seeing life as "a journey down a spiral staircase in which we traverse, often again and again, albeit at different 'elevations,' many psychological territories we have traveled before" (Shneidman, 1989, p. 684). Older persons need a safe place to review their lives as the intensity of their ambitious strivings and the narcissistic gratifications of an earlier time are transformed. This process helps establish the attitude of what Erikson (1950) called generativity; that is, a concern with guiding the next generation. One must take personal stock of oneself and modify one's narcissistic aspirations (Kahana, 1978; Sandler, 1978). Open discussions with one's loved ones or primary clinician, or even a psychodynamic psychotherapy process, promote the sense of interiority or introspection that is crucial in late life.

PATIENT GUIDELINES FOR COPING WITH AGING

1. Have a positive outlook and focus on what you can do, not on what you can't do. Women sense that the best of life is only for the young. But you can grow, and even thrive, over your entire lifespan. As Maggie Kuhn, the founder of the Gray Panther Movement, wrote:

   Old age is not a disaster. It is a triumph over disappointment, failure, loss, illness. When we reach this point in life, we have great experience with failure. I always know that if one of the things I have initiated falters or fails, it won't be the end. I'll find a way to learn from it and begin again. When I was younger, I took failure much more seriously.

   (Kuhn et al., 1991, p. 214)

2. Look after your physical and emotional well-being. The two most frequent emotional problems affecting older women are depression and anxiety. If you feel sad, blue, or fearful, speak up and seek help. If you begin to lose interest in activities that used to be important, have difficulty sleeping, or don't enjoy being with people who used to matter to you, you may be suffering from a form of clinical depression. Newer, safer medications and psychotherapy are bringing relief to more and more older people, helping them lead full, active lives. Unfortunately, thousands of older adults with symptoms of depression do not get the help they need because they fail to tell the doctor all of their complaints. Diagnosis is frequently missed.

3. Expand your social network. Older women are more likely to live alone than are older men. They underreport potentially serious symptoms but tend to overuse the medical system for less serious, but troublesome, complaints. They also tend to receive less social support as they grow older. Women in their senior years are likely to have survived a number of losses, sometimes even the loss of a spouse. These losses increase their risk of physical illness and emotional stress, unless they reach out for other support. Increasing your social ties promotes emotional well-being and health. Positive attachments reduce the risk of infection and other diseases.

4. Stay active. A good diet, daily exercise, and regular visits with your doctor are important preventive health measures. Physical exercise and strength training

not only reduce your chances of developing osteoporosis (which can lead to fractures and a host of other medical problems), but they also improve cognition and mood. Overall, women have a more constructive attitude about taking care of their health than men. This may be one important factor in their living, on average, 7 years longer than men.

5. As much as possible, try not to worry about getting Alzheimer's disease. If you have a family history of the disease, you should visit with your physician about how to maintain your cognitive health by staying mentally active and by taking hormone, vitamin, or herbal supplements. You will want to review any specific risk factors before initiating medication. Worrying about developing a condition such as Alzheimer's disease can sap the energy you need to confront real issues that you can do something about (e.g., exercising, ensuring your economic well-being). Do not accept inaccurate myths about aging. Many women maintain an active and invigorating sexual life, even though our society has a bias against viewing older people as sexual.

6. You may have read the inaccurate statement that women are more susceptible to dementia than men. It is true that there are more women than men with Alzheimer's disease. But women are at greater risk for getting the disease *only* because they live longer than men.

7. Learn from other women who have gone before you. There are a number of excellent books (see end of chapter) and documentary videotapes that will give you some excellent examples about how others have gone about living a full and highly productive life as they grew older. Finding interesting things to do and staying in control as you "ripen" are essential factors in maintaining psychological and physical health.

ADDITIONAL GUIDELINES FOR PRIMARY CARE CLINCIANS

1. Rule out any treatable causes of cognitive decline (e.g., medical illness, depression). Help your patients focus on the concept of successful, healthy aging so that they feel empowered to continue to grow over each phase of the life cycle.

2. Keep an open ear for symptoms of emotional problems. Late-life mental disorders have a significant negative impact on the survival of older patients (see Zubenko et al., 1997). Underdiagnosis and undertreatment of depression are particularly common.

3. Capitalize on identifying depressed patients in your practice and initiate appropriate antidepressant medication at an adequate dose. Encourage adequate follow-up. When using psychotropic medications in the elderly population, physicians can easily underprescribe, with subtherapeutic doses, or overprescribe, leading to drug toxicity. Increase the dose in small increments and do not hesitate to refer to a psychiatrist if the patient does not quickly respond to a trial of two different antidepressant medications in adequate dosages. Keep an up-to-date pharmacotherapy reference available for the latest dosage recommendations.

4. Combine drug therapy for depression with psychotherapy in the elderly. Many of these patients must adapt to difficult life situations that require

emotional support and development of coping skills. They must also deal with the losses associated with growing older. By all means, improve your patients' understanding of depressive illness through systematic education, helping them learn about options for treatment that will improve their quality of life.

5. If you treat the older depressed patient without specialty referral, begin by using the safer antidepressants (e.g., SSRIs; nefazodone). The tricyclics, although inexpensive and of proven efficacy, have the major side effects of hypotension, cardiac toxicity, and anticholinergic toxicity. In addition to constipation, anticholinergic toxicity causes some frail elderly to fall. In one important study of medically ill, depressed patients (Koenig et al., 1997), 60% of them received no antidepressants at any time, and 50% received a benzodiazepine that potentially exacerbated the depression while leaving them at risk for falls, hip fractures, and other accidents. Depression is a very treatment-responsive illness, and you are in an excellent position to identify and manage it.

6. Assess the risk for suicide. In the elderly, suicide is closely associated with untreated major depressive illness. Physicians should ask about suicidal thoughts in all older patients who present with symptoms of depression. A majority of depressed suicide victims had seen their primary care physician during their last month of life; 39% during the last week (Lebowitz et al., 1997).

7. Listen for complaints of persistent sleep disturbance. An important clue to recognizing depression in older women in a primary care setting is a relatively common, treatment-resistant insomnia (Mendelson, 1997). The complaint of poor sleep is more common in older women than in men. If hypnotic medication is used in an elderly patient, a shorter-acting benzodiazepine or the nonbenzodiazepine zolpidem is preferable because of the decreased likelihood of residual daytime sedation (see Chapter 7). If the patient is also depressed, consider a low dose of a sedating antidepressant such as trazodone. There is a wide range of normal variation in the need for sleep, but it is important to distinguish patients with insomnia from those who are able to manage on as little as 2 or 3 hours of sleep per night. Most older people need and get 8 hours of sleep. Their sleep needs do not change, but their sleeping patterns do. Consequently, they may be sleeping less at night but napping more during the day. Ask the patient about her sleep habits, checking for any lack of feeling refreshed from sleep, not just the total number of hours spent in bed at night. (A patient may wake up at 3 a.m. because she went to bed at 8 p.m.) In the elderly person, sleep disturbance may be related to medical illness (e.g., sleep apnea, hypothyroidism, obesity) or medication (e.g., metoprolol). In some persons, insomnia may be a prodromal indication of psychiatric illness such as major depression, generalized anxiety disorder, or obsessive-compulsive disorder (see Chapters 1, 2, and 7).

8. Remember that older patients do suffer from eating disorders and/or addictions. Inquire about the use of addictive substances (e.g., alcohol, benzodiazepines) in the comprehensive history. Brief and extended periods of exposure to benzodiazepines have been associated with an increased risk of motor

vehicle crashes in some elderly populations (Hemmelgarn, et al., 1997). Try to minimize their long-term use or at least discourage driving.

9. In the patient with cognitive decline, consider the use of estrogen therapy. Although estrogen has not been shown conclusively to be effective in the prevention or treatment of Alzheimer's disease, in some women it appears to improve cognition or to reduce the severity of the dementia.

10. Remember that more women than men have Alzheimer's disease as a result of women's longer lifespans. Because most caregivers are women, the overall impact of the disease is greater for women than for men. Be sure to offer your patient hope by keeping her apprised of the newest research on drug trials (e.g., nonsteroidal antiinflammatory agents, antioxidants), which in some cases appear to retard the progression of Alzheimer's disease.

11. Although no treatment has yet been found to arrest the degenerative process in all patients, consider use of the acetylcholinesterase inhibitors, tacrine HCl (Cognex) or donepezil (Aricept). Keep the patient and family involved by encouraging them to join an Alzheimer's association in your local community or other support groups. Without giving false hope for a cure, be sure to acknowledge that other cholinesterase inhibitors and cholinergic agonists are in clinical trials and may be of benefit to their loved ones.

12. Empathize with the psychological needs of family members and caregivers of the elderly in your practice and help them make realistic plans for their loved one. The majority of elderly patients, including those with Alzheimer's disease, receive most of their care from an informal family network that is the first line of defense against institutionalization but bears the burden alone. Because caregiving is stressful, caregivers have increased physical and psychological morbidity themselves. They benefit from your encouragement not to relinquish opportunities for socialization and recreation. Their task is to learn to care for themselves while they care for others, and your advice is a crucial motivator.

13. Be alert to the burdens of the "sandwich generation" (i.e., women who have responsibilities for caring for their own families as well as their aging parents) in your practice. Many adults (primarily women) care for older parents, have marriage and childcare responsibilities, and are employed outside the home. These caregivers are subject to job and family conflicts and are prone to develop depression or depressive-related symptoms (see McCann et al., 1997). The primary care clinician can help by encouraging these women to take care of themselves. Caregivers cannot provide care unless they have an emotional and physical reservoir inside themselves to draw on. You might suggest that these caregivers look to alternative or decreased work schedules whenever possible to free up some time for themselves. Finding alternatives to meeting the elderly person's every emotional and financial need might start with the caregiver attending a support group meeting where she is reminded that she cannot give to others what she does not have in herself to give.

14. Use the tendency for women to report symptoms as a positive asset in your practice. Their readiness to solicit advice may be a result of gender socialization patterns. Women tend to report more symptoms because, as the primary caregiver in most family groups, they learn coping strategies that alert them to illness and prepare them to provide care for others (see Leventhal, 1994).

This means that women in your practice tend to take your advice and to engage in a variety of health practices or strategies you recommend.

15. You might consider framing the attention a woman places on her body as a positive form of self-monitoring that she has acquired over the course of her life. Women's primary responsibilities for child and family care have poised them "to be the experts at monitoring and coping with somatic problems" (Leventhal, 1994, p. 31). The woman's psychosocial role, and not a tendency to "be a hypochondriac," is what propels her to use health care and to engage in preventive behavior as a way of controlling the worries of her family members.

16. Help the patient and her caregiver to prepare for death (see Chapter 9).

17. Remember that aged patients are involved in a "life review," a process of recalling experiences and memories of "past successes and failures to arrive at some sort of balance sheet. The crisis of age is the acceptance of this balance sheet" (Mayerson, 1976, p. 267). Listening to the patient's story, as much as possible within the confines of a busy practice, is an enormously supportive gesture. It helps the patient maintain ego strength and a sense of personal integrity because the clinician shows respect and pleasure for past successes.

The clinician's function for the elderly patient is one of a "champion" who helps face down "incapacity in death"; the physician also becomes an "intimate friend" who "takes up the slack in a natural succession as meaningful others depart" (Mayerson, 1976, p. 262) through relocation, incapacitation, or death. The clinician also gains perspective and insights into his or her own life by conversing with elderly patients.

SUMMARY

Growing older is more often a women's issue because older women outnumber older men by 6 million, and this difference increases with advancing age. These women naturally want to stay healthier, to lead more active lives, and, in essence, to be "truly alive" all their lives. They seek the services of their primary care clinician (and mental health providers) to achieve all of those goals. There is a growing list of activities, pharmacologic remedies, and therapeutic opportunities to help such patients live more meaningfully and with fewer ills. But many treatable conditions still remain undiagnosed. This chapter addresses some of the most common and potentially treatable disorders of the elderly and offers directives about how to be helpful to the patient, her family members, and other caregivers.

Recognition of cognitive dysfunction, mood impairment, substance misuse, eating irregularities, and behavioral disturbances will increasingly become a part of the daily practice of most primary care clinicians. Age-related physiologic factors need to be taken into consideration in the drug treatment of elderly persons, whose age places them at higher risk for adverse effects and drug interactions. Improving compliance and taking into consideration self-medication, multiple medications, and certain functional impairments are all crucial to the overall health of the elderly patient.

The primary care clinician also must attend to important psychological issues.

Each woman in her final years is faced with making a life review; that is, reviewing her entire life and making an assessment of her goals, failures, and accomplishments. Although the medical literature has pointed out the longer life expectancy of women and has commented extensively on the medical and psychological consequences of those who live alone, it has paid relatively little attention to helping patients actually adapt by making new and meaningful changes. This task has fallen on the shoulders of the healing community. Women must be encouraged by their primary care clinicians to stay active and involved all their lives. Finding a safe space where they can also engage in open dialogue about their lives is often indicated, particularly when the patient suffers an acute loss or setback or simply has trouble dealing with the vicissitudes of aging.

The clinician must also pay attention to the needs of caregivers of the elderly. Many adults and children treasure their time with elder relatives, thriving on their guidance and wisdom and craving the opportunity to learn about family history and the "olden days" when the parent or grandparent was in the position the younger person is in now. This time for reminiscence with loved ones permits the older person to make the crucially important journey of "life review." But attending to others also takes its toll, no matter how much the role is cherished. The greater the need the elderly person has for guidance, the greater the caregiver feels taxed or drained by the onus of responsibility. Increasingly, the "young old" care for the "old old," and these relatives and friends are usually women themselves. Without the gentle confrontation and empathic concern of the primary care clinician, these caregivers will so burden themselves that they will be at risk for emotional difficulties or physical disease as they relinquish opportunities for socialization and become isolated.

The primary care clinician who stays attuned to the broad scope of issues affecting the physical and emotional well-being of the older patient and her caregivers can help improve quality of life for both parties. As in so much of medicine, the crux of the matter lies not in making an extraordinary diagnosis of a rare disease or in carrying out some new, innovative, or radical treatment. Rather, the task lies in diagnosing the most common conditions (e.g., depression) and making use of widely available treatments. But in the seemingly banal or insignificant also lies the sublime opportunity to make a real difference in the life of another person. Understanding the psychological issues that older women and their caregivers confront in the final decades of life promotes their life-affirming and creative adaptational opportunities. Inevitably, the clinician also learns in the process, particularly by listening to the interesting and human stories the patient has to tell. Working with aging patients thus provides unique insights for the clinician over the course of an entire professional life. These opportunities should be cherished for what they teach us about health, fortitude, and resilience.

Resources for the Patient and Her Family

Doress-Worters PB, Siegal DL: *The New Ourselves, Growing Older: Women Aging with Knowledge and Power,* rev. ed. New York, Touchstone, 1987/1994.
  This is perhaps the most well-known, important, encyclopedic paperback about growing older. In addition to its comprehensive, interesting, easily read suggestions about medical problems, finances, sexuality, and relationships, a lengthy section is devoted to available resources for older persons (e.g., books, articles, support groups, organiza-

tions). *Emphasis is placed on how to live fully and enthusiastically in one's later years. Practical suggestions for those who care for the elderly are also fully described. A key aspect of this book is its authoritative summaries and positive images of aging. Pertinent sections may be recommended by your clinician. Such information can be empowering, thus strengthening your doctor-patient relationship and fortifying your own compliance and self-reliance (hence reducing your need to call on your doctor so frequently).*

Weaver F: *I'm Not as Old as I Used to Be: Reclaiming Your Life in the Second Half.* New York, Hyperion, 1997.

Weaver F: *The Girls with the Grandmothers' Faces: A Celebration of Life's Potential for Those Over Fifty-five.* New York, Hyperion, 1996.

Frances Weaver fulfilled her lifelong dream of becoming a writer after her physician-husband's death. It is hard to imagine how any reader who glances at even a few pages of these autobiographic sketches will not feel energized and inspired. She views growing older as a time of multiple opportunities when grasped with fierceness and passion. Weaver consciously made efforts to master new activities such as learning to use a computer, traveling by herself, and expanding her circle of friends, because she believes "the sincere desire to lead a productive, interesting life at any age depends upon our own imagination and acceptance of new ideas" (1996, p. 13).

Both of these widely available and acclaimed books are actually quite witty and wonderful for any man or woman from midlife on who needs an appropriately placed kinesthetic boot in the gluteus maximus to even begin to consider making a change. The Girls with the Grandmothers' Faces addresses topics such as widowhood, dealing with the travails of adult children, traveling alone, sexuality, and changes in one's physical appearance. I'm Not as Old as I Used to Be goes into more depth about the challenges of grief and widowhood and recommends finding pleasure in everyday opportunities such as kite flying, college classes for audit or credit, dance lessons, or mastering the word processor. Chances are that many older women have already found these books: They are national best-sellers for very good reason. Weaver's advice will also help clinicians to keep a positive attitude about their practice and their own aging. Because she is such a natural optimist, Weaver grasps the potential of the individual to grow psychologically and spiritually over the course of the entire life cycle. None of us has to be "as old as we used to be."

Resource for Caregivers

Mace NL, Rabins PV: *The Thirty-Six Hour Day,* rev. ed. Baltimore, MD, Johns Hopkins University Press, 1991 (softcover edition: Warner Books, NY). Original edition published in 1981.

This now-classic guide for caregivers has been endorsed by the Alzheimer's Disease and Related Disorders Association of America. It describes exactly what to do with a myriad of problems that inevitably arise when a loved one has been diagnosed with dementia. Topics range from dealing with the initial work-up to the final phases of the illness, with special emphasis on problems in independent living (e.g., when the patient can no longer manage money, drive safely, live alone, make good decisions). The authors explain the common behavioral and medical problems that a caregiver is likely to face and give straightforward suggestions about how to get proficient help. It is often difficult for clinicians to fully appreciate the ravages of a particular disease unless they have experienced it themselves. Consequently, they often give advice that misses the mark—not because they don't care, but because they don't know what to say. This book helps clinicians enter the world of the dementia patient and her family, so as to become better equipped to offer meaningful suggestions and empathically respond to their concerns. To understand exactly what patients and families are going through, and how to help them, by all means read this book.

Additional Resources for Primary Care Clinicians

Berman PL, Goldman C (eds.): *The Ageless Spirit*. New York, Ballantine, 1992.

In order to grasp what a life well lived can actually be for your older patients, read these essays based on a series of interviews with elderly authors, actors, comedians, and activists. The book is a compendium of wisdom about how meaningful the later years can be, right up to the very end of life. Full of humor and rock-hard insights, this book can also be recommended to patients. Its value to the clinician lies in its rollicking coverage of the physiologic and psychological metamorphosis of growing older in a manner that eclipses the colorless prose of most medical texts.

National Institute on Aging/National Institute of Health Annual Progress Report on Alzheimer's Disease. NIH Publication no. 97-4014. Silver Spring, MD, U.S. Department of Health and Human Services, 1997.

This yearly summary of the most recent findings of modern medicine's ability to delay the progression of symptoms of Alzheimer's disease is a worthwhile reference to have in the office. Although it is thorough, it is also nontechnical enough to be of value to many patients and their families. Particular highlights are the brief reviews of the most current neuropathologic discoveries about the brain, advances in identifying genetic risk factors and diagnosing Alzheimer's disease, and future research directions, including therapeutics. Primary care clinicians will be able to give the most up-to-date scientific information about treatments that families ask about (e.g., herbal remedies, estrogen replacement, selegiline, vitamin E). Special attention is placed on how to get extra support for families who are giving care. For example, adult daycare for dementia patients is becoming available in more and more communities. It is recommended to reduce stress and improve well-being for those caregivers who must function with the constant worry and strain of a loved one with Alzheimer's disease. The book lists many places, Alzheimer's Society branches, and support groups where families can get concrete and salutary assistance.

Sodeman WA: *Instructions for Geriatric Patients*. Philadelphia, WB Saunders, 1995.

To help patients, family members, and caregivers understand illness and comply with treatment, this book of simple instruction sheets can be photocopied in the office and handed directly to the patient at the end of a visit. The instruction sheets cover a range of medical issues (e.g., genitourinary problems, skin diseases, rheumatic and orthopedic problems, infections) but mental health concerns are not given short shrift. Attention is given to recognition and treatment of depression, delirium, dementia, sleep disturbances, and eating disorders. A final, brief section on legal issues addresses questions of advance directives, living wills, and durable powers of attorney. Sections on memory aids and driving tips are applicable to many seniors and those who are primarily responsible for their day-to-day care.

References

Alexopoulos GS: The treatment of depressed demented patients. *J Clin Psychiatry* 1996;57(Suppl 14):14–20.

Alexopoulos GS, Silver JM, Kahn DA, et al.: *Treatment of Agitation in Older Persons with Dementia: The Expert Consensus Guideline Series. A Postgraduate Medicine Special Report*. Minneapolis, McGraw-Hill, 1998.

Arieti S, Bemporad J: *Severe and Mild Depression: The Psychotherapeutic Approach*. New York, Basic Books, 1978.

Barry PP: Health care of the elderly woman. In: Carr PL, Freund KM, Somani S (eds.): *The Medical Care of Women*, pp. 663–672. Philadelphia, WB Saunders, 1995.

Beck D, Casper R, Andersen A: Truly late onset of eating disorders: a study of 11 cases averaging 60 years of age at presentation. *Int J Eat Disord* 1996;20:389–395.

Berman PL, Goldman C: *The Ageless Spirit*. New York, Ballantine, 1992.

Clark F, Azen SP, Zemke R: Occupational therapy for independent-living older adults: a randomized controlled trial. *JAMA* 1997;278:1321–1326.

Cole SA: Behavioral disturbances in Alzheimer's disease. *Patient Care* 1995;29:121–131.

Comfort A: *A Good Age.* New York, Crown, 1976.

Cullen P, Abid F, Patel A, et al.: Eating disorders in dementia. *Int J Geriatr Psychiatry* 1997;12:559–562.

Cullum CM, Rosenberg RN: Memory loss: When is it Alzheimer disease? *JAMA* 1998;279:1689–1690.

Delaney S, Delaney AE: *Having Our Say: The Delaney Sisters' First 100 Years.* New York, Kodansha International, 1993.

Diagnostic and Statistical Manual of Mental Disorders, 4th ed. Washington, DC, American Psychiatric Association, 1994.

Duffey JD, Coffey CE: Depression in Alzheimer's disease. *Psychiatr Ann* 1996;26:269–273.

Doress-Worters PB, Siegal DL: *The New Ourselves, Growing Older: Women Aging with Knowledge and Power,* rev. ed. New York, Touchstone, 1994. (Original publication, 1987.)

Erikson EH: *Childhood and Society.* New York, Norton, 1950.

Finkel SI: Efficacy and tolerability of antidepressant therapy in the old age. *J Clin Psychiatry* 1996;57(Suppl 5):23–28.

Flint AJ, Rifat SL: Two-year outcome of psychotic depression in late life. *Am J Psychiatry* 1998;155:178–183.

Flitcraft A: Violence, abuse, and assault over the life phases. In: Wallis L (ed.): *Textbook of Women's Health,* pp. 249–259. Philadelphia, Lippincott-Raven, 1998.

Folly Theatre. *Jazz Program.* Kansas City, MO, April 18, 1998.

Forrest KY, Bunker CH, Songer TJ, et al.: Driving patterns and medical conditions in older women. *J Am Geriatr Soc* 1997;45:1214–1218.

Gatz M, Harris, JR, Turk-Charles S: The meaning of health for older women. In: Stanton AL, Gallant SJ (eds.): *The Psychology of Women's Health: Progress and Challenges in Research and Application,* pp. 491–529. Washington, DC, American Psychological Association, 1995.

Gillum R: Review of *Having Our Say: The Delaney Sisters' First 100 Years. The Pharos* 1997;60:50.

Harris MJ: Psychosis in late life: spotting new-onset disorders in your elderly patients. *Postgrad Med* 1997;102:139–142.

Hemmelgarn B, Suissa S, Huang A, et al.: Benzodiazepine use and the risk of motor vehicle crash in the elderly. *JAMA* 1997;278:27–31.

Hudson MF: Elder mistreatment: its relevance to older women. *J Am Med Womens Assoc* 1997;52:142–146.

Jeste DV: Psychiatry of old age is coming of age. *Am J Psychiatry* 1997;154:1356–1358.

Jeste DV, Eastham JH, Lacro JP, et al.: Management of later life psychosis. *J Clin Psychiatry* 1996;57(Suppl 3):39–45.

Jung CG: The stages of life. In: Campbell J (ed.): *The Portable Jung,* pp. 3–22. New York, Penguin, 1978. (Original publication, 1930.)

Kahana RJ: Psychoanalysis in later life: discussion. *J Geriatr Psychiatry* 1978;11:3–49.

Khachaturian ZS: Plundered memories. *The Sciences* 1997;37:18–26.

Koenig HG, George LK, Meador KG: Use of antidepressants by nonpsychiatrists in the treatment of medically ill hospitalized depressed elderly patients. *Am J Psychiatry* 1997;154:1369–1375.

Kuhn M, Long C, Quinn L: *No Stone Unturned: The Life and Times of Maggie Kuhn.* New York, Ballantine Books, 1991.

Lake JT, Grossberg GT: Management of psychosis, agitation, and other behavioral problems in Alzheimer's disease. *Psychiatr Ann* 1996;16:274–279.

LeBars PL, Katz MM, Berman N, et al.: A placebo-controlled, double-blind randomized trial of an extract of *Ginkgo biloba* for dementia. *JAMA* 1997;278:1327–1332.

Lebowitz D, Pearson JL, Schneider LS, et al.: Diagnosis and treatment of depression in late life: consensus statement update. *JAMA* 1997;278:1186–1190.

Leiblum SR, Segraves RT: Sex and aging. In: Oldham JM, Riba MD (eds.): *Review of Psychiatry,* vol 14, pp. 677–696. Washington, DC, American Psychiatric Press, 1995.

Leventhal EA: Gender and aging: women and their aging. In: Adesso VJ, Reddy DM, Fleming R (eds.): *Psychological Perspectives on Women's Health,* pp. 11–35. Washington, DC, Taylor & Francis, 1994.

Lewis L: Transference and countertransference in psychotherapy with adults having traumatic brain injury. In: Langer KG, Laatsch L, Lewis L (eds.): *Psychotherapeutic Interventions with Brain Injury and Stroke Patients: A Clinicians' Treatment Resource* (in press).

Lewis L, Athey G, Eyman JE, et al.: Psychological treatment of adult psychiatric patients with traumatic frontal lobe injury. J *Neuropsychiaty Clin Neurosci* 1992;4:323–330.

Lewis L, Langer KG: Symbolization in psychotherapy with patients who are disabled. *Am J Psychother* 1994;48:231–239.

Mace NL, Rabins PV: *The Thirty-six Hour Day*, rev. ed. Baltimore, MD, Johns Hopkins University Press, 1991 (softcover edition: Warner Books, NY). Original edition published in 1981.

Mayerson EW: *Putting the Ill at Ease*. Hagerstown, MD, Harper & Row, 1976.

McCann JJ, Hebert LE, Bennett DA, et al.: Why Alzheimer's disease is a women's health issue. *J Am Med Womens Assoc* 1997;52:132–137.

Mendelson W: A 96-year-old woman with insomnia. *JAMA* 1997;277:990–996.

Morrison-Bogorad M, Phelps C, Buckholtz W: Alzheimer disease research comes of age: the pace accelerates. *JAMA* 1997;277:837–840.

Morse RM: Substance abuse among the elderly. *Bull Menninger Clin* 1988;52:259–268.

Nadien M: Aging women: issues of mental health and maltreatment. In: Sechzer JA, Pfafflin SM, Denmark FL, et al. (eds.): *Women and Mental Health*, pp. 129–145. New York, New York Academy of Sciences, 1996.

National Institute on Aging/National Institute of Health Annual Progress Report on Alzheimer's Disease. NIH Publication no. 97-4014. Silver Spring, MD, U.S. Department of Health and Human Services, 1997.

Newhouse PA: Use of serotonin selective reuptake inhibitors in geriatric depression. *J Clin Psychiatry* 1996;57(Suppl 5):12–22.

Noyes MA: Pharmacotherapy for elderly women: *J Am Med Womens Assoc* 1997;52:138–141, 158.

Olshansky SJ, Carnes BA, Grahm D: Confronting the boundaries of human longevity. *American Scientist* 1998;861:52–61.

Oxman TE: Antidepressants and cognitive impairment in the elderly. *J Clin Psychiatry* 1996;57(Suppl 5):38–44.

Penninx BWJH, Guralnik JM, Ferrucci L: Depressive symptoms and physical decline in community-dwelling older persons. *JAMA* 1998;279:1720–1726.

Post SG, Whitehouse PJ, Binstock RH, et al.: The clinical introduction of genetic testing for Alzheimer's disease: an ethical perspective. *JAMA* 1997;277:832–836.

Prager D: *Happiness Is a Serious Problem*. New York, NY, HarperCollins, 1998.

Pruyser P: Creativity in aging persons. *Bull Menninger Clin* 1987;51:425–535.

Roberts RE, Kaplan GA, Shema SJ: Does growing old increase the risk for depression? *Am J Psychiatry* 1997;154:1384–1390.

Rothschild AJ: The diagnosis and treatment of late-life depression. *J Clin Psychiatry* 1996;57(Suppl 5):5–11.

Sandler AM: Psychoanalysis in later life: problems in the psychoanalysis of an aging narcissistic patient. *J Geriatr Psychiatry* 1978;11:5–36.

Sano M, Ernesto C, Thomas RG, et al.: A controlled trial of selegiline, alpha-tocopherol or both as treatment for Alzheimer's disease. *N Engl J Med* 1997;336:1216–1222.

Schneider LS, Small GW: Clinical developments in Alzheimer's disease. *J Clin Psychiatry* 1996;57(Suppl 14):3–42.

Shneidman E: The Indian summer of life: a preliminary study of septuagenarians. *Am Psychol* 1989;44:684–694.

Sherrill JT, Frank E, Geary M: Psychoeducational workshops for elderly patients with recurrent major depression and their families. *Psychiatr Serv* 1997;48:76–81.

Small GW, Rabins PV, Barry PP, et al.: Diagnosis and treatment of Alzheimer's disease and related disorders: consensus statement of the American Association of Geriatric Psychiatry, the Alzheimer's Association, and the American Geriatrics Society. *JAMA* 1997;278:1363–1371.

Sodeman WA: *Instructions for Geriatric Patients*. Philadelphia, WB Saunders, 1995.

Sunderland T: Treatment of the elderly suffering from psychosis and dementia. *J Clin Psychiatry* 1996;57(Suppl 9):53–56.

Tariot PN: Treatment strategies for agitation and psychosis in dementia. *J Clin Psychiatry* 1996;57(Suppl 14):21–29.

Thompson LW: Cognitive-behavioral therapy and treatment for late-life depression. *J Clin Psychiatry* 1996;57(Suppl 5):29–37.

Wallerstein J, Blakeslee S: *The Good Marriage: How and Why Love Lasts*. Boston, Houghton Mifflin, 1995.

Weaver F: *I'm Not as Old as I Used to Be: Reclaiming Your Life in the Second Half*. New York, Hyperion, 1997.

Weaver F: *The Girls with the Grandmothers' Faces: A Celebration of Life's Potential for Those Over Fifty-five.* New York, Hyperion, 1996.

Yaffe K, Sawaya G, Lieberburg I, et al.: Estrogen therapy in postmenopausal women: effects on cognitive function and dementia. *JAMA* 1998;279:688–695.

Zerbe KJ: *The Body Betrayed: Women, Eating Disorders, and Treatment.* Washington, DC, American Psychiatric Press, 1993. (Softcover edition: *The Body Betrayed: A Deeper Understanding of Women, Eating Disorders, and Treatment.* Gürze Books, Carlsbad, CA, 1995.)

Zisook S: Depression in late life. Special considerations in treatment. *Postgrad Med* 1996;100:161–172.

Zubenko GS, Mulsant BH, Sweet RA, et al.: Mortality of elderly patients with psychiatric disorders. *Am J Psychiatry* 1997;154:1360–1368.

Afterword

What factors are included in, and to some extent foster, a particular woman's mental well-being? Anne Morrow Lindbergh (1955), writing at midlife from the perspective of overcoming deep grief and hoping to find ways to reconcile tensions facing women (the multiple obligations to one's family, spouse, and career), saw an individual's coming of age as learning to stand alone. The process is never a comfortable one. Attributes once important need to be shed. Growth is inevitably characterized to some extent by loss; nevertheless, it holds out the potential for positive transformation. She writes

One might be free for growth of mind, heart, and talent; free at last for spiritual growth; free of the clamping sunrise shell. Beautiful as it was, it was a closed world one had to outgrow . . . . And the time may come when—comfortable and adaptable as it is—one may outgrow even the oyster shell (p. 88).

Contemporary psychiatrists and psychoanalysts might quibble with Lindbergh's emphasis on self-sufficiency. The capacity to form attachments, learn from others, sustain commitments, and be truly interdependent in a healthy way is now considered the cornerstone of personal well-being. But few mental health professionals would have trouble with the notion that every woman needs time and space to be herself, to grow, and to see her own individual spirit flourish.

Psychotherapists witness that outgrowing of the oyster shell on a daily basis, when patients terminate personal treatment and move on—in hopes of engaging more constructively in their lives. In a sense, the protective shell of the therapy process can be relinquished when the patient has the "inside answers" herself—those intangible qualities and affirming opportunities that she sought when first beginning treatment. In a sense, she takes in the best aspects of the therapist, so that she is able to move on.

In this book, I have reviewed how a rapidly emerging body of research supports the notion that gender differences play a major role in the psychosocial and biological manifestations of mental health and mental illness. Clearly, the emotional problems that affect women at particular stages of life are a major public health problem in the United States and all over the world. Some of the disorders that are more common among women include anxiety disorders, depression, eating disorders, and posttraumatic stress disorder. Women also have unique psychosocial responses to bereavement and loss, medical illness, and aging. Primary clinicians are called on first to heal an individual woman's wounded spirit and then to use the facts known about gender differences and responses to treatment to help the patient initiate the process that will ultimately permit the growth of mind, heart, and talent that Anne Morrow Lindbergh so eloquently describes.

In all likelihood, additional research will help primary care clinicians and mental health professionals address their patients' emotional problems with treatments that take gender into account. For example, while some mental illnesses linked to the reproductive system may be controlled by hormonal factors and hence treated with replacement therapy, patients with other disorders may better respond to one class or group of medications. As we have seen even now, knowledge about gender differences as related to drug metabolism, gastric emptying time, weight and body composition, and potential side effects plays a crucial role in the prescribing of specific psychotropic medications. Even the pharmaceutical industry has begun to take gender into account in testing new drugs and offering recommendations on dosage, duration, and treatment (Blumenthal, 1996). The value of this research will likely reduce human suffering, helping the patient negotiate a more comfortable and adaptable affiliation with the outside world and especially with herself.

In the future, it is also likely that gender-specific psychotherapies will be prescribed. Drawing on the psychosocial differences between men and women, these treatments will help us to explain more fully the greater prevalence of some disorders in women and why each gender is predisposed to specific developmental and life cycle problems. Regardless of the psychotherapeutic approach, likely topics for exploration will be women's interpersonal relationships and patterns of interaction, generally poor self-esteem and inferior social status, and response to adverse and traumatic events. The guarantee of adequate access to health care and health insurance will also require sensitive long-range planning. For example, women currently are more inclined to take advantage of preventive and screening services than men. They also tend to be more active in their role as a patient. Women are also more likely, however, to be uninsured, underinsured, and responsible for higher co-payments and other restrictions than men (Nadelson, 1998).

Primary care clinicians must remain aware of these rapidly evolving trends that affect the health and well-being of women in their practice. As evidence continues to mount, indicating that psychotherapy is cost-effective for a wide range of emotional and physical problems, a closer alliance between primary care and psychiatry is likely to flourish. Such a renaissance might even permit a fuller integration between pharmacologic and psychosocial treatment strategies than what has occurred to date. Individuals will no doubt always find doctor-patient rapport vital to recovery.

Whatever additional tools science is able to provide, when the patient can be appreciated and understood for all her unique strengths and limitations, the growth of mind, heart, talent . . . and spirit are bound to occur. The doctor-patient relationship has always been at the heart of the matter and should be the best of what we clinicians do. The therapeutic process works from both the outside in and the inside out. Small wonder it cannot be captured well by research protocols or quantified by double-blind studies. Important as these tools are, the beauty of healing has always been in its mystery, the ineluctable yearning of human beings to heal, to outgrow even the oyster shell of the most stultifying malady that engulfs them.

Today psychoanalysts have many terms for this process; we call it "listening to the patient's narrative" or "entering into the intersubjective space." It all really means the hearing of the patient's story, the giving of appropriate attention to the tears, smiles, nuances, gestures, genuine thank you's, and the unspoken feelings the patients cannot yet quite put into words. It is being there for her, one day at a time, one problem at a time, one story at a time. The value of listening in medicine has been appreciated for centuries because it works. It still does!

References

Blumenthal SJ: Women's mental health: The new national focus. *Ann NY Acad Sci* 789;1996:1–16.
Lindbergh AM: *Gift from the Sea.* New York, Signet Books, 1955.
Nadelson CC: Gender and health policy. *Harv Rev Psychiatry* 1998;5:340–343.

General Resources for Patients

Baron-Faust R: *Mental Wellness for Women.* New York, William Morrow & Company, 1997.

> Ms. Baron-Faust wrote this excellent summary about women's mental health needs in conjunction with physicians at the New York University Medical Center Women's Service and its department of psychiatry. Topics include addiction, trauma and violence, personality disorders, anxiety and mood disorders, and hormone replacement therapy. The strengths of this book lie in its cogent summaries of the biochemistry of illness and cognitive-behavioral interventions. Although a woman with a particular disorder will likely turn to a book that discusses her particular concerns, those who want a broad-based, comprehensive reference for the bookshelf will be delighted by this resource. It may also be of particular interest to care extenders or to young people who want an authoritative guide about the developments in psychiatry over the past 10 years.

Carlson KJ, Eisenstat SA, Ziporyn T: *The Harvard Guide to Women's Mental Health.* Cambridge, MA, Harvard University Press, 1996.

> This award-winning, authoritative guide answers the questions that women most commonly have about their general medical health and physical ailments. Some excellent sections are devoted specifically to premenstrual syndrome, menopause, rape and domestic violence sequelae, substance abuse, stress, and depression. This book has received a great deal of acclaim.

Carlson KJ, Eisenstat SA, Ziporyn T: *The Women's Concise Guide to Emotional Well-being.* Cambridge, MA, Harvard University Press, 1997.

> This book is basically an abridged edition of *The Harvard Guide to Women's Mental Health.* It tackles the psychiatric issues of depression and anxiety, eating disorders, schizophrenia, violence, sexual dysfunction, and stress management over the life cycle. Patients can quickly read the brief summaries and have a sense of the latest treatments. The authors wrote their sections as answers to questions (Are there ways to prevent postpartum depression? How can a woman protect herself against sexual harrassment?) that are quite user friendly.

Miller SB: *When Parents Have Problems: A Book for Teens and Older Children with an Abusive, Alcoholic, or Mentally Ill Parent.* Springfield, IL, Charles C Thomas, 1995.

> Parents who struggle with a mental illness often wonder how they can help their children. This unique resource is written for teens whose parents are trying to cope with a range of mild to severe emotional issues. The author is a clinical psychologist who understands and empathizes with her audience—those who have been affected by parental suffering, neglect, or crisis while growing up. This highly recommended reference helps young people to understand the nature of the specific issues they face, learn to deal with reactions they have to them, and begin to find sources of help that can be both supportive and affirming.

Roukema RW: *What Every Patient, Family, Friend, and Caregiver Needs to Know About Psychiatry.* Washington, DC, American Psychiatric Press, 1998.

Although not specifically devoted to women's mental health, this popular press guide to the diagnosis and treatment of emotional illness is state of the art. Section topics include Normal Development and the Life Cycle, The Genetics of Psychiatric Illness, The Major Psychiatric Syndromes, and The Basics of Treatment. This text can be recommended to families and friends who have a question about psychiatric illness or to anyone who simply wants to learn more. Its clear prose, well-executed summaries, and case examples make for a lively and engaging read.

Slupik RI: *American Medical Association's Complete Guide to Women's Health.* New York, Random House, 1996.

This comprehensive and well-written guide to staying healthy for life (e.g., nutrition, fitness, stress management) provides excellent summaries on the major mental health concerns of women. An extensive section on sexual and reproductive health and pregnancy makes this a particularly excellent reference for women, from young adulthood through menopause.

Vaughan SC: *The Talking Cure: The Science Behind Psychotherapy.* New York, Grosset/Putman, 1997.

For any individual contemplating the start of psychotherapy and wanting to learn more about how and why it works, this new reference is a superlative guide. The accounts of actual psychotherapeutic sessions that describe the process of treatment are refreshingly candid and engrossing to read. The author, herself a psychiatrist and psychoanalyst at Columbia University, then reviews the latest scientific findings about how the brain works and in what ways psychotherapy may actually modify it. A deeper understanding of what ultimately decreases emotional pain and improves the quality of life for individuals who decide to engage in "the talking cure" emerges. This book is likely to become a classic reference for individuals who embark on psychotherapy or psychoanalysis and want to learn and to understand more about themselves.

Index

Note: Page numbers followed by (t) refer to tables.

353